ORAL AND MAXILLOFACIAL SURGERY CLINICS
of North America

The Neck

ERIC J. DIERKS, DMD, MD, FACS
R. BRYAN BELL, DDS, MD, FACS
Guest Editors

RICHARD H. HAUG, DDS
Consulting Editor

August 2008 • Volume 20 • Number 3

SAUNDERS
An Imprint of Elsevier, Inc.
PHILADELPHIA LONDON TORONTO MONTREAL SYDNEY TOKYO

W.B. SAUNDERS COMPANY
A Division of Elsevier Inc.

1600 John F. Kennedy Blvd., Suite 1800, Philadelphia, PA 19103-2899

http://www.oralmaxsurgery.theclinics.com

ORAL AND MAXILLOFACIAL SURGERY
CLINICS OF NORTH AMERICA
August 2008
Editor: John Vassallo; j.vassallo@elsevier.com

Volume 20, Number 3
ISSN 1042-3699
ISBN-13: 978-1-4160-6328-5
ISBN-10: 1-4160-6328-5

© 2008 Elsevier ▪ All rights reserved.

This journal and the individual contributions contained in it are protected under copyright by Elsevier, and the following terms and conditions apply to their use:

Photocopying

Single photocopies of single articles may be made for personal use as allowed by national copyright laws. Permission of the Publisher and payment of a fee is required for all other photocopying, including multiple or systematic copying, copying for advertising or promotional purposes, resale, and all forms of document delivery. Special rates are available for educational institutions that wish to make photocopies for non-profit educational classroom use. For information on how to seek permission visit www.elsevier.com/permissions or call: (+44) 1865 843830 (UK)/(+1) 215 239 3804 (USA).

Derivative Works

Subscribers may reproduce tables of contents or prepare lists of articles including abstracts for internal circulation within their institutions. Permission of the Publisher is required for resale or distribution outside the institution. Permission of the Publisher is required for all other derivative works, including compilations and translations (please consult www.elsevier.com/permissions).

Electronic Storage or Usage

Permission of the Publisher is required to store or use electronically any material contained in this journal, including any article or part of an article (please consult www.elsevier.com/permissions). Except as outlined above, no part of this publication may be reproduced, stored in a retrieval system or transmitted in any form or by any means, electronic, mechanical, photocopying, recording or otherwise, without prior written permission of the Publisher.

Notice

No responsibility is assumed by the Publisher for any injury and/or damage to persons or property as a matter of products liability, negligence or otherwise, or from any use or operation of any methods, products, instructions or ideas contained in the material herein. Because of rapid advances in the medical sciences, in particular, independent verification of diagnoses and drug dosages should be made.

Although all advertising material is expected to conform to ethical (medical) standards, inclusion in this publication does not constitute a guarantee or endorsement of the quality or value of such product or of the claims made of it by its manufacturer.

Oral and Maxillofacial Surgery Clinics of North America (ISSN 1042-3699) is published quarterly by Elsevier Inc., 360 Park Avenue South, New York, NY 10010-1710. Months of issue are February, May, August, and November. Business and Editorial Offices: 1600 John F. Kennedy Blvd., Suite 1800, Philadelphia, PA 19103-2899. Customer Service Office: 6277 Sea Harbor Drive, Orlando, FL 32887-4800. Periodicals postage paid at New York, NY and additional mailing offices. Subscription prices are $244.00 per year for US individuals, $358.00 per year for US institutions, $113.00 per year for US students and residents, $282.00 per year for Canadian individuals, $418.00 per year for Canadian institutions, $307.00 per year for international individuals, $418.00 per year for international institutions and $144.00 per year for Canadian and foreign students/residents. To receive student/resident rate, orders must be accompanied by name or affiliated institution, date of term, and the *signature* of program/residency coordinator on institution letterhead. Orders will be billed at individual rate until proof of status is received. Foreign air speed delivery is included in all *Clinics* subscription prices. All prices are subject to change without notice. **POSTMASTER:** Send address changes to *Oral and Maxillofacial Surgery Clinics of North America*, Elsevier Periodicals Customer Service, 6277 Sea Harbor Drive, Orlando, FL 32887-4800. **Customer Service: 1-800-654-2452 (US). From outside of the US, call 1-407-563-6020. Fax: 1-407-363-9661. E-mail: JournalsCustomerService-usa@elsevier.com.**

Reprints. For copies of 100 or more of articles in this publication, please contact the Commercial Reprints Department, Elsevier Inc., 360 Park Avenue South, New York, New York, 10010-1710; Tel.: (+1) 212-633-3813, Fax: (+1) 212-462-1935, and E-mail: reprints@elsevier.com.

Oral and Maxillofacial Surgery Clinics of North America is covered in MEDLINE/PubMed (*Index Medicus*).

Printed in the United States of America.

THE NECK

CONSULTING EDITOR

RICHARD H. HAUG, DDS, Professor of Oral and Maxillofacial Surgery; and Executive Associate Dean, University of Kentucky, College of Dentistry, Lexington, Kentucky

GUEST EDITORS

ERIC J. DIERKS, DMD, MD, FACS, Attending Surgeon and Fellowship Director in Head and Neck Oncologic Surgery, Oral and Maxillofacial Surgery Service, Legacy Emanuel Hospital and Health Center; Clinical Professor of Oral and Maxillofacial Surgery, Oregon Health & Science University; and Head & Neck Surgical Associates, Portland, Oregon

R. BRYAN BELL, DDS, MD, FACS, Attending Surgeon and Director of Resident Education, Oral and Maxillofacial Surgery Service, Legacy Emanuel Hospital and Health Center; Clinical Associate Professor of Oral and Maxillofacial Surgery, Oregon Health & Science University; and Head & Neck Surgical Associates, Portland, Oregon

CONTRIBUTORS

JAMES C. ANDERSON, MD, Assistant Professor of Radiology and Chief, Division of Neuroradiology, Department of Radiology, Oregon Health & Science University, Portland, Oregon

LEON A. ASSAEL, DMD, Professor and Chairman, Department of Oral and Maxillofacial Surgery, Oregon Health & Science University, Portland, Oregon

SHAHROKH C. BAGHERI, DMD, MD, Chair of Oral and Maxillofacial Surgery, Northside Hospital; Clinical Assistant Professor of Oral and Maxillofacial Surgery, Emory University School of Medicine; and Private Practice, Atlanta Oral and Facial Surgery, Atlanta, Georgia

R. BRYAN BELL, DDS, MD, FACS, Attending Surgeon and Director of Resident Education, Oral and Maxillofacial Surgery Service, Legacy Emanuel Hospital and Health Center; Clinical Associate Professor of Oral and Maxillofacial Surgery, Oregon Health & Science University; and Head & Neck Surgical Associates, Portland, Oregon

JOHN F. CACCAMESE Jr., DMD, MD, FACS, Assistant Professor and Program Director, Department of Oral and Maxillofacial Surgery, University of Maryland Medical System; and Assistant Clinical Professor, Department of Pediatrics, University of Maryland Medical System, Baltimore, Maryland

JEFF W. CHEN, MD, PhD, FACS, Neurological Surgeon and Director of Neurotrauma, Legacy Emanuel Hospital, Portland, Oregon

ALLEN CHENG, DDS, Resident, Department of Oral & Maxillofacial Surgery, University of California, San Francisco, California

JAMES I. COHEN, MD, PhD, Department of Otolaryngology/Head and Neck Surgery, Oregon Health & Science University, Portland, Oregon

DOMENICK P. COLETTI, DDS, MD, Assistant Professor and Division Chief, Department of Oral and Maxillofacial Surgery, University of Maryland Medical System, Baltimore, Maryland

ERIC J. DIERKS, DMD, MD, FACS, Attending Surgeon and Fellowship Director in Head and Neck Oncologic Surgery, Oral and Maxillofacial Surgery Service, Legacy Emanuel Hospital and Health Center; Clinical Professor of Oral and Maxillofacial Surgery, Oregon Health & Science University; and Head & Neck Surgical Associates, Portland, Oregon

RUI FERNANDES, DMD, MD, FACS, Assistant Professor, Division of Oral & Maxillofacial Surgery and Section of Surgical Oncology, Department of Surgery, University of Florida College of Medicine, Jacksonville, Florida

DAVID L. HIRSCH, DDS, MD, Assistant Professor, Department of Oral and Maxillofacial Surgery, New York University College of Dentistry; and New York University School of Medicine, New York, New York

JON D. HOLMES, DMD, MD, FACS, Private Practice, Oral and Facial Surgery of Alabama; and Assistant Clinical Professor, University of Alabama at Birmingham, Birmingham, Alabama

JAMES A. HOMAN, MD, Neuroradiology Fellow, Oregon Health & Science University, Portland, Oregon

H. ALI KHAN, DMD, MD, Private Practice, Atlanta Oral and Facial Surgery, Atlanta, Georgia

JASON LEE, DDS, Fellow in Microvascular Reconstructive Surgery, Division of Oral & Maxillofacial Surgery, Department of Surgery, University of Florida College of Medicine, Jacksonville, Florida

DIMITRIOS NIKOLARAKOS, BDSc, MBBS, FRACDS(OMS), Fellow, Head and Neck Surgery, Legacy Emanuel Hospital and Health Center, Portland, Oregon

ROBERT A. ORD, DDS, MD, FRCS, FACS, Professor and Chair, Department of Oral and Maxillofacial Surgery, University of Maryland Medical Center, Baltimore College of Dental Surgery, Baltimore, Maryland

TIMOTHY M. OSBORN, DDS, MD, Resident, Department of Oral and Maxillofacial Surgery, Oregon Health & Science University, Portland, Oregon

JASON K. POTTER, MD, DDS, Private Practice, Plastic and Maxillofacial Surgery; and Adjunct Assistant Professor, Department of Oral and Maxillofacial Surgery, Baylor College of Dentistry, Dallas, Texas

PETER A. ROSA, DDS, MD, Chief Resident, Department of Oral and Maxillofacial Surgery, New York University College of Dentistry; and New York University School of Medicine, New York, New York

ANDREW R. SALAMA, DDS, MD, Assistant Professor, Department of Oral and Maxillofacial Surgery, University of Maryland Medical Center, Baltimore College of Dental Surgery, Baltimore, Maryland

KELLI D. SALTER, MD, PhD, Department of General Surgery, Oregon Health & Science University, Portland, Oregon

BRIAN L. SCHMIDT, DDS, MD, PhD, FACS, Associate Professor and Residency Program Director, Department of Oral & Maxillofacial Surgery, University of California, San Francisco, California

DAVID S. VERSCHUEREN, DMD, MD, Resident, Department of Oral and Maxillofacial Surgery, Oregon Health & Science University, Portland, Oregon

THE NECK

CONTENTS

Preface xi
Eric J. Dierks and R. Bryan Bell

Dedication xiii
Eric J. Dierks and R. Bryan Bell

GENERAL CONSIDERATIONS

Radiographic Correlation with Neck Anatomy 311
James C. Anderson and James A. Homan

>The anatomy of the head and neck is an important set of knowledge for the oral and maxillofacial surgeon. Current imaging techniques and the exquisite detail that they provide are frequently the first glimpse at disease and important to surgical planning. CT and MRI are the primary modes of neck imaging and are complimentary in the information that they provide. This article reviews the current methods of anatomic imaging and the current methods of analysis of the region by radiologists.

Neck Masses: Evaluation and Diagnostic Approach 321
Jason Lee and Rui Fernandes

>Oral and maxillofacial surgeons frequently deal with patients who present with an unknown neck mass. Formulation of a differential diagnosis is essential and requires that the surgeon bring to bear a host of skills to systematically arrive at a definitive diagnosis and ensure that the correct treatment is rendered. This article highlights some of the skills needed in the workup of neck masses and reviews some of the available techniques that aid in achieving the correct diagnosis.

NON-NEOPLASTIC DISORDERS

Congenital Neck Masses 339
Peter A. Rosa, David L. Hirsch, and Eric J. Dierks

>Congenital neck lesions reflect abnormal embryogenesis in head and neck development. A thorough knowledge of embryology and anatomy is critical in the diagnosis and treatment of these lesions. The appropriate diagnosis of these lesions is necessary to provide appropriate treatment and long-term follow up, because some of these lesions may undergo malignant transformation or be harbingers of malignant disease.

Deep Space Neck Infection: Principles of Surgical Management 353
Timothy M. Osborn, Leon A. Assael, and R. Bryan Bell

Knowledge of the management of infections of the deep spaces of the neck is essential to the daily practice of oral and maxillofacial surgery. Timely decisions must be made through the acute course of the disease. Interventions must be performed with the appropriate surgical skill. The surgeon must decide on medical and surgical management, including antibiotic selection, how to employ supportive resuscitative care, when to operate, what procedures to perform, and how to secure the airway. To make these decisions the surgeon must understand the anatomy of the region and the etiology of infection, appropriate diagnostic workup, and medical and surgical management. This article provides a review of these pertinent topics.

Deep Neck Infections: Clinical Considerations in Aggressive Disease 367
John F. Caccamese Jr. and Domenick P. Coletti

Deep neck infections are common and occur as a consequence of several etiologies. Antibiotic therapy, interventional radiology, and patient support modalities have become increasingly sophisticated, although surgery continues to be the mainstay of treatment for most patients. Today, neck infections are rarely life threatening when sound and timely management is applied.

Cervical Spine Injuries 381
Jeff W. Chen

This article describes the anatomy of the cervical spine and the most common types of fractures associated with the cervical spine. Cervical spinal cord syndromes are also reviewed because such syndromes discovered during neurologic examinations frequently provide the first clue that there is an underlying spinal cord injury. Because most associated maxillofacial and spinal injuries occur in the setting of motor vehicle accidents, it is particularly important for the maxillofacial surgeon to be cognizant of the injuries, particularly in the context of the need for facial/cranial surgery. Appropriate measures are necessary to immobilize or fixate the spine before surgery to avoid exacerbating the spinal injury.

Penetrating Neck Injuries 393
Shahrokh C. Bagheri, H. Ali Khan, and R. Bryan Bell

The modern approach to patients presenting with penetrating injuries to the neck requires the cautious integration of clinical findings and appropriate imaging studies for formulation of an effective, safe, and minimally invasive modality of treatment. The optimal management of these injuries has undergone considerable debate regarding surgical versus nonsurgical treatment approaches. More recent advances in imaging technology continue to evolve, providing more accurate and timely information for the management of these patients. In this article the authors review both historic and recent articles that have formulated the current management of penetrating injuries to the neck.

Management of Laryngeal Trauma 415
R. Bryan Bell, David S. Verschueren, and Eric J. Dierks

Fractures of the larynx are uncommon injuries that may be associated with maxillofacial trauma. Clinicians treating maxillofacial injuries should be familiar with the signs and symptoms of laryngeal fractures and with proper airway management. A timely evaluation of the larynx, rapid airway intervention, and proper surgical repair are essential for a successful outcome.

NON-SQUAMOUS NEOPLASMS

Thyroid Disorders: Evaluation and Management of Thyroid Nodules 431
James I. Cohen and Kelli D. Salter

> Although thyroid nodules are a common clinical entity, few (5% to 10%) are malignant and require surgical treatment. Most nodules are discovered incidentally in patients undergoing surveillance for medical reasons unrelated to thyroid disorders. Therefore, a systematic approach to their evaluation is important to avoid unnecessary surgery. High-resolution ultrasonography and fine-needle aspiration have resulted in substantial improvements in diagnostic accuracy, cost reductions, and higher malignancy yield at the time of surgery. In this article, the authors present practical guidelines and a suggested management strategy for the effective diagnosis and management of incidentally discovered thyroid nodules.

Clinical Implications of the Neck in Salivary Gland Disease 445
Andrew R. Salama and Robert A. Ord

> Neck manifestations from salivary gland tissue are most commonly related to inflammation and obstruction of the glands. However, various benign and malignant processes are also seen along a continuum of clinical presentation and behavior. Preoperative diagnostics, including imaging and fine needle aspiration, are key elements in treatment planning, even in the absence of absolute histologic confirmation of tumors. Benign tumor implants in the neck can be managed with conservative surgery, whereas aggressive surgical management, including neck dissection and adjuvant therapy, is generally advocated for malignancy.

SQUAMOUS CELL CARCINOMA

Neck Dissection: Nomenclature, Classification, and Technique 459
Jon D. Holmes

> Lymph node status is the single most important prognostic factor in head and neck cancer because lymph node involvement decreases overall survival by 50%. Appropriate management of the regional lymphatics, therefore, plays a central role in the treatment of the head and neck cancer patients. Performing an appropriate neck dissection results in minimal morbidity to the patient, provides invaluable data to accurately stage the patient, and guides the need for further therapy. The purposes of this article are to present the history and evolution of neck dissections, including an update on the current state of nomenclature and current neck dissection classification, describe the technique of the most common neck dissection applicable to oral cavity cancers, and discuss some of the complications associated with neck dissection. Finally, a brief review of sentinel lymph node biopsy will be presented.

Management of the N0 Neck in Oral Squamous Cell Carcinoma 477
Allen Cheng and Brian L. Schmidt

> Oral squamous cell carcinoma (SCC) has an unpredictable capacity to metastasize to the neck, an event that dramatically worsens prognosis. Metastasis occurs even in earlier stages when no neck lymph node involvement is clinically detectable (N0). Management of the N0 neck, namely when and how to electively treat, has been debated extensively. This article presents the controversies surrounding management of the N0 neck, and the benefits and pitfalls of different approaches used in evaluation and treatment. As current methods of assessing the risk for occult metastasis are insufficiently accurate and prone to underestimation of actual risk, and because selective neck dissection (SND) is an

effective treatment and has minimal long-term detriment to quality of life, the authors believe that all patients who have oral SCC, excluding lip SCC, should be prescribed elective treatment of the neck lymphatics. However, this opinion remains controversial. Because of the morbidity of radiation therapy and because treatment of the primary tumor is surgical, elective neck dissection is the preferred treatment. In deciding the extent of the neck dissection, several retrospective studies and one randomized clinical trial have shown SND of levels I through III to be highly efficacious.

Management of the Node-Positive Neck in Oral Cancer 499
Dimitrios Nikolarakos and R. Bryan Bell

Surgery continues to play a prominent role in the management of patients with loco-regionally advanced squamous cell carcinoma of the upper aerodigestive tract. Most evidence supports the use of comprehensive neck dissection for node-positive disease and suggests that planned neck dissection following definitive radiation therapy and chemoradiation therapy is unnecessary in the great majority of patients with node-positive neck disease who exhibit a complete response. Evidence for less aggressive therapy is much less compelling in patients with bulky adenopathy. For such patients, there is growing enthusiasm for selective or even super-selective neck dissection for surgical salvage. Finally, when cervical disease is so advanced as to involve the carotid artery, evidence continues to portend a dismal prognosis.

SURGICAL TECHNIQUE

Tracheotomy: Elective and Emergent 513
Eric J. Dierks

Tracheotomy has been practiced since ancient times and continues to be a crucial procedure. Contemporary elective adult tracheotomy is described in detail. Intra-operative and postoperative complications can arise with elective tracheotomy. Pediatric and obese patients require special consideration when undergoing a tracheotomy. The emergency cricothryroidotomy and "slash" tracheotomy are discussed. Continuing education regarding advances in tracheotomy procedures is advised.

Preparation of the Neck for Microvascular Reconstruction of the Head and Neck 521
Jason K. Potter and Timothy M. Osborn

Reconstruction of congenital, developmental, or acquired head and neck defects remains a significant challenge for the oral and maxillofacial surgeon. Microvascular free tissue transfer has several advantages over nonvascularized bone grafts and pedicled soft tissue flaps that currently make it the modality of choice for the reconstruction of extirpative defects of the head and neck. Preoperative planning must include detailed attention to the technical aspects of the microvascular procedure. This includes a thorough understanding of the vascular anatomy of the patient's neck; vascular anatomy of the various flaps including pedicle lengths; and a knowledge of how to facilitate microvascular surgery in the neck and to manage complicating factors in the difficult neck.

Index 527

FORTHCOMING ISSUES

November 2008

Head and Neck Manifestations of Systemic Disorders
Sidney L. Bourgeois, Jr, DDS, *Guest Editor*

February 2009

Complications of Cosmetic Facial Surgery
Joseph Niamtu III, DMD, *Guest Editor*

May 2009

Current Controversies in Maxillofacial Trauma
A. Omar Abubaker, DMD, PhD and
Daniel M. Laskin, DDS, MS, *Guest Editors*

PREVIOUS ISSUES

May 2008

Orofacial Pain and Dysfunction
Ramesh Balasubramaniam, BDSc, MS and
Gary D. Klasser, DMD, *Guest Editors*

February 2008

Practice Management
M. Todd Brandt, DDS, MD, *Guest Editor*

November 2007

Topics in Bone and Bone Related Disorders
Mark R. Stevens, DDS, *Guest Editor*

THE CLINICS ARE NOW AVAILABLE ONLINE!

Access your subscription at:
http://www.theclinics.com

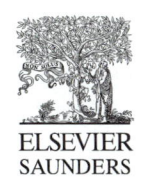

Preface

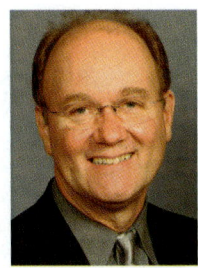

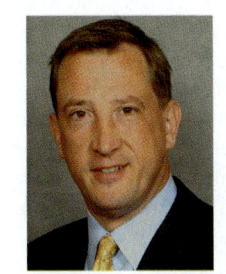

Eric J. Dierks, DMD, MD, FACS   R. Bryan Bell, DDS, MD, FACS
Guest Editors

> Learning is not attained by chance, it must be sought for with ardor and attended to with diligence.
>
> Abigail Adams (1744–1818)

The American Association of Oral and Maxillofacial Surgeons defines oral and maxillofacial surgery as the specialty of dentistry that includes the "diagnosis, surgical and related treatment of diseases, injuries and defects involving both the functional and esthetic aspects of the hard and soft tissues of the head, mouth, teeth, gums, jaws and **neck**" [emphasis added]. In preparing this issue of the *Oral and Maxillofacial Clinics of North America*, we recognize that the training of American oral and maxillofacial surgeons in the surgical and nonsurgical management of conditions affecting the neck is varied. We also recognize that our relatively young surgical specialty continues to mature as it advances the education of its members through formal fellowship training in head and neck oncologic surgery, cranio-maxillofacial trauma, pediatric cleft and craniofacial surgery, and esthetic surgery. As the profession matures, there is and will be a need for all oral and maxillofacial surgeons to be familiar with, if not proficient in, the management of a wide variety of cervical disorders.

The neck contains seven different organ systems and is one of the most complex anatomic regions in the human body. Any or all of these systems may be affected by a variety of congenital, developmental, and acquired abnormalities, so an interdisciplinary approach to treatment often is necessary. Multiple surgical specialties overlap in this critical area; in addition to oral and maxillofacial surgery they include otolaryngology, plastic surgery, neurosurgery, and thoracic surgery, as well as general surgery and its subspecialties of vascular, trauma, and endocrine surgery. To provide a contemporary and concise review of cervical disorders, we have invited practitioners of a number of these allied disciplines whose areas of expertise complement those of the oral and maxillofacial surgeon to contribute their experience. We are deeply indebted to all the authors for their excellent and timely contributions and gratefully acknowledge the sacrifice of time and energy that is necessary to generate a quality product.

"To whom much is given, much is expected." Both of us have been fortunate in our personal and professional lives to be surrounded by individuals who have made indelible impressions on us through their confidence, industry, mentorship, friendship, support, and love. We are each beholden to our professional fathers: Don A. Hay, Gene R. Huebner, Timothy A. Turvey, Raymond P. White, Bryce E. Potter, and Eric J. Dierks (RBB), and to Edwin Granite, Brian Alpert, and William Meyerhoff (EJD). We thank our colleagues, Leon Assael, Robert Myall, Kevin Arce, William B. Long, for their guidance and support; and our parents, William and Sherry Bell and Al and Harriett Dierks, for their stimulation and inspiration. To our wives, Heidi Bell and Barbara Dierks, we owe everything.

Eric J. Dierks, DMD, MD, FACS
Oral and Maxillofacial Surgery Service
Legacy Emanuel Hospital and Health Center
Department of Oral and Maxillofacial Surgery
Oregon Health & Science University
Head and Neck Surgical Associates
1849 NW Kearney, Suite 300
Portland, OR 97209

E-mail address: dierksej@hnsa1.com

R. Bryan Bell, DDS, MD, FACS
Oral and Maxillofacial Surgery Service
Legacy Emanuel Hospital and Health Center
Department of Oral and Maxillofacial Surgery
Oregon Health & Science University
Head and Neck Surgical Associates
1849 NW Kearney, Suite 300
Portland, OR 97209

E-mail address: bellb@hnsa1.com

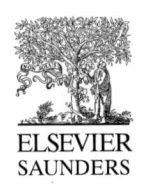

Dedication

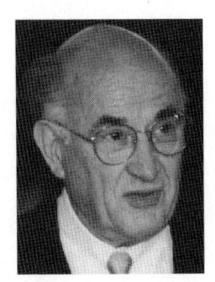

William H. Bell, DDS

We respectfully dedicate this edition of the *Oral and Maxillofacial Surgery Clinics* to Dr. William H. Bell, who, in different ways and at different points in our careers, served as a continual source of inspiration. In the late 1960s, Dr. Bell contributed to the transformation of our American specialty from that of oral surgery to one of oral and maxillofacial surgery through his landmark research on the biologic basis for the Le Fort I osteotomy. His subsequent textbooks provided a detailed description of the surgical correction of dentofacial deformities and served as a reference for thousands of surgeons in multiple disciplines across the globe. It is a testament to his meticulous attention to detail and passionate pursuit of excellence that in many ways these books remain contemporary 40 years after their publication. He has devoted his life to improving the human condition through patient care and to the advancement of surgery through research and education. Now in his sixth decade as an oral and maxillofacial surgeon, at a time when our specialty is again evolving, he continues to expand our collective horizons through his teaching and international outreach. It is our hope that the fire that burns in him will ignite the spirits of generations of surgeons to come for the betterment of patients whom it is our privilege to serve.

Eric J. Dierks, DMD, MD, FACS
R. Bryan Bell, DDS, MD, FACS

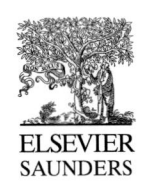

Radiographic Correlation with Neck Anatomy

James C. Anderson, MD*, James A. Homan, MD

Division of Neuroradiology, Department of Radiology, Oregon Health & Science University, 3181 S.W. Sam Jackson Park Road, Mail Code L340, Portland, OR 97239-3098, USA

The anatomy of the head and neck is an important set of knowledge for the oral maxillofacial surgeon. Current imaging techniques and the exquisite detail that they provide are frequently the first glimpse at disease and important to surgical planning. CT and MRI are the primary modes of neck imaging and are complimentary in the information that they provide. This article reviews the current methods of anatomic imaging and the current methods of analysis of the region by radiologists.

Imaging

CT

Although CT has long been one of the primary methods of imaging the head and neck, current scanners have several advantages over the previous generations of scanners. Multidetector spiral (helical) scanners now are composed of an array of detector elements mounted in a gantry that can continually rotate while the table and patient move through the scanner. This has largely replaced the "step-and-shoot" process of earlier CT scanners. This configuration allows extremely rapid acquisition of a volume data set. The practical advantage is less motion artifact from the rapid scan and a data set that allows for multiplanar manipulation after data acquisition. Postprocessing in the coronal or sagittal planes (and into any other nonstandard plane) and into three-dimensional volume-rendered images and various slice thicknesses allows depiction of the anatomy in ways that can help visualize anatomy, disease, and provide insight into surgical approaches [1]. Intravenous iodinated contrast enhancement is generally used to help identify vascular structures and potentially contrast enhancing pathology.

Although contrast-enhanced CT provides excellent detail of the vasculature of the neck, allowing one to evaluate both the venous and arterial systems, CT angiography is performed to provide additional resolution and detail to the vasculature. Multidetector CT scanners allow for rapid high-resolution acquisition of data timed to correspond to the contrast bolus passing through the arterial system of the neck. This method has developed to a point where CT angiography challenges catheter angiography as the initial method to evaluate the vasculature of the neck [2,3].

MRI

MRI examinations of the neck are generally customized for the anatomic area of interest and the clinical history. Different techniques, coils, and sequences can be used for areas adjacent to the skull base versus the infrahyoid region. Because of the large number of variables that can be manipulated during scanning, customization and careful attention to scan quality are vital to obtain information that is clinically useful.

Although there is no clear superiority of MRI or CT, MRI does have the advantage in the area of soft tissue contrast. Depiction of normal soft tissue anatomy and pathologic process is excellent with MRI. The relative lack of dental artifact on MRI gives it the advantage when evaluating the oral cavity and to some extent the oral pharynx and adjacent regions. CT data can be markedly degraded by the streak artifacts from dental

* Corresponding author.
 E-mail address: andejame@ohsu.edu
 (J.C. Anderson)

1042-3699/08/$ - see front matter © 2008 Elsevier Inc. All rights reserved.
doi:10.1016/j.coms.2008.02.001

hardware. Although there are methods of scanning off plane to reduce the area affected by the artifact, this involves additional scanning and increased radiation exposure. Previously stated advantages of MRI to image in multiple planes has been lessened somewhat by the advent of multidetector spiral CT scanners, which allow manipulation of the data into alternate planes to the usual transverse plane [4].

Contrast use in MRI with gadolinium-based compounds is generally safe, although awareness of the possibility of contrast reactions and for nephrogenic systemic fibrosis in patients with impaired renal function, which is a relatively new concern, should be considered [5].

Neck anatomy

The complexity of neck anatomy has led to various means of organizing the structures for analysis. One of the more entrenched methods is based on the location of and spread of squamous cell cancer of the mucosa in the head and neck. This uses the terms "nasopharynx," "oral pharynx," "hypopharynx," and "larynx" to divide the neck into locations of the primary disease. This method of division defines the areas by the directly visualized mucosa and anatomic structures. Radiographically, these areas can be defined and the extent of deep tissue invasion of squamous cell cancer can be evaluated [6].

The nasopharynx is defined anteriorly by the nasal choana and posteriorly by the prevertebral musculature, upper cervical spine, and inferior clivus. The lateral borders are the mucosal surfaces including the fossa of Rosenmüller and the eustachian tube. The inferior extent is the soft palate and the imaginary line extending posteriorly from the hard and soft palate [6].

The oral pharynx is defined superiorly by the soft palate, and anteriorly by the ring of structures composed of the posterior tongue (circumvallate papilla), the anterior tonsil pillars, and the soft palate. The inferior extent is the epiglottis and glossoepiglottic fold and the phyngoepiglottic fold. Posteriorly, the superior and middle constrictor muscles are the border [6].

The hypopharynx or laryngopharyx is the area inferior to the inferior margin of the oral pharynx, and posterior to the larynx. It extends inferiorly to the lower border of the cricoid cartilage (Fig. 1) [6,7].

Although these definitions and divisions are useful in the staging and evaluation of squamous

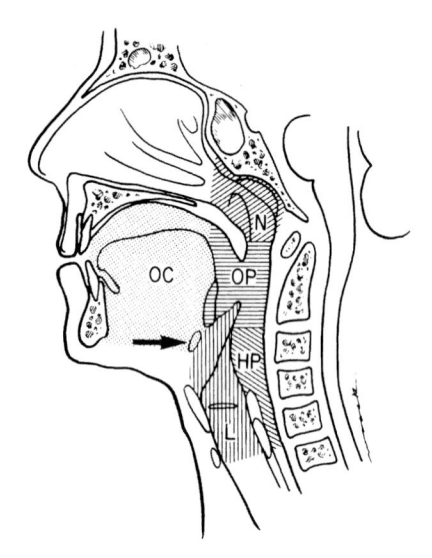

Fig. 1. Normal upper aerodigestive tract. This sagittal upper aerodigestive tract illustrates its major subdivisions: the nasopharynx (N), oropharynx (OP), oral cavity (OC), hypopharynx (HP), and larynx (L). Only the most cephalad aspect of the larynx and hypopharynx is above the hyoid bone (*arrow*). This traditional method of subdivision for the upper aerodigestive tract follows along the lines of the primary sites in the extracranial head and neck where squamous cell carcinoma is found. This traditional terminology remains central to the staging issued in squamous cell carcinoma of the upper aerodigestive tract.

cell carcinoma, they do little to help with the remainder of the anatomy deep to the mucosal surfaces when imaged in the traditional transverse plane of the cross-sectional imaging of CT and MRI.

Spaces

Because of the transverse plane in which CT imaging has long been viewed, radiologists have used various methods to describe the region in a manner that allows accurate communication of both the anatomy and the disease processes of the head and neck. Unfortunately, there have been debates about the terminology and definition of the fascia of the neck; it is difficult to define a single agreed on method for separating the regions of the neck [6–10].

The method described next is primarily based on a system refined by Harnsberger. Although this may only be one of many methods, it has somewhat simplified the analysis of the neck when imaged in the transverse plane. In this method the fascial planes of the head and neck are used to divide the region into definable areas and as a means of systematically analyzing the complex anatomy to help communicate the imaging findings between colleagues. This spatial method of analysis has both an anatomic basis and is a relatively systematic way to evaluate the neck in the transverse plane on CT and MRI. This method divides the neck into the suprahyoid and infrahyoid neck and then further divides regions by the anatomic fascial planes. In this algorithm, the facial structures are divided into the sinonasal region, the orbit, and the oral cavity (Fig. 2). The remainder of the structures of the face and neck are divided into spaces using the fascia as defining structures. The spaces of the suprahyoid neck are pharyngeal mucosal space, parapharyngeal space, masticator space, parotid space, carotid space, retropharyngeal space, danger space, and perivertebral space. Additionally, there are the anatomic locations associated with the oral cavity including the sublingual and submandibular spaces. Each of these spaces contains a definable set of structures and is easily identified on cross-sectional imaging and facilitates communication between radiologists and clinicians [7].

Suprahyoid spaces

The sublingual space is located in the floor of the mouth with the mandible defining the anterolateral border, the mylohyoid the inferiorly, hyoid posteriorly, and oral mucosa superiorly. The sublingual glands, deep lobes and ducts of the submandibular glands, lingual arteries, nerves and veins, V3 branches from the trigeminal nerve, genioglossus, geniohyoid, styloglossus, palatoglossus, hyoglossus, and fat are contained within the sublingual space. Of pathologic importance, the posterior margin of the sublingual space freely communicates with the submandibular and parapharyngeal spaces. A common description of the sublingual space is the "horizontal horseshoe."

The submandibular space lies superior to the hyoid and inferiolateral to the mylohyoid muscle and freely communicates with the sublingual space. This space contains the superficial lobes of the submandibular glands, anterior bellies of the diagastric muscles, and level 1A and 1B lymph nodes. This space is also referred to as the "vertical horseshoe" [11].

The pharyngeal mucosal space is defined by the mucosal surfaces of the nasopharynx, oropharynx, and suprahyoid hypopharynx. The mucosal surfaces of the oral cavity can be included, but more commonly, the oral cavity is considered its own space. The immediate submucosa is also included; this space contains mucosa, lymphoid tissue, minor salivary glands, and some muscular tissue. MRI is considered the imaging modality of choice for this space to evaluate for lesions that cannot be directly visualized or for invasion deep to the submucosa (Fig. 3) [12].

The parapharyngeal space is a primarily fat-filled space extending from skull base to hyoid bone. This space is defined in various ways by various authors. Some authors divide this space into the prestyloid and poststyloid compartments; others include portions of the deep parotid and muscular tissue of the masticator. The primary area of debate on this space in the literature is whether the carotid sheath and its fascial layers are the posterior border. For the purposes of this article, however, the definition of this space is the one used by Harnsberger, which limits the

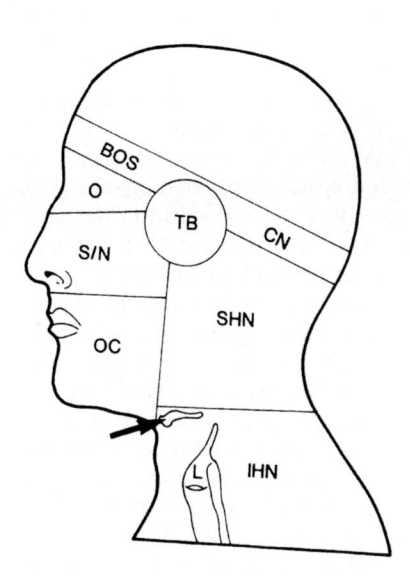

Fig. 2. The "head and neck man." In teaching and writing about the extracranial head and neck area the discussion is usually divided by the major anatomic regions shown in this drawing. The suprahyoid neck (SHN) represents the deep core tissues posterior to the sinonasal (S/N) and oral cavity (OC) areas. Below the level of the hyoid bone (*arrow*) the infrahyoid neck (IHN) can be seen. A distinct area within the infrahyoid neck is the larynx (L). BOS, base of skull; CN, cranial nerves; O, orbit; TB, temporal bone.

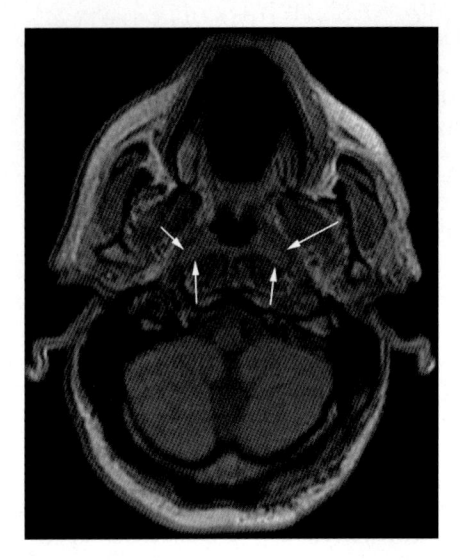

Fig. 3. T1-wieghted transverse MRI at the level of the nasopharynx in the suprahyoid head and neck. The pharyngeal mucosa is well seen (*arrows*) as distinct from the fat and musculature deep to the mucosal surface.

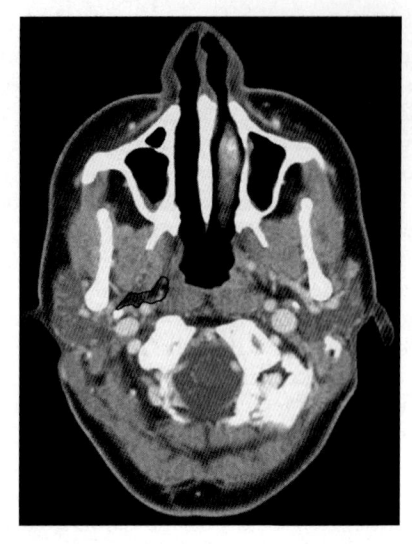

Fig. 4. Transverse CT image through the nasopharynx. Outlined in black is the parapharyngeal space as defined by Harnsberger. This fat-filled structure is centrally located between the other spaces of the neck and is helpful in determining location of origin of masses.

definition of the parapharyngeal space as the primarily fatty-filled space that does not include parotid tissue, mucosa, muscle, bone, or nodes. The posterior border is the carotid space. The margins are limited medially by the middle layer of the deep cervical fascia and laterally by a slip of the superficial layer of the deep cervical fascia separating it from the masticator and parotid. The contents of the parapharyngeal space defined in this manner are fat, vascular tissue, nerves, and rare rests of salivary gland tissue (Fig. 4) [12,13].

The primary importance of the parapharyngeal space radiographically is that it serves as a marker to determine the location or origin of other pathology in the neck because it tends to be displaced away from the site of origin of any mass. Displacement of the parapharyngeal space laterally implicates a lesion in the pharyngeal mucosa, posteriorly implicates the masticator space, anteriorly implicates the carotid space, anterolaterally implicates the retropharyngeal space, and medial displacement implicates the lesion resides in the parotid space.

The masticator space is defined by the superficial layer of the deep cervical fascia (investing fascia). Medially, this extends from the deep edge of the pterygoid muscles from the mandible to attach on the skull base medial to foramen ovale. Laterally the fascia tracts along the superficial masseter muscle to the zygomatic arch, then over the temporalis muscle. This more superior extent (superior to the zygomatic arch) has been termed the "temporal fossa" or space; however, this is an anatomic designation only and no fascia separates these portions of the masticator space. Radiologists may refer to this area as the superior masticator space or the suprazygomatic masticator space; these are equivalent to the term "temporal fossa." The common term "infratemporal fossa" is also part of the masticator space, being the portion between the pterygopalatine fossa medially and the zygomatic arch laterally. Also of note, the parotid duct is superficial to the fascia and is not in the masticator space (Fig. 5) [14,15].

The parotid space is defined as the parotid gland and the structures that are within it, such as the facial nerve, vessels, and the intraparotid lymph nodes. CT is used to evaluate for stone disease and some acute infections; however, MRI is the modality of choice for imaging for masses, perineural tumor spread, and autoimmune diseases (Fig. 6) [16].

The carotid space is surrounded by the carotid sheath, which has components of the investing and pretracheal layers of fascia. Within the carotid sheath are the common and internal carotid arteries, internal jugular vein, vagus nerve, and other nervous tissue, and some deep cervical lymph nodes. The carotid space extends from the

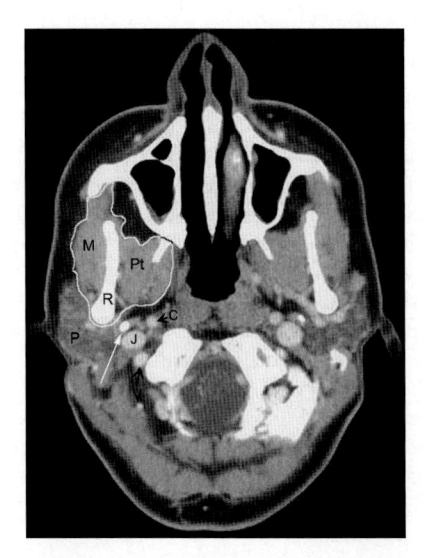

Fig. 5. Transverse CT image through the nasopharynx. Outlined in white is the masticator space, which on this image consists of the masseter muscle (M), mandibular ramus (R), and pterygoid muscules (Pt). Adjacent structures include the parotid (P), styloid process (*white arrow*), internal carotid artery (C), internal jugular vein (J), and vertebral artery (V).

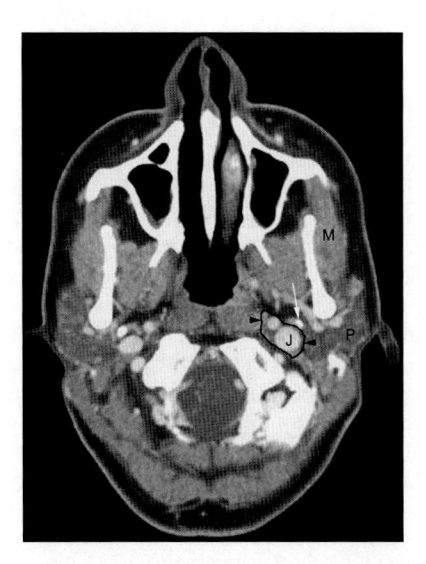

Fig. 7. Transverse CT image through the nasopharynx. The carotid space is outlined in black and indicated by the black arrowheads. The styloid process (*white arrow*) lies anterior to the internal jugular vein (J). Masseter muscle (M) and parotid (P) are indicated.

skull base to the mediastinum and is in both the suprahyoid and infrahyoid neck (Fig. 7) [7,17].

The retropharyngeal space and danger space can be discussed together because they are situated between the prevertebral layer of the deep cervical fascia and the buccopharyngeal fascia. It is limited by the carotid sheaths lateral and also extends from skull base to mediastinum. It is primarily a potential space filled with loose connective tissue; however, in the suprahyoid portion there are lymph nodes present, most notably the lateral retropharyngeal nodes or nodes of Rouvière [18,19].

The perivertebral space is the area defined by the prevertebral fascia, which encloses the bony vertebra and surrounding muscles. This space is divided into an anterior and posterior portion by fascia that attaches to the transverse processes of the vertebral bodies. This space extends both suprahyoid and infrahyoid [20].

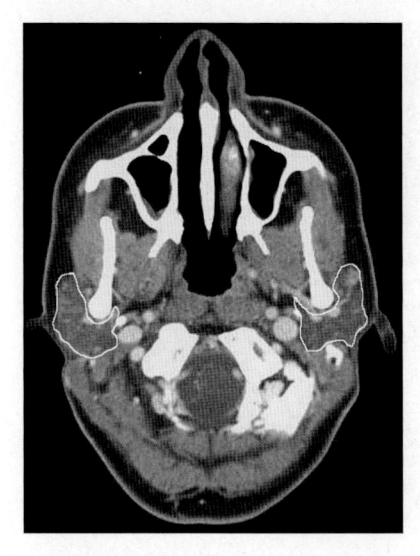

Fig. 6. Transverse CT image through the nasopharynx. The partotid spaces are outlined in white bilaterally. This space consists of the parotid gland, vessels, facial nerve, and intraparotid lymph nodes.

Infrahyoid

The infrahyoid neck can also be defined by the anatomic facial planes and correlated with the usual surgical approaches to these areas. The traditional approach to these areas is the surgical and gross dissection triangles. These triangles are less easily defined and visualized using cross-sectional imaging viewed in the transverse plane. Confusion often ensues when transverse images are viewed and attempted to be interpreted using the anterior and posterior triangles as anatomic areas. An alternate method of analysis that is based on the cross-sectional images and fascially defined spaces and can then be translated into the triangle vernacular has been devised. This continues the terminology and method developed for the suprahyoid neck [21].

The anterior triangle is defined by the sternocleidomastoid muscle as the posterior and lateral border, the midline is the medial border, and the inferior border is the clavicle. The triangle is further divided by the hyoid bone into a suprahyoid and infrahyoid components. The suprahyoid components of the submental and sublingual triangles are not discussed here. The infrahyoid components are further divided by the superior belly of the omohyoid muscle into the muscular and carotid triangles.

The posterior triangle is defined anteromedially by the sternocleidomastoid muscle, posteriorly by the trapezius muscle, and inferiorly by the clavicle. It is further divided by the inferior belly of the omohyoid into the occipital and supraclavicular triangles [19].

The spatial analysis of the infrahyoid neck uses the anatomic fascial planes to define five spaces, two of which are unique to the infrahyoid anatomy and the other three are continuations from the suprahyoid neck. These spaces are the visceral space, carotid space, retropharyngeal space, perivertebral space, and posterior cervical space. The carotid, retropharyngeal, and perivertebral spaces have been discussed previously (Fig. 8).

The visceral space is enclosed by the pretracheal layer of the deep cervical fascia, or to avoid confusion the visceral layer, because it surrounds the tracheal, esophagus, and thyroid (Fig. 9). This extends from the hyoid into the thorax. Posteriorly the visceral layer blends with the buccopharyngeal fascia and laterally with the carotid sheath [21].

The posterior cervical space is essentially the primarily fat-filled space, with some lymph nodes and the spinal accessory nerve, which lies between the perivertebral space posteromedially, the carotid space anteromedially, and the investing layer of the deep cervical fascia surrounding the sternocleidomastoid muscle laterally. This space is predominantly infrahyoid in location, although a small portion does extend superior to the hyoid. This space is essentially equivalent to the posterior triangle [19,21].

Lymphatic system

The use of imaging in the evaluation of the cervical lymphadenopathy for neoplastic, inflammatory, and infectious processes is frequently encountered in current medical practice. It is critical for the interpreting radiologist and consulting surgeon to have a comprehensive knowledge base and understanding of the normal cervical lymphatic anatomy.

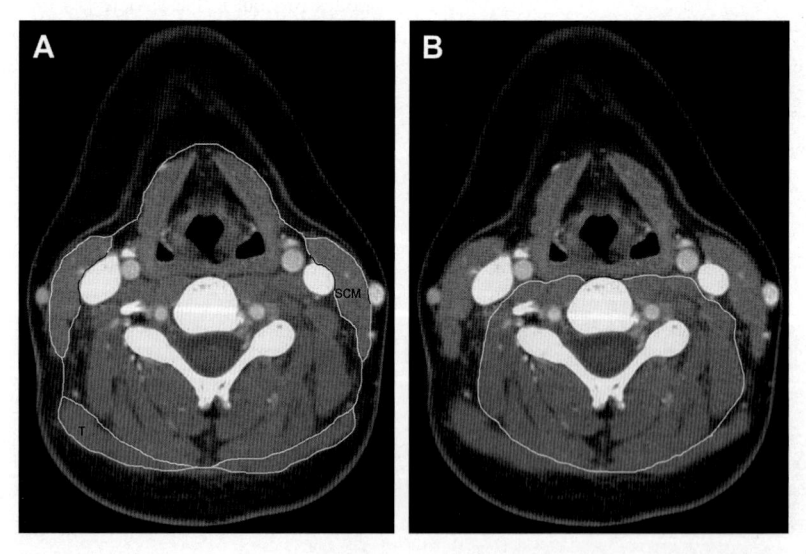

Fig. 8. (*A*) Transverse CT image through the infrahyoid neck. The investing fascia is highlighted and demonstrates it splitting around the sternocleidomastoid muscle (SCM) and the trapezius muscle (T). (*B*) Transverse image through the infrahyoid neck. The prevertebral fascia is highlighted. This fascia defines the perivertebral space, which is both suprahyoid and infrahyoid in location, extending from skull base into the thoracic region.

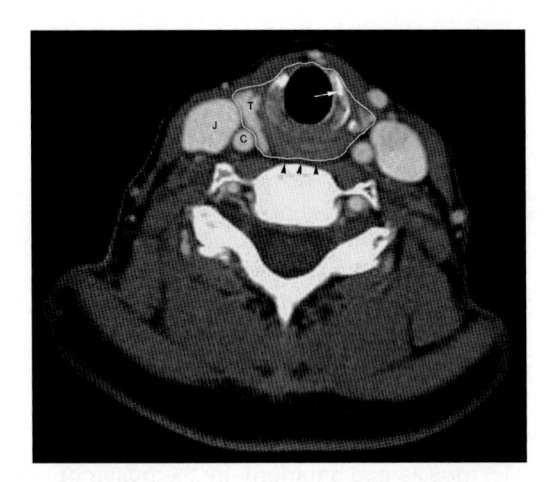

Fig. 9. Transverse image through the infrahyoid neck at the level of the cricoid cartilage (*white arrow*). The prevertebral layer of the deep cervical fascia (or visceral fascia) is highlighted in white. This fascia encircles the thyroid gland (T), larynx, and esophagus. Posterior to the visceral space is the retropharyngeal space (*black arrowheads*), which is seen as a thin dark line of fat between the esophagus and the vertebral body. C, carotid artery; J, internal jugular vein.

The cervical lymphatic system demonstrates characteristic drainage patterns that involve numerous chains and clusters. These patterns of drainage were categorized into zones for prognostic importance and reproducible anatomic localization for neck dissection. The system currently in place is the revised Neck Dissection Classification by the American Head and Neck Society and American Academy of Otolarynogology-Head and Neck Surgery that divides the cervical lymphatic system into separate levels [22].

Currently, the system organizes each side of the neck into six levels, with levels I, II, and V further subclassified secondary to additional pathologic importance. Level I lymph nodes include the submental and submandibular groups. The submental nodal group (level IA) is bounded by the triangle formed by the anterior belly of the diagastric and hyoid bone and receives drainage from the floor of the mouth, anterior oral tongue, lower lip, and mandibular alveolar ridge. The submandibular nodal group (level IB) is bounded by the triangle formed by the anterior bellies of the diagastric, stylohyoid, and body of the mandible. This level receives drainage from the oral cavity, midface soft tissues, submandibular gland, and anterior nasal cavity.

Level II is the upper jugular lymph nodes including the jugulodigastric node, which are bounded by the skull base, hyoid bone, stylohyoid muscle, and the posterior border of the sternocleidomastoid muscle. This level is subclassifed into IIA and IIB by a vertical plane created by the spinal accessory nerve. Level IIA is anterior and level IIB is posterior to the spinal accessory nerve. The drainage received by this level includes oral cavity, nasal cavity, nasopharynx, oropharynx, hypopharynx, larynx, and parotid gland.

Level III is the middle jugular nodes and delineated by the hyoid, cricoid cartilage, posterior sternocleidomastoid muscle, lateral sternohyoid muscle, common carotid, and internal carotid. Lymph drainage into this level is from the oral cavity, nasopharynx, oropharynx, hypopharynx, larynx, and parotid gland.

Level IV is the lower jugular nodes and located within the borders created by the cricoid cartilage, clavicle, lateral sternohyoid, common carotid, and posterior sternocleidomastoid muscle. Hypopharynx, thyroid, esophagus, and larynx all drain into this nodal group.

Level V posterior triangle group are inferior to the spinal accessory nerve and transverse cervical artery and bounded by the trapiezus muscle, posterior sternocleidomastoid muscle, and clavicle. This level is also separated into VA spinal accessory nodes from VB transverse cervical-supraclaviclular nodes by a horizontal line extending from the cricoid. Drainage is from the nasopharynx, oropharynx, and cutaneous structures from the neck and posterior scalp.

The final group is the level VI anterior compartment, which includes the prelaryngeal, prethyroid, and pretracheal and paratracheal nodal groups. This compartment is bounded by the hyoid, suprasternal notch, and lateral boundaries of the common carotid arteries. These nodes receive drainage from the thyroid gland, larynx, piriform sinus, and esophagus.

Lymph nodes not located within these regions are designated by their specific anatomic location. Examples include retropharyngeal, parotid, buccinator, postauricular, malar, mandibular, infraorbital, and suboccipital groups.

Radiographic-based lymph node classification

Unfortunately, not all of the designated anatomic boundaries are radiographically apparent. Radiologists have devised substitutes that approximate the surgical landmarks (Box 1). The stylohyoid muscle and spinal accessory nerve are examples with

Box 1. Radiographic-based lymph node classification

Level I nodes are contained superiorly by the mylohyoid muscle, inferiorly by the lower body of the hyoid bone, and anteriorly by an imaginary coronal line at the posterior margin of the submandibular gland on axial imaging. Level I nodes are further subdivided into IA and IB.

Level IA (submental) nodes are those level I nodes contained laterally by the medial aspects of the anterior diagastric muscles, superiorly by the mylohyoid, and inferiorly by the lower body of the hyoid.

Level IB (submandibular) nodes are level I nodes contained superiorly by the mylohyoid, inferiorly by the lower body of the hyoid, medially by the medial aspects of the anterior diagastric muscles, and posteriorly by a coronal line at the posterior aspects of the submandibular gland.

Level II (upper jugular) nodes are contained superiorly by the skull base from the margin of the jugular fossa and inferiorly to the lower body of the hyoid. The anterior border is the imaginary coronal line that extends from the posterior edge of the submandibular gland. The posterior border is an imaginary coronal line at the posterior aspect of the sternocleidomastoid muscle on axial imaging. Any lymph nodes medial to an imaginary sagittal line through the carotid artery are referred to as "retropharyngeal" and not level II. Level II nodes are subclassified into IIA and IIB.

Level IIA nodes are anterior, lateral, medial, and posterior but inseparable from the internal jugular vein.

Level IIB nodes lie posterior to the internal jugular vein separated by a visible fat plane.

Level III (middle jugular) nodes are contained superiorly by the lower body of the hyoid and inferiorly by the lower margin of the cricoid cartilage. These nodes also lie anterior to the posterior border of the sternocleidomastoid muscle and medial to the common and internal carotid arteries.

Level IV (lower jugular) nodes are contained superiorly by the lower margin of the cricoid, inferiorly by the clavicle, anterolateral by an oblique line from the posterior margin of the sternocleidomastoid, and medially by the common carotid artery.

Level V nodes are contained posteriorly by a coronal line on axial imaging from the anterior margin of the trapezius muscle and anteriorly by the posterior margin of the sternocleidomastoid from the skull base to the clavicle. Level V nodes are also subdivided into VA and VB nodes.

Level VA (spinal accessory) nodes are level V nodes superior to a horizontal line from the lower margin of the cricoid cartilage to the skull base.

Level VA (transverse cervical/ supraclavicular) nodes are those level V nodes that lie inferior to the lower margin of the cricoid and clavicle.

Level VI (anterior compartment) nodes are contained superiorly by the lower body of the hyoid and inferiorly by the sternal manubrium. These nodes also lie medial to an imaginary sagittal line through the common and internal carotid arteries.

the posterior submandibular gland and fat plane posterior to the internal jugular vein being the radiographic correlates, respectively [23,24].

Summary

This article reviews the anatomy of the head and neck with regards to its radiology. A brief discussion of the current imaging modalities is provided. The various methods of visualizing, analyzing, and communicating this complex region of anatomy are correlated.

References

[1] Imhof H, Czerny C, Dirisamer A. Head and neck imaging with MDCT. Eur J Radiol 2003;45(Suppl 1):S23–31.

[2] Brant-Zawadzki M, Heiserman JE. The roles of MR angiography, CT angiography, and sonography in vascular imaging of the head and neck. AJNR Am J Neuroradiol 1997;18(10):1820–5.

[3] Hollingworth W, Nathens AB, Kanne JP, et al. The diagnostic accuracy of computed tomography angiography for traumatic or atherosclerotic lesions of the carotid and vertebral arteries: a systematic review. Eur J Radiol 2003;48(1):88–102.

[4] Wippold FJ. Head and neck imaging: the role of CT and MRI. J Magn Res Imaging 2007;25:453–65.

[5] Grobner T, Prischl FC. Gadolinium and nephrogenic systemic fibrosis. Kidney Int 2007;72:260–4.

[6] Greene FL, Page DL, Fleming ID, et al, editors. AJCC cancer staging handbook. 6th edition. 2002. American Joint Committee on Cancer, Springer: New York, Online access STAT!Ref accessed Nov. 2007. p. 47–60.

[7] Harnsberger HR. Introduction to the suprahyoid neck. In: Harnsberger HR, editor. Handbook of head and neck imaging. 2nd edition. St Louis (MO): Mosby; 1995. p. 3–28.

[8] Som PM, Curtin HD. Fasciae and spaces. In: Som PM, Curtin HD, editors. Head and neck imaging. 3rd edition. St. Louis (MO): Mosby; 1996. p. 738–46.

[9] Accioli de Vasconcellos JJ, Britto JA, Henin D, et al. The fascial planes of the temple and face: an enbloc anatomic study and a plea for consistency. The British Association of Plastic Surgeons 2003;56:623–9.

[10] Wendell-Smith CP. Fascia: an illustrative problem in international terminology. Surg Radiol Anat 1997;19:273–7.

[11] Smoker WR. Normal anatomy of the neck. In: Som PM, Curtin HD, editors. Head and neck imaging. 3rd edition. St Louis (MO): Mosby; 1996. p. 711–37.

[12] Harnsberger HR. The parapharyngeal space and the pharyngeal mucosal space. In: Handbook of head and neck imaging. 2nd edition. St Louis (MO): Mosby; 1995. p. 29–45.

[13] Som PM, Curtin HD. Parapharyngeal space. In: Som PM, Curtin HD, editors. Head and neck imaging. 3rd edition. St. Louis (MO): Mosby; 1996. p. 915–51.

[14] Harnsberger HR. The masticator space. In: Harnsberger HR, editor. Handbook of head and neck imaging. 2nd edition. St Louis (MO): Mosby; 1995. p. 46–59.

[15] Moore KL, Dalley AF. Head. In: Moore KL, Dalley AF, editors. Clinically oriented anatomy. 4th edition. Philadelphia: Lippincott Williams & Williams; 1999. p. 916–23.

[16] Harnsberger HR. The parotid space. In: Harnsberger HR, editor. Handbook of head and neck imaging. 2nd edition. St Louis (MO): Mosby; 1995. p. 60–74.

[17] Harnsberger HR. The carotid space. In: Harnsberger HR, editor. Handbook of head and neck imaging. 2nd edition. St Louis (MO): Mosby; 1995. p. 75–88.

[18] Harnsberger HR. The retropharyngeal space. In: Harnsberger HR, editor. Handbook of head and neck imaging. 2nd edition. St Louis (MO): Mosby; 1995. p. 89–104.

[19] Moore KL, Dalley AF. Neck. In: Moore KL, Dalley AF, editors. Clinically oriented anatomy. 4th edition. Philadelphia: Lippincott Williams & Williams; 1999. p. 995–1081.

[20] Harnsberger HR. The perivertebral space. In: Harnsberger HR, editor. Handbook of head and neck imaging. 2nd edition. St Louis (MO): Mosby; 1995. p. 105–19.

[21] Harnsberger HR. The infrahyoid neck: normal anatomy and pathology of the head and neck from the hyoid bone to the clavicles. In: Harnsberger HR, editor. Handbook of head and neck imaging. 2nd edition. St Louis (MO): Mosby; 1995. p. 151–98.

[22] Robbins KT, Clayman G, Levine PA, et al. Neck dissection classification update. Arch Otolaryngol Head Neck Surg 2002;128(7):751–8.

[23] Som PM. Lymph nodes. In: Som PM, Curtin HD, editors. Head and neck imaging. 3rd edition. St Louis (MO): Mosby; 1996. p. 772–93.

[24] Krestan C, Herneth AM, Formanek M, et al. Modern imaging lymph node staging of the head and neck region. Eur J Radiol 2006;58:360–6.

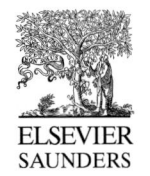

Neck Masses: Evaluation and Diagnostic Approach

Jason Lee, DDS[a], Rui Fernandes, DMD, MD, FACS[b],*

[a]*Division of Oral & Maxillofacial Surgery, Department of Surgery, University of Florida College of Medicine, Jacksonville, FL, USA*
[b]*Division of Oral & Maxillofacial Surgery, and Section of Surgical Oncology, Department of Surgery, University of Florida College of Medicine, Jacksonville, FL, USA*

Oral and maxillofacial surgeons frequently deal with patients who present with an unknown neck mass. Formulation of a differential diagnosis is essential and requires that the surgeon bring to bear a host of skills to systematically arrive at a definitive diagnosis and ensure that the correct treatment is rendered. This article highlights some of the skills needed in the workup of neck masses and reviews some of the available techniques that aid in achieving the correct diagnosis.

Clinical evaluation

The way you talk with a patient while taking a history lays the foundation for good care. By listening and responding skillfully and empathically, you learn what is bothering the patient and what symptoms he or she has experienced. You also may learn what the patient thinks the trouble may be, how or why it happened, and what outcome is hoped for or feared. As you listen to the story of an illness, moreover, you begin to formulate a range of possible diagnoses. By asking additional questions, you can fill in the gaps in the patient's initial account and test some of your diagnostic hypotheses... [1].

The history and physical examination is the cornerstone of medicine. The surgeon must continually strive to improve on this skill through deliberate and systematic manipulation of the history and physical. In stressing the importance of history-taking, Sir William Osler said: "If you listen to your patient, they will tell you their diagnosis" [1].

History and review of systems

The chief complaint provides the foundation for the evaluation of the patient and directs the examination. Once this data have been obtained, the history of the present illness should be examined further because it is valuable for the development of the initial diagnostic impressions. Characteristics of the mass, such as the location, growth rate, and presence of pain, provide clues to the nature of the problem. For example, a long-standing nonpainful mass with slow or insignificant changes points toward a benign process. Associated symptoms, such as referred pain, changes in voice quality, difficulty swallowing, and epistaxis, should be discussed with the patient and can give clues to the origin of the mass. The surgeon should also question the patient regarding systemic symptoms. Although such symptoms may be uncommon, they can suggest metastatic disease, especially if neurologic and pulmonary complaints are present. The classic "B signs" of lymphoma are fever, night sweats, and weight loss.

The clinician not only has to consider the present illness, but the patient's sex, age, social history, occupational exposure, travel history, and past surgical and medical history. For example, it is not too uncommon for patients to present to a surgeon with a neck mass only a few months after another physician removed a skin cancer from the patient's face or neck.

---

* Corresponding author. Department of Surgery, University of Florida College of Medicine, 653-1 West 8th Street, Jacksonville, FL 32246
E-mail address: rui.fernandes@jax.ufl.edu (R. Fernandes).

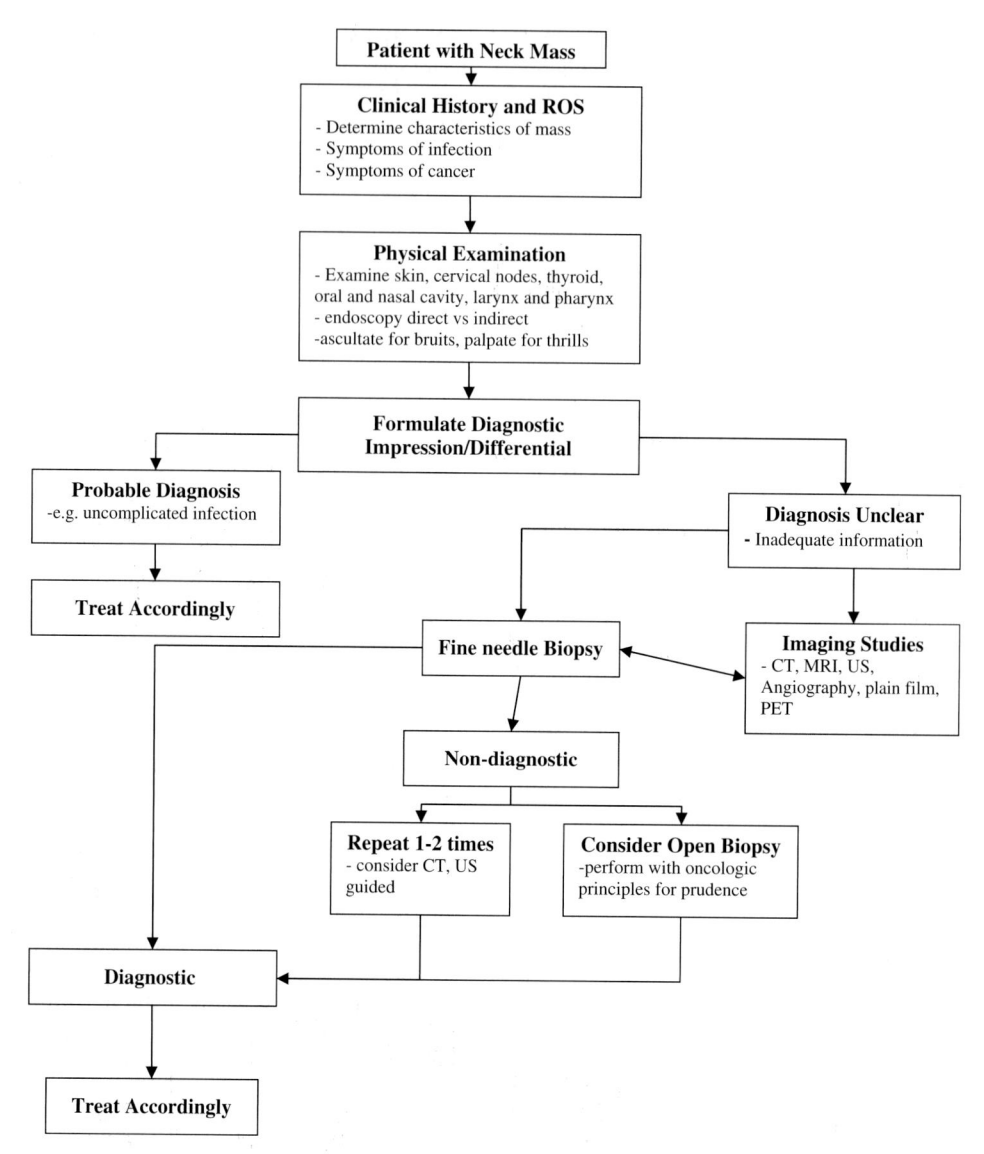

Fig. 1. Algorithm for assessment of a neck mass. *Abbreviations:* PET, positron emission tomography; ROS, review of system; US, ultrasound.

course of antibiotic therapy poses a treatment dilemma to the clinician. The incidence of malignancy is lower in children than in adults, with mesenchymal tumors representing 90% of the lesions found in children [17]. Torsiglieri and colleagues [18] reviewed 455 pediatric FNABs and found 55% congenital lesions, 27% inflammatory, 5% noninflammatory benign lesions, 3% benign neoplasms, and 11% malignancies, the most common being lymphoma. Several studies have reported the efficacy and safety of FNAB in the pediatric population [19,20]. The psychologic trauma of an FNAB to the patient and the parents has to be weighed against the risks and benefits of traditional open biopsy under general anesthesia.

FNAB is a valuable diagnostic tool in the evaluation of a neck mass in both the pediatric and adult patient. Its low overall cost, low associated morbidity, and high accuracy put it at the top of the diagnostic algorithm. However, despite their positive attributes, FNABs are not

> **Box 1. Limited differential for a neck mass**
>
> *Nonneoplastic*
> Congenital
>   Thyroglossal duct cyst
>   Branchial cleft cyst
>   Hemangiomas
>   Lymphangioma (cystic hygroma)
>   Layngoceole
>   Dermoid
> Infectious
>   Acute lymphadenitis
>   Abscess
>   Tuberculosis
>   Cat scratch disease
>
> *Neoplastic*
> Benign
>   Lipoma
>   Salivary
>   Pleomorphic adenoma
>   Warthin's tumor
>   Thyroid goiter
>   Paragangliomas (eg, carotid body tumors)
> Malignant
>   Salivary
>   Mucoepidermoid
>   Adenoid cystic
>   Thyroid carcinoma
>   Metastatic carcinoma
>   Sarcoma
>   Lymphoma

infallible and should never replace sound clinical judgment.

Imaging studies

Imaging is frequently employed to help determine the exact location and other characteristics of the disease process among patients who present with a neck mass. The only exception may be someone with an obvious inflammatory or infective process where empiric treatment may be started, followed by re-evaluation. CT and MRI have proven to be indispensable tools in evaluating a patient with a neck mass and can be used to complement one another. In principle, imaging complements the physical examination, and axial and coronal sectional studies are based on anatomy and the changes that occur with pathology.

CT and MRI studies can also complement one another. An important consideration is context of the study (eg, after-operation, following earlier procedures).

The use of imaging in the determination of head and neck malignancies is vital for determining the origin, extent, and thus resectability of the mass. Imaging of the cervical lymphatics alters the estimated clinical stage in 20% to 30% of patients [21].

CT scan

CT is probably the most widely used imaging study in the head and neck, outside the neurocranium. It has the advantages of wide availability, speed, relatively low cost, and good spatial resolution. It is excellent at separating fat from muscle, and bone is well imaged. However, its ability to separate muscle and tumor is not as good. Spiral (helical) CT is quickly becoming the mainstay in many medical centers [22]. The advantages of spiral CT are a result of the continuous rotation of the x-ray tube and the detector as the patient moves through the gantry. This allows rapid scanning of large volumes of tissue during quiet respiration; a reduction in the amount of intravenous contrast needed, as well as the amount of motion artifact; and multiplanar and three-dimensional reconstruction [23–25]. CT can be particularly valuable in the head and neck pathology patient because many of these patients have significant comorbidities, such as chronic obstructive pulmonary disease, and cannot handle their secretions. Therefore, breath-holding and long scanning time are not well tolerated.

MRI

Although MRI has several favorable characteristics for the evaluation of the head and neck, its superiority compared with CT has not been established [26,27]. There is, however, a distinct advantage in its soft tissue capabilities and it is useful when the distinction between the mass and surrounding soft tissue is poor. Metallic dental restorations do not significantly degrade the MRI image. Many different techniques are available for image enhancement on MRI. In general, T1-weighed images relate to how quickly nuclei return to their base state. This type of image takes less time to produce and fat appears bright and cerebrospinal fluid dark. T2-weighted images relate to the loss of phase coherence and typically take longer to acquire. These images produce cerebrospinal fluid that is bright and fat that is darker. Gadolinium-enhanced images can also improve the clarity of margins of many lesions and, because gadolinium is a noniodinated medium, it is considered safer in patients with renal impairment and a history of allergic reactions [28,29]. Additional techniques, such as fast-spin echo and fat suppression, produce sharper images in shorter times and allow for better delineation of tissues. For example, in fast spin echo T2 images, fat does not appear dark, and distinguishing between fat and fluid (eg, hemorrhage) is difficult. Fat suppression techniques obliterate the signal from fat, producing an image where fluid is bright and fat is dark. This technique can also be applied to gadolinium-enhanced T1 images where the lesion abuts fatty tissues and the extent of the mass is obscured because both are bright [30].

In patients with cancer of the head and neck, nodal involvement has significant prognostic value. Studies in the late 80s by Mancuso and colleagues [31] and Som [32] illustrated the use of CT in detection of nodal metastasis. Radiographic abnormalities that may indicate a pathologic process include nodal enlargement beyond maximal normal size, clusters of ill-defined nodes, and distinctive nodal shapes. Although shape and size are no longer considered reliable, round nodes tend to be neoplastic and elliptic nodes tend to be normal or hyperplastic [33]. Contrast-enhanced CT is thought to be superior to MRI in the detection of central nodal necrosis [27]. With the development of fat suppression techniques, gadolinium enhancement, field strength, high-resolution microimaging, and stylized surface coils, MRI has been reported to be comparable to CT in central nodal necrosis detection [26,34]. MRI is also preferred for targeted imaging of a primary site, such as base of tongue, salivary glands, and the base of the skull, especially when perineural extension is a concern [35]. Another recent advance is that of the use of MRI imaging to identify pathologic nodes using supermagnetic iron oxide nanoparticles that accumulate in normal functioning nodes, giving an intense signal. The goal is to improve sensitivity in detecting smaller metastatic nodes from reactive nodes [36].

Positron emission tomography

Positron emission tomography (PET) is another modality for evaluating the patient with a neck mass, especially if metastatic disease is high on the differential. PET is a functional study based on the uptake of 18-fluorodeoxyglucose in cells proportional to their rate of glycolysis [37]. PET scans have the ability to survey the whole body and detect primary tumors that would not otherwise be visualized. It routinely is used to detect an occult primary and in the evaluation of recurrent disease after treatment [38,39]. Traditionally, the widespread use of PET has been limited because of its expense, its poor spatial resolution, and its limited availability. Other limitations are its inability to detect lesions smaller than 5 to 10 mm and the physiologic uptake of laryngeal and oropharyngeal muscles, resulting in unwanted false positives [40,41]. Recently, PET has been combined with other modalities, such as CT, providing anatomic and functional information. Several studies have reported improved detection of primary and metastatic disease when PET combined with CT was compared with PET, CT, and MRI alone [42,43].

Ultrasound

Ultrasound is another study that is readily available, inexpensive, noninvasive, and accurate. Conventional B-mode ultrasound has been used with success as an examination tool in the evaluation of benign, inflammatory, vascular, and malignant lesions, as well as in the evaluation and surveillance of thyroid nodules [44–47]. It also can be used in both the pre- and postoperative phases of treatment. Other techniques, such as contrast-enhanced color Doppler sonography, have also been investigated to give information about blood flow to lymph nodes. Moritz and colleagues [48] showed that characterization of hilar vessels with branching indicated lymphadenitis and predominately peripheral vessels indicated malignancy with very high sensitivities and specificities. The limitation of ultrasound is that it is highly operator-dependent and many radiologists inexperienced in ultrasound prefer CT or MRI. Ultrasound is commonly used to direct FNAB techniques to improve the diagnostic yield [49,50]. Ultrasound is widely used in Europe for neck mass evaluation and many European oral-maxillofacial surgery clinics employ ultrasound as an adjunct to physical examination.

Angiography

Vascular lesions should be considered when dealing with a mass in the head and neck, especially in the pediatric population [51]. Clinical examination is often sufficient for diagnosis when all or a portion of the lesion is superficial. However, the extent of the lesion is often underestimated [52,53]. Deeper lesions of the neck require imaging and sometimes the study itself can diagnose the lesion. For example, angiography of carotid body tumors demonstrates their pathognomonic lyre signs (bowing of the external and internal carotid arteries) [54]. Imaging can also be essential for treatment feasibility, preoperative planning, and sometimes diagnosis. The combined use of angiography, CT, and MRI has been described for evaluating hemangiomas, lymphangiomas, arteriovenous malformations, and paragangliomas. In general, MRI is considered to give the most diagnostic information regarding tissue characterization and extension of vascular lesions [54,55]. CT and plain radiographic studies are valuable when intraosseous involvement is suspected. However, care must be taken with lesions involving the mandible because on plain radiography vascular malformations are difficult to distinguish from benign odontogenic tumors, such as ameloblastomas or myxomas [56]. Both CT and magnetic resonance angiography can be used for three-dimensional reconstruction. These can be helpful in preoperative planning and in some situations can eliminate the need for angiography [57,58]. Catheter angiography is valuable when large vascular connections are suspected or when preoperative delineation of feeding and draining vessels for surgery and embolization is needed. Catheter angiography does not, however, demonstrate the involvement of the lesion with the surrounding tissue [59,60].

Common neck masses

The following is a short list of common neck masses that may be encountered by the surgeon.

Nonneoplastic masses

Nonneoplastic masses in the neck may be separated into two broad categories: congenital or infectious. The following is a brief description of entities that may be placed in the differential of neck masses.

Congenital

Congenital masses are those that were present since birth. They may have enlarged over a period of time but the common thread is the presentation at birth.

Lymphangiomas (cystic hygromas)

The old term for cervical lymphangioma is cystic hygroma. This entity results from a malformation of the lymphatic system in the cervical region that leads to proliferation of the vessels in the region and a subsequent mass. These masses may encompass a large area of the neck without true localization to a specific site. Lymphangiomas may be subdivided into macrocystic versus microcystic. This distinction is based on the predominant size of the cystic spaces within the lesion and may impact on the treatment and resolution of the lesion. Macrocystic lesions are more susceptible to the sclerosing agent OK432 (picibanil).

Branchial cleft cysts

Branchial cleft cysts originate from entrapped squamous epithelium and lymphoid tissues during development of the branchial grooves. There are multiple types of branchial cleft cysts ranging from type I to type IV. The most common branchial cleft cyst is the type II (second branchial cleft). The location of the second branchial cleft cyst is in the upper neck deep to the sternocleidomastoid muscle with its anterior sinus often exiting anterior to the muscle. These cysts often present during the younger years of development with the majority presenting before 10 years of age. One can occasionally see these cysts in adults, often after an infection resulting in a rapid enlargement of the cyst and pain. These cysts are often confused with large necrotic cystic nodes from tonsilar cancer.

Thyroglosal duct cysts

The most common developmental cyst found in the neck is the thyroglossal duct cyst [61]. This cyst originates from a lack of degeneration of the cystic track from the migration of the thyroid gland in the neck during development. As such, the track may be found anywhere from the foramen cecum up to the pyramidal lobe of the thyroid. During development, as the thyroid descends in the neck, it is close to the developing hyoid bone (Reichert's cartilage). Given this fact, the track of the cyst may be present in front, back, or through the central portion of the hyoid bone. The typical presentation of the thyroglossal duct cyst is a large mass in the midline of the neck that moves with swallowing or protrusion of the tongue. The lesion may also present as a lateral or paramedian mass. A common clinical scenario is that of a young person with a recent upper respiratory track infection and a new neck mass.

The resection of these cysts entails the complete removal of the mass and its track along with the central portion of the hyoid bone as described by Sistrunk [62] (Fig. 2).

Vascular lesions

Virchow [63] described the first anatomic pathologic classification of vascular lesions. Our current understanding was greatly expanded by the work of Mulliken and Glowacki [64], who classified vascular lesions as hemangiomas and vascular malformations. Hemangiomas are present at birth and rapidly proliferate in the first years of life, followed by a slow involution. Vascular malformations are present at birth but may not be evident and show proportionate growth. Hemangiomas typically are classified as capillary, cavernous, and capillary-cavernous. These lesions are more common in females (3:1) and 60% are located in the head and neck [65,66]. A large majority of these lesions are not treated because of their tendency for spontaneously involution. However 40% to 50% of these have residual telangectasias, scarring, or atrophic skin that needs treatment. Immediate therapeutic intervention is necessary in patients with lesions that compromise the airway, visual or auditory function, and feeding [67]. Many different treatment modalities have been described, including steroids, cryotherapy, embolization, sclerotherapy, laser, and surgery [68]. Vascular lesions are classified by the type of vessel involved and their intravascular flow (ie, high versus low). Capillary, lymphatic, and venous malformations are classified as "low flow." Arterial, arteriovenous malformations and arteriovenous fistulas are considered "high flow" [64]. Generally, treatment consists of laser, or embolization, or both, followed by surgery [68].

Infectious

Infectious processes may also account for enlargement/masses in the neck. These lesions may appear as localized or diffuse. Other causes,

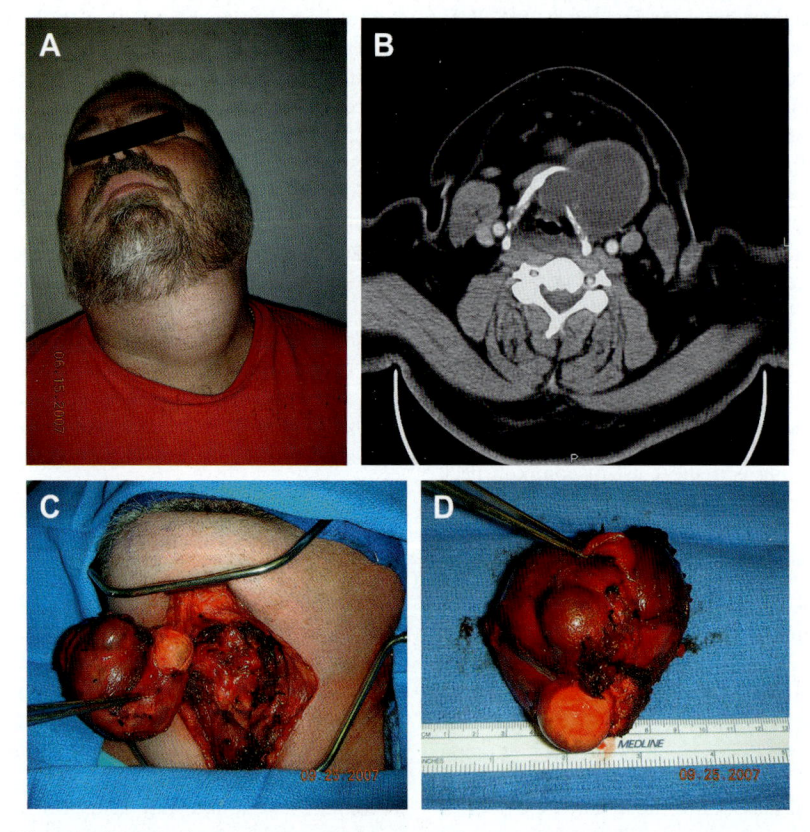

Fig. 2. (*A*) Adult male with enlarging neck mass. (*B*) CT scan of the central neck mass revealing the large cystic mass in the central neck consistent with a thyroglossal duct cyst. (*C*) Surgical resection of the mass via a Sistrunk procedure. (*D*) Surgical specimen.

aside from the routine abscesses originating from odontogenic sources or folliculitis, include tuberculosis and cat scratch disease (CSD).

Tuberculosis

During the past 2 decades, tuberculosis was a relatively rare disease. However, with the continued progression of the HIV and AIDS, a rise in the number of cases has been noted in the western hemisphere. Tuberculosis has and continues to be a major health problem for the developing world. When present in the neck, this disease is referred to as scrofula.

Cat scratch disease

The causative organism of CSD is the gram-negative bacterium Bartonella henselae. CSD is one of the common reasons for infectious cervical lymphadenopathy both in adults and children. Usually 3 to 10 days after contact with an infected cat, often a newly acquired kitten, a small papule appears followed by a prolonged period of regional lymphadenopathy [69]. The workup for CSD includes a thorough history and physical examination and can be confirmed by serology (IgG or IgM antibodies against *Bartonella*) or bartonella DNA. The treatment for CSD is supportive care. A course of antibiotic, often a cephalosporin, may be employed for patients with painful or abscessed lymph nodes.

Neoplastic masses

Benign lesions

Tumors in the neck may originate from any tissues present in the neck. As such, the tumors include salivary gland tumors (originating from the submandibular gland or tail of the parotid gland), nerve sheath and nerve tumors, lipomas, vascular tumors, and others. This simple but often forgotten fact will aid in the formulation of a good differential diagnosis for the surgical trainee.

Lipomas

Benign lipomatous tumors have been subclassified according to their histologic features and growth pattern into classic lipomas (solitary or multiple), fibrolipoma, angiolipoma, infiltrating lipoma, intramuscular lipoma, hibernoma, pleomorphic lipoma, lipoblastomatosis, and diffuse lipoblastomatosis [70,71]. Further classification has also been done according to either size or weight. A tumor is classified as a giant lipoma if the size is greater than 10 cm in one dimension or the weight greater than 1000 g [72]. Lipomas may present in the neck as large isolated masses present for long periods of time without much change over the years. The treatment of these benign tumors is a simple excision. Recurrence of these tumors is rare (Figs. 3 and 4).

Carotid body tumors

A carotid body tumor is a type of a paraganglioma. Paragangliomas represent vascular neoplastic tumors that arise from chemoreceptors located in the walls of blood vessels or are associated with specific nerves [73]. The tissue of origin of these tumors denotes the name given to the tumors. They range from carotid body tumors to jugular paragangliomas. The common presentation of a carotid body tumor is a neck mass that does not move in a superior-inferior direction but does in the anterior-posterior direction. The mass may be pulsatile or present with a bruit. Angiography used to be the primary imaging modality for carotid body tumors. This study would give a characteristic appearance referred to as the lyre sign. Today MR or CT scans may be used to obtain this information. The treatment for these tumors is surgical resection whenever possible, depending on tumor size and patient comorbidities (Fig. 5).

Thyroid nodules and goiters

Goiter, the Latin term for throat, describes an enlargement of the thyroid gland. The type of goiter can be classified based on its epidemiologic, etiologic, functional, or morphologic factors. Iodine deficiency is the most common factor contributing to the development of goiter. However, other factors that can play a role include elevated thyrotropin, advanced age, pregnancy, and exposure to lithium. Also, a variant of Hashimoto's thryoiditis is associated with goiters, as is Graves' disease, and nutritional goitrogens (eg, cassava) [74]. The World Health Organization has also graded goiters from 0 to 2 or 3, based on palpation and size of the goiter. Treatment is based on functional disease or compressive symptoms (to surrounding nerves, vessels, or organs). Goiters also can be substernal, graded from I to III, depending on the position in the mediastinum, necessitating the appropriate presurgical planning [75]. In the United States, surgery is the mainstay of treatment but radioactive iodine can be used instead [76,77] (Fig. 6).

Thyroid nodules can also present a challenge to the clinician. Although most thyroid nodules are benign, evaluation needs to be done to rule out

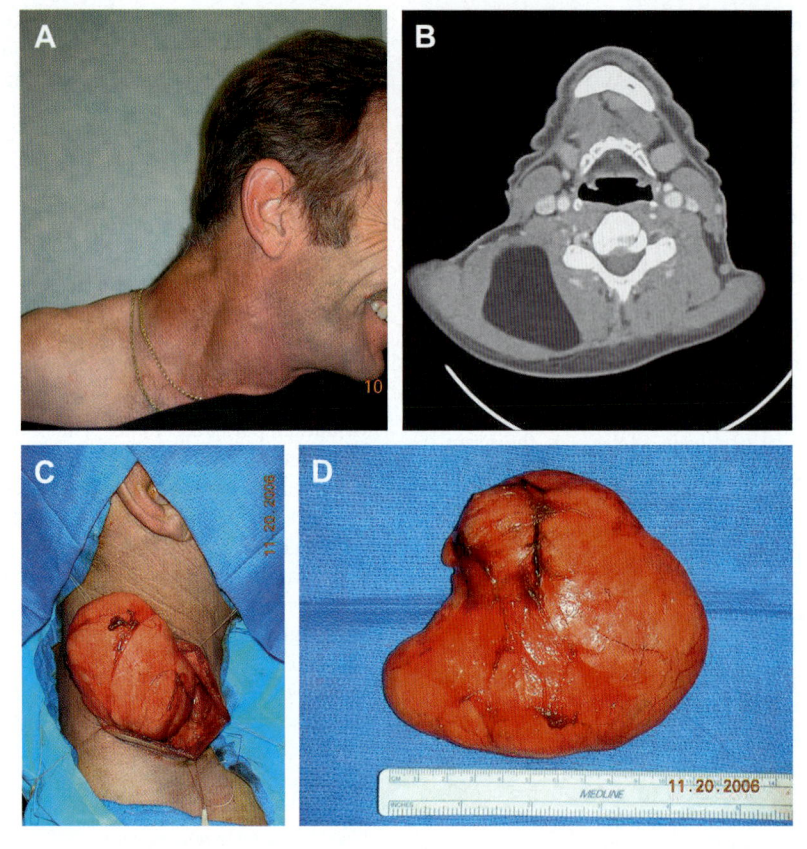

Fig. 3. (*A*) Patient with a right neck mass in level V. (*B*) CT scan of the mass revealed a large mass consistent with a lipoma. (*C*) Surgical exposure and delivery of the mass. (*D*) Surgical specimen.

cancer. The workup varies depending on the surgeon and the patient's presentation. Such factors as stability and size of nodule, age, sex, and history of irradiation all influence the risk of malignancy [78]. The workup generally consists of fine needle aspiration (principal tool), ultrasound, thyroid function tests, and scintigraphy.

Malignant neoplasms

Much like benign tumors of the neck, malignant neoplasms can originate from any tissues in the region, or may present secondary to metastasis from distant sites. The possibilities range from metastatic carcinomas (eg, lung, colon, breast) to salivary gland malignancies (Fig. 7). An asymmetric, asymptomatic mass in the neck, especially in adults, is always considered a malignancy until proven otherwise. The occurrence of a malignant process in these lesions is approximately 30% [79,80]. We present a short list of malignant neoplasms that can present in the neck.

Upper aerodigestive tract cancer

Upper aerodigestive tract cancers include lesions arising from the oral cavity, nasopharynx, hypopharynx, and the larynx. These cancers represent about 3% of all cancers. It is predicted that in 2008, 47,560 men and women will be diagnosed with this disease. About 90% of these will be epithelial in nature [81]. Alcohol and tobacco are the common etiologic factors in the development of this disease. Recent studies have shown that there is also a link with the human papilloma virus. The oral cavity is the most common site for primary tumors of the head and neck, with the tongue and floor of the mouth predominating. Several factors influence the presence of regional metastasis, such as depth of invasion (>2 mm), site, and stage. As many as 30% of patients present with cervical involvement and

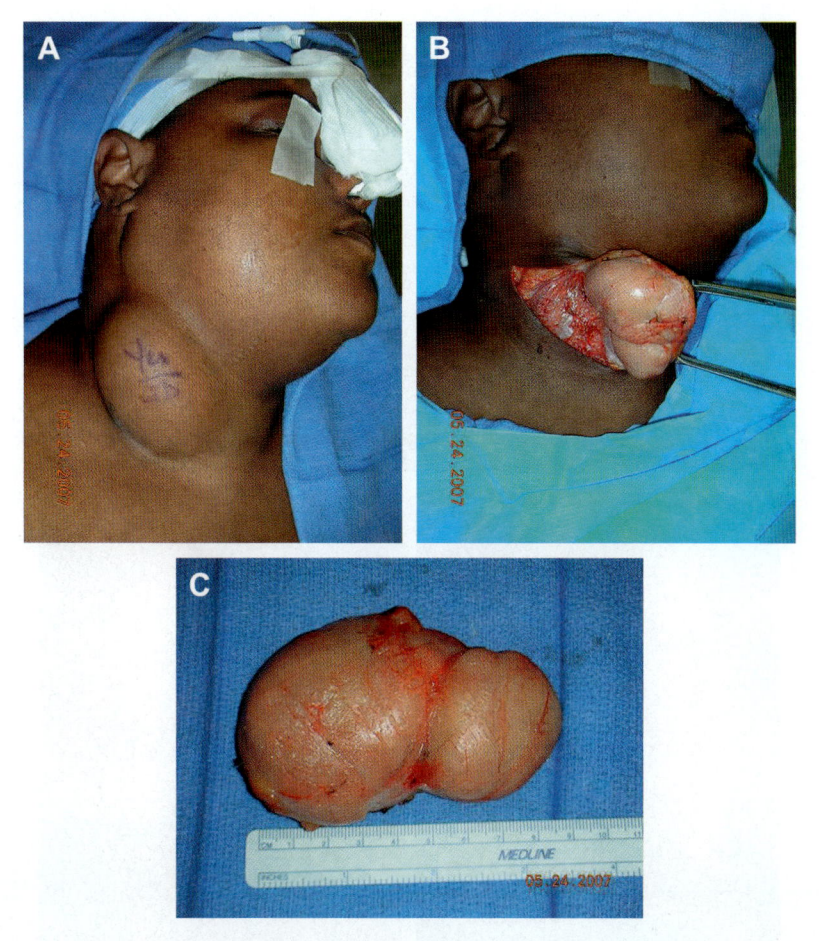

Fig. 4. (*A*) A young woman with a long-standing, enlarging neck mass consistent with a lipoma. (*B*) Surgical delivery of the mass. Note the superficial location of the mass. (*C*) Surgical mass.

up to 45% of patients harbor occult metastasis, usually in levels I, II, or III [82,83]. Nasopharyngeal carcinoma is relatively rare in the United States. However, because of the propensity of nasopharyngeal carcinoma for cervical metastasis, which has been reported as high as 87%, it should not be overlooked [82,83]. Oropharyngeal carcinomas most commonly arise at the tonsil and base of tongue and, because of the abundant lymphoid tissue in this subsite (Waldeyer's ring), lymphomas often present here as well. Depending on the subsite, there is a 15% to 75% rate of cervical node involvement and bilateral metastasis is common [82,83]. Large cystic metastasis from this subsite is common and can be mistakenly diagnosed and treated as a branchial cleft cyst. As a result, high-risk "unknown primary" patients should undergo tonsillectomy and blind biopsy. The hypopharynx extends from the hyoid to the postcricoid area and is divided into three subsites: (1) the pyriform sinus (the most common site), (2) the lateral/posterior pharyngeal walls, and (3), the postcricoid area. Cervical involvement is high and the prognosis is quite poor with these tumors. Laryngeal tumors are divided into (1) supraglottic, (2) glottic, and (3) subglottic categories. Cancers of the glottis are most common and have the best prognosis. Cervical involvement varies with the subsite and is highest with supraglottic carcinomas. Supraglottic cancers tend to present later because the area is difficult to examine and symptoms (eg, voice hoarseness) don't arise as early as with glottic cancers. Treatment of upper aerodigestive tract cancers depends on the subsite and involves multimodality therapy consisting of surgery, radiation, and chemotherapy.

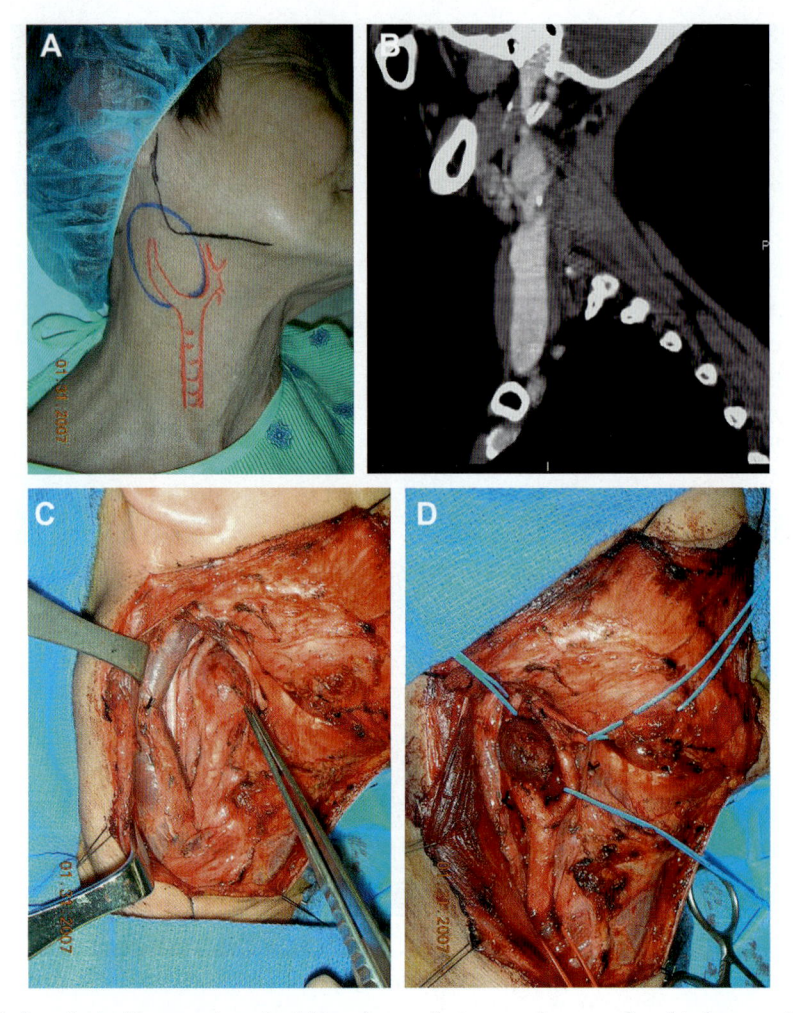

Fig. 5. (*A*) Elderly patient with a symptomatic right neck mass that, on workup, was found to be a carotid body tumor. (*B*) CT of the tumor showed the characteristic displacement of the tumor between the internal and external carotid branch. (*C*) Exposure of the tumor taking care to have superior and inferior control of the vessels. (*D*) Near-complete removal of the tumor without ligation of the vessels and preservation of the nerves.

Skin cancer

Skin cancers are the most common malignancy in the United States, where basal cell carcinoma (BCCA) and squamous cell carcinoma (SCCA) represent the majority of lesions treated. These malignancies are highly curable and rarely metastasize: 0.1% for BCCA and 2% to 5% for SCCA [84,85]. However, specific pathologic features represent an increased likelihood of cervical spread that should be respected by the clinician. Like other head and neck malignancies, lymphatic spread is associated with decreased survival [85]. For BCCA, most patients with metastatic disease have the morphea or basosquamous form, demonstrate perineural invasion, and are prone to multiple local recurrences. The risk of regional nodal involvement for SCCA increases with multiple recurrences, increased thickness, increased size (larger than 2 cm), more poorly differentiated tumors, perineural invasion, and tumor locations in scars, burns, and certain sites (eg, temple, ear, lips) [84–87].

Melanoma, although less common than the aforementioned skin cancers, has a mortality rate that far surpasses that of SCCA and BCCA. In 2008, 62,480 new cases will be diagnosed and 8420 men and women will die of melanoma [81]. Several staging factors, including depth of invasion, site, ulceration, macrometastasis, and number of positive nodes, should be considered when

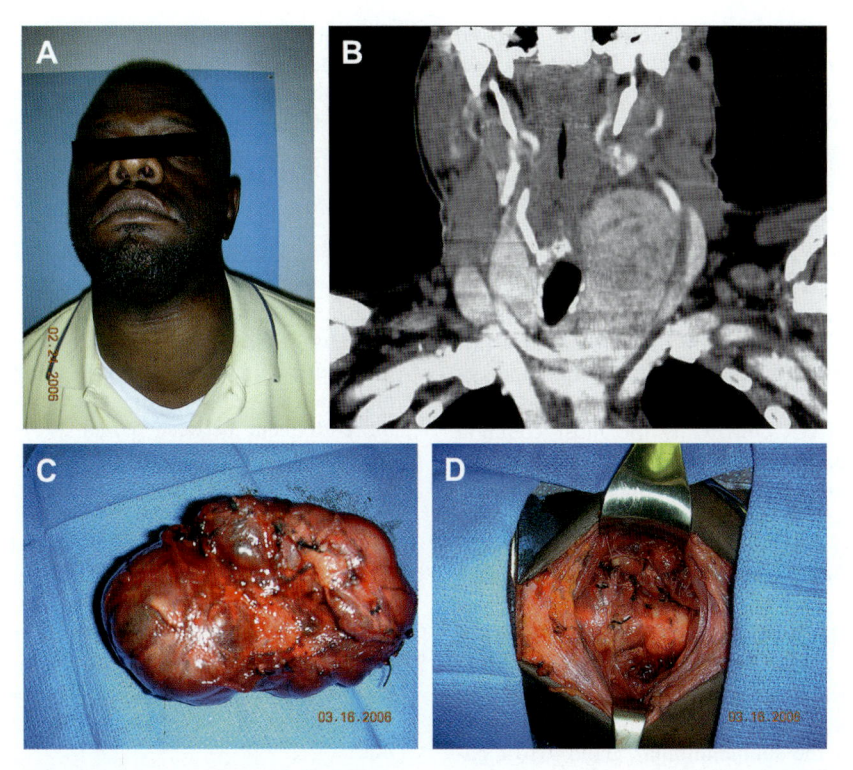

Fig. 6. (*A*) Patient with large anterior neck mass with greater extension to the right neck. (*B*) Coronal CT of the neck reveals a large thyroid goiter with significant deviation of the great vessels and the airway. (*C*) Surgical specimen of the goiter. Note the large lobulated mass. (*D*) Neck surgical bed after removal of the goiter.

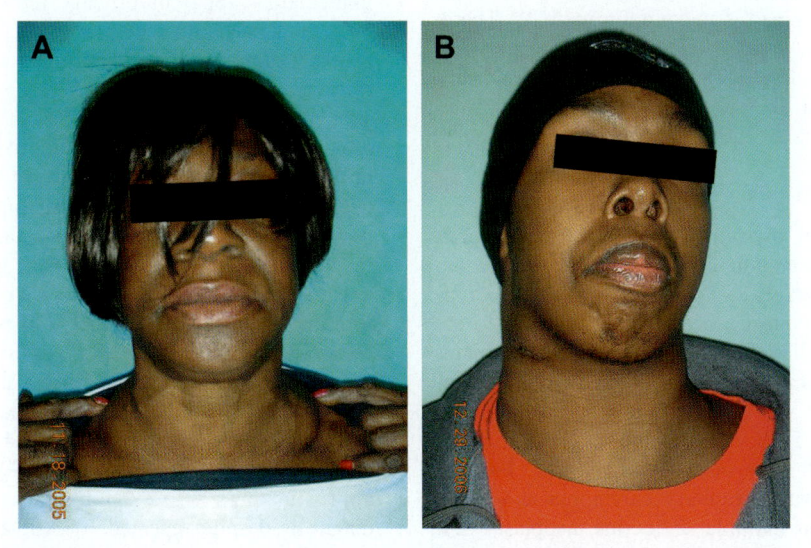

Fig. 7. (*A*) Patient with multiple bilateral lower neck nodes. Workup consisting of fine needle aspiration and CT scan revealed the neck nodes to be metastatic lung carcinoma. (*B*) Young man with known carcinoid tumor developed numerous neck nodes, which were found to be metastatic nodes on open biopsy.

choosing the appropriate therapy [88]. Mucosal melanoma in the head and neck is rare but highly aggressive and lethal. The most common sites are the nose, paranasal sinuses, oral cavity, and nasopharynx. These areas should be evaluated in patients with cervical lymphadenopathy and no primary skin lesions.

Salivary gland tumors

The clinician should be familiar with several malignant tumors that occur in the salivary glands. The most common that present as a primary or metastatic lesion in the neck are mucoepidermoid carcinoma (MEC) and adenoid cystic carcinoma (ACC). MEC is the most common salivary gland malignancy and the second most common malignancy of the submandibular gland. MEC is divided into low, intermediate, and high grades, depending on the ratio of mucin, intermediate, or epithelial cells. Compared to low-grade MEC, high-grade lesions tend to present at a later stage; have higher incidence of nodal involvement, recurrence, and distant metastasis; and promise lower chances of survival [89]. ACC is the second most common salivary gland tumor and the most common in the submandibular gland. Most patients present between 30 and 70 years of age. Three histologic subtypes exist: cribiform, tubular, and solid. ACC has a tendency for perineural spread, most often affecting the facial nerve or V2 or V3 of the trigeminal nerve. Perineural spread can be centripetal (toward brain) or centrifugal (peripheral), the former making resection difficult. Lymphatic spread is uncommon in ACC. Therefore, a mass in the neck would likely represent the primary lesion. Prognosis is time-dependent and survival does not plateau at 5 years. Even after 20 years mortality continues to increase.

Thyroid cancer

In general, thyroid cancer presenting as a neck mass is uncommon and the prognosis is good, with the notable exception of anaplastic carcinoma. The typical cancers of the thyroid are the well-differentiated carcinomas (WDTCs), medullary carcinoma, anaplastic carcinoma, and lymphoma. The WDTCs are papillary and follicular carcinoma. Follicular carcinoma also includes Hurthle cell and insular carcinomas. Patients diagnosed with medullary carcinoma should be screened for multiple endocrine neoplasia 2A, multiple endocrine neoplasia 2B, and familial medullary carcinoma. Treatment depends on the cancer and the institution and involves some or all the following interventions: total or subtotal thyroidectomy, neck dissection, radioiodine ablation, chemotherapy, and radiation therapy. A detailed discussion thyroid nodule evaluation is presented in another article of this volume.

Lymphoma

Cervical adenopathy is among the most common presenting symptoms in lymphoma, occurring in 75% of Hodgkin's and 30% to 40% of non-Hodgkin's patients. It is the most common malignancy in childhood, representing 10% of all malignancies [90]. Hodgkin's lymphomas are more frequent between 5 and 30 years of age, whereas the non-Hodgkin's forms occur later in life [91]. The nodes tend to be softer, more rubbery, and more mobile than those associated with metastatic carcinoma. Extranodal involvement is seen in the head and neck most often in Waldeyer's ring and tends to be the non-Hodgkin's type. Diagnosis is usually achieved by fine needle aspiration followed by open biopsy confirmation. Therapy depends on the type and stage and consists of chemotherapy, or radiation, or both.

Unknown primaries

Carcinomas from an unknown primary represent a small group of malignancies that pose a significant challenge to the clinician. Patients with malignant cervical adenopathy with no immediately apparent primary represent 3% to 10% of all head and neck cancers [92]. Most of the primary tumors occur in the upper aerodigestive tract, but primary sites in the lungs, abdomen, skin, and urinary tract are possible [93]. Generally, if a patient presents with mid- to high-jugular nodes, the clinician should suspect a head and neck origin versus an isolated supraclavicular node, which may be indicative of a primary below the clavicles, such as in the lungs or gastrointestinal tract. The literature reports that the primary tumor is found in 10% to 40% of patients. The most common site for the origin of the primary tumor is the palatine tonsil (35%), base of tongue (26%), lung (17%), and nasopharynx (9%). Other sites, such as the esophagus, skin, and larynx, contribute between 1% and 4% [94–97]. However, approximately 1% to 2% of primary tumors elude diagnosis despite repeated FNAB, imaging, and directed oropharyngeal biopsies [96]. Generally, the workup consists of physical examination; imaging, including PET scan; biopsy of an affected node; directed biopsy of the upper aerodigestive tract; at least ipsilateral tonsillectomy; and panendoscopy.

References

[1] Bates B. A guide to physical examination and history taking. 6th edition. Philadelphia: J.B. Lippincott Company; 1995. p. 1.
[2] Suen JY, Goepfert H. Standardization of neck dissection nomenclature. Head Neck Surg 1987;10: 75–7.
[3] Shah JP, Strong E, Spiro RH, et al. Surgical grand rounds. Neck dissection: current status and future possibilities. Clin Bull 1981;11:25–33.
[4] Fleming ID, Cooper JS, Henson DE, et al. AJCC cancer staging manual. Philadelphia: Lippincott-Raven, 1997.
[5] Robbins KT, Medina JE, Wolf GT. Standardizing neck dissection terminology. Arch Otolaryngol Head Neck Surg 1991;117:601–5.
[6] Petrivic Z, Arsovic N, Trivic A. Selective neck dissection for N0 neck supraglottic carcinoma. Int Congr Ser 2003;1240:853–8.
[7] Martin H, Morfit HM. Cervical node metastases as the first symptom of cancer. Surg Gynecol Obstet 1944;78:133–59.
[8] Martin HE, Ellis EB. Biopsy of needle puncture and aspiration. Ann Surg 1930;92:160–81.
[9] Spearman M, Curtin H, Dusenbury D, et al. Computed tomography—directed fine needle aspiration of the skull base parapharyngeal and infratemporal fossa masses. Skull Base Surg 1995;5(4):199–205.
[10] Smith EH. The hazards of fine-needle aspiration biopsy. Ultrasound Med Biol 1984;10:629–34.
[11] Smallman LA, Young JA, Oates J, et al. Fine needle aspiration cytology in the management of ENT patients. J Laryngol Otol 1988;102:909–13.
[12] Engzell U, Zajicek J. Aspiration biopsy of tumors of the neck. I. Aspiration biopsy and cytologic findings in 100 cases of congenital cysts. Acta Cytol 1970;14: 51–75.
[13] Ramzy I, Rone R, Shantz HD. Squamous cells in needle aspirates of subcutaneous lesions: a diagnostic problem. Am J Clin Pathol 1986;85:319–24.
[14] Burgess KL, Hurtwick RWJ, Bedard YC. Metastatic squamous carcinoma presenting as a neck cyst. Differential diagnosis from inflamed branchial cleft cyst in fine needle aspirates. Acta Cytol 1993;37: 494–8.
[15] Warson F, Blommaert D, DeRoy G. Inflamed branchial cyst: a potential pitfall is aspiration cytology. Acta Cytol 1986;30:201–2.
[16] Hehn ST, Grogen TM, Miller TP. Utility of fine needle aspiration as a diagnostic technique in lymphoma. J Clin Oncol 2004;22:3046–52.
[17] May M. Neck masses in children: diagnosis and treatment. Ear Nose Throat J 1978;7:136–58.
[18] Torsiglieri AJ, Tom LW, Ross AJ 3rd, et al. Pediatric neck masses: guidelines for evaluation. Int J Pediatr Otorhinolaryngol 1988;16(3):199–210.
[19] Ramadan HH, Wax MK, Boyd CB. Fine needle aspiration of head and neck masses in children. Am J Otolaryngol 1997;18(6):400–4.
[20] Liu ES, Bernstien JM, Sculerati N, et al. Fine needle aspiration biopsy of pediatric head and neck masses. Int J Pediatr Otorhinolaryngol 2001;60:135–40.
[21] Stevens MH, Harnsberger HR, Mancuso AA, et al. Computer tomography of cervical lymph nodes. Staging and management of head and neck cancer. Arch Otolaryngol 1985;111:735–9.
[22] Kerbele M, Kenn W, Hahn D. Current concepts in imaging laryngeal and hypolaryngeal cancer. Eur Radiol 2002;12:1672–83.
[23] Spreer J, Krahe T, Jung G, et al. Spiral versus conventional CT in routine examinations of the neck. J Comput Assist Tomogr 1995;19:905–10.
[24] Mukherji SK, Castillo M, Huda W, et al. Comparison of dynamic and spiral CT for imaging the glottic larynx. J Comput Assist Tomogr 1995;19:899–904.
[25] Suojanen JN, Mukherji SK, wippold FJ. Spiral CT of the larynx. AJNR Am J Neuroradiol 1994;15:1579–82.
[26] King AD, Tse GM, Yeun EH, et al. Necrosis in metastatic neck nodes: diagnosis accuracy of CT, MR imaging and US. Radiology 2004;230:720–6.
[27] Yousem DM, Som PM, Hackney DB, et al. Central nodal necrosis and extracapsular neoplastic spread in cervical lymph nodes: MR versus CT imaging. Radiology 1992;182:753–9.
[28] Vogl T, Dresel S, Juergens M, et al. MR imaging with Gd-DTPA in lesions of the head and neck. J Otolaryngol 1993;22:220–30.
[29] Hudgins PA, Gussack GS. MR imaging in the management of extracranial malignant tumors of the head and neck. Am J Roentgenol 1992;159:161–9.
[30] Lewin JS, Curtin HD, Ross JS, et al. Fast spin echo imaging of the neck: comparison with conventional spin echo, utility of fat suppression, and evaluation of tissue contrast characteristics. AJNR Am J Neuroradiol 1994;15:1351–7.
[31] Mancuso AA, Harnsberger HR, Muraki AS, et al. Computed tomography of cervical and retropharyngeal lymph nodes: normal anatomy, variants of normal, and applications in staging of head and neck cancers. Radiology 1984;152:749–53.
[32] Som PM. Lymph nodes of the neck. Radiology 1987; 165:593–600.
[33] Atula T, Varpula MJ, Kurki TJI, et al. Assessment of cervical lymph node status in head and neck cancer patients: palpation, computed tomography, and low field magnetic resonance imaging compared with ultra-sound guided fine-needle aspiration cytology. Eur J Radiol 1997;25(2):152–61.
[34] King AD, Tse GMK, Yuen EH, et al. Comparison of CT and MR imaging for the detection of extranodal neoplastic spread in metastatic neck nodes. Eur J Radiol 2004;230:720–6.

[35] Wippold FJ 2nd. Head and neck imaging: the role of CT and MRI. J Magn Reson Imaging 2007;25: 453–65.
[36] Mack MG, Balzer JO, Straub R, et al. Superparamagnetic iron oxide—enhanced MR imaging of head and neck lymph nodes. Radiology 2002;222: 239–44.
[37] Phelps ME. Inaugural article: positron emission tomography provides molecular imaging of biological processes. Proc Natl Acad Sci U S A 2000;97: 9226–33.
[38] Rege SD, Maass A, Chaiken L, et al. Use of positron emission tomography with fluoro-deoxyglucose in patients with extracranial head and neck cancers. Cancer 1994;73:3047–58.
[39] Greven KM, Williams DW 3rd, Keyes JW Jr, et al. Can positron emission tomography distinguish tumor recurrence from irradiation sequelae in patients treated for larynx cancer? Cancer J Sci Am 1997;3: 353–7.
[40] Blodgett TM, Fukui MB, Snyderman CH, et al. Combined PET-CT in the head and neck: part1. Physiologic, altered physiologic and artifactual FDG uptake. Radiographics 2005;25:897–912.
[41] Fukui MB, Blodgett TM, Snyderman CH, et al. Combined PET-CT in the head and neck: part 2. Diagnostic uses and pitfalls of oncologic imaging. Radiographics 2005;25:897–912.
[42] Ng SH, Yen TC, Chang JTC, et al. Prospective study of [18] fluorodeoxyglucose positron emission tomography and computed tomography and magnetic resonance imaging in oral cavity squamous cell carcinoma with palpably negative neck. J Clin Oncol 2006;24(27):4371–6.
[43] Branstetter BF 4th, Blodgett TM, Zimmer LA, et al. Head and neck malignancy: Is PET/CT more accurate than PT or CT alone? Radiology 2005;235: 580–6.
[44] Quraishi MS, O'Halpin DR, Blayney AW. Ultrasonography in the evaluation of neck abscesses in children. Clin Otolaryngol Allied Sci 1997;22(1):30–3.
[45] Bruneton JN, Normand FN, Balu-Maesro C, et al. Lymphomatous superficial lymph nodes: US detection. Radiology 1987;165:233–5.
[46] Cooper DS, Doherty GM, Haugen BR, et al. Management guidelines for patients with thyroid nodules nad differentiated thyroid cancer. Thyroid 2006;16: 109–42.
[47] Ahuja AT, Richards P, Wong KT, et al. Accuracy of high resolution sonography compared with magnetic resonance imaging in the diagnosis of head and neck venous vascular malformations. Clin Radiol 2003;58:869–75.
[48] Moritz JD, Ludwig A, Oestmann JW. Contrast-enhanced color Doppler sonography for evaluation of enlarged cervical lymph nodes in head and neck tumors. Am J Roentgenol 2000;174:1279–84.
[49] Knappe M, Louw M, Gregor RT. Ultrasonography-guided fine-needle aspiration for the assessment of cervical metastases. Arch Otolaryngol Head Neck Surg 2000;126:1091–6.
[50] Sack MJ, Weber RS, Weinstein GS, et al. Image-guided fine-needle aspiration of the head and neck: five years' experience. Arch Otolaryngol Head Neck Surg 1998;124:1155–61.
[51] Watson WL, McCarthy WD. Blood and lymph vessel tumor: a report of 1056. Surg Gynecol Obstet 1940;71(5):569–88.
[52] Kaban LB, Mulliken JB. Vascular lesions of the maxillofacial region. J Oral Maxillofac Surg 1986; 4(3):163–6.
[53] Gelbert F, Riche MC, Reizine D, et al. MR imaging of head and neck vascular malformations. J Magn Reson Imaging 1991;1(5):579–84.
[54] Westerband A, Hunter GC, Cintora I, et al. Current trends in the detection and management of carotid body tumors. J Vasc Surg 1998;28:84–92.
[55] Yonetsu K, Nakayama E, Miwa K, et al. Magnetic resonance imaging of oral and maxillofacial angiomas. Oral Surg Oral Med Oral Pathol 1993;76(6): 783–9.
[56] Flis CM, Connor SE. Imaging of head and neck venous malformations. Eur Radiol 2005;15:2185–93.
[57] Randoux B, Marro B, Koskas F, et al. Carotid artery stenosis: prospective comparison of CT, three-dimensional gadolinium-enhanced MR, and conventional angioagraphy. Radiology 2002;223(2):586–7.
[58] Perkins JA, Sidhu M, Manning SC, et al. Three-dimensional CT angiography of vascular tumors of the head and neck. Int J Pediatr Otorhinolaryngol 2004;69(3):319–25.
[59] Welsh D, Hengerer AS. The diagnosis and treatment of intramuscular hemangioma of the masseter muscle. Am J Otolaryngol 1980;1:186–90.
[60] Stanley RJ, Cubillo E. Nonsurgical treatment of arteriovenous malformations of the trunk and limb by transcatheter arterial embolization. Radiology 1975; 115(3):609–12.
[61] Al-Khateeb TH, Al Zoubi F. Congenital neck masses: a descriptive retrospective study of 252 cases. J Oral Maxillofac Surg 2007;65:2242–7.
[62] Sistrunk WE. The surgical treatment of cysts of the thyroglossal tract. Ann Surg 1920;71:121–4.
[63] Virchow R. Angiome. In: Virchow R, editor. Die krankheiten geschwulste. Berlin: August Hirswald; 1863. p. 306–425.
[64] Mulliken JB, Glowacki J. Hemangiomas and vascular malformations of infants and children: a classification based on endothelial characteristics. Plast Reconstr Surg 1988;69:412–22.
[65] Bowers RE, Graham EA, Tomlinson KM. The natural history of the strawberry nevus. Arch Dermatol 1960;82:667–80.
[66] Enjolras O, Riche MC, Merland JJ, et al. Management of alarming hemangiomas in infancy: a review of 25 cases. Pediatrics 1990;85:491–8.
[67] Low DW. Hemangiomas and vascular malformations. Semin Pediatr Surg 1994;3(2):40–61.

[68] Werner JA, Dunne AA, Folz BJ, et al. Current concepts in the classification, diagnosis, and treatment of hemangiomas and vascular malformations of the head and neck. Eur Arch Otorhinolaryngol 2001;258:141–9.

[69] Ridder GJ, Boedeker CC, Technau-Ihling K, et al. Cat-scratch disease: otolaryngologic manifestations and management. Otolaryngol Head Neck Surg 2005;132:353–8.

[70] Salvatore C, Antonio B, Del Vecchio W, et al. Giant infiltrating lipoma of the face: CT and MR imaging findings. AJNR Am J Neuroradiol 2003;24: 283–6.

[71] Copcu E, Sivrioglu N. Posterior cervical giant lipomas. Plast Reconstr Surg 2005;115:2156–7.

[72] Sanchez MR, Golomb FM, Moy JA, et al. Giant lipoma: case report and review of the literature. J Am Acad Dermatol 1993;28:266–8.

[73] Perskey MS, Setton A, Niimi Y, et al. Combined endovascular and surgical treatment of head and neck paragangliomas—a team approach. Head Neck 2002;24:423–31.

[74] Meier C. Non toxic goiters. In: Randolph GW, editor. Surgery of the thyroid and parathyroid glands. Philadelphia: Saunders; 2003.

[75] Shahian DM, Rossi RL. Posterior mediastinal goiter. Chest 1988;94:599–602.

[76] Hermus AR, Huysmans DA. Treatment of benign nodular thyroid disease. N Engl J Med 1998;338: 1438–47.

[77] Maurer AH, Charles ND. Radioiodine treatment for non-toxic multinodular goiter. J Nucl Med 1999;40:1313–6.

[78] Ross SR. Evaluation and nonsurgical management of the thyroid nodule. In: Randolph GW, editor. Surgery of the thyroid and parathyroid glands. Philadelphia: Saunders; 2003.

[79] Jereczek-Fossa BA, Jassem J, Orecchia R. Cervical lymph node metastasis of squamous cell carcinoma from and unknown primary. Cancer Treat Rev 2003;30:135–64.

[80] Koivunen P, Laranne J, Virtaniemi J, et al. Cervical metastasis of unknown origin: a series of 72 patients. Acta Otolaryngol 2002;122:569–74.

[81] Ries LAG, Melbert D, Kraphcho M, et al, editors. SEER cancer statistics review 1975–2005. Bethesda (MD): National Cancer Institute; based on November 2007 SEER data submission, posted to the SEER website, 2008. Available at: http://seer.cancer.gov/csr/1975_2005/.

[82] Lindberg R. Distribution of cervical lymph node metastasis from squamous cell of the upper respiratory and digestive tract. Cancer 1972;29: 1446–9.

[83] Shah JP. Patterns of cervical lymph node metastasis from squamous cell carcinomas of the upper aerodigestive tract. Am J Surg 1990;160(4):405–6.

[84] Lo JS, Snow SN, Reizner GT, et al. Metastatic basal cell carcinoma: report of 12 cases with a review of the literature. J Am Acad Dermatol 1991;24:715–9.

[85] Rowe DE, Carroll RJ, Day CL Jr. Prognostic factors for local recurrence, metastasis, and survival rates in squamous cell carcinoma of the skin, ear, and lip. Implications for treatment modality selection. J Am Acad Dermatol 1992;26:976–90.

[86] Randle HW. Basal cell carcinoma. Identification and treatment of the high-risk patient. Dermatol Surg 1996;22:255–61.

[87] Barksdale SK, O'Connor N, Barnhill R. Prognostic factors for cutaneous squamous cell and basal cell carcinoma. Determinants of risk of recurrence, metastasis, and development of subsequent skin cancers. Surg Oncol Clin N Am 1997;6:625–38.

[88] Balch CM, Buzaid AC, Soong SJ, et al. Final version of the American Joint Committee on Cancer staging system for cutaneous melanoma. J Clin Oncol 2001; 19:3635–48.

[89] Hicks MJ, el-Naggar AK, Flaitz CM, et al. Histocytologic grading of mucoepidermoid carcinoma of major salivary glands in prognosis and survival: a clinicopathologic and flow cytometric investigation. Head Neck 1995;17:89–95.

[90] Bonilla JA, Healy GB. Management of malignant head and neck tumors in children. Pediatr Clin North Am 1989;36:1443–50.

[91] Dailey SH, Sataloff RT. Lymphoma. An update on evolving trends in staging and management. Ear Nose Throat J 2001;80:164–70.

[92] Adams JR, O'Brien CJ. Unknown primary squamous cell carcinoma of the head and neck: a review of diagnosis, treatment and outcomes. Asian J Surg 2002;25:188–93.

[93] Talmi YP, Wolf GT, Hazuka M, et al. Unknown primary of the head and neck. J Laryngol Otol 1996;110:353–6.

[94] Altman E, Cadman E. An analysis of 1539 patients with cancer of unknown primary site. Cancer 1986; 57:120–4.

[95] Chepeha D, Koch W, Pitman K. Management of unknown primary tumor. Head Neck 2003;25:499–504.

[96] Gunthinas-Linhius O, Klussman P, Dinh S, et al. Diagnostic work-up and outcome of cervical metastasis from an unknown primary. Acta Otolaryngol 2006;126:536–44.

[97] Hass I, Hoffman TK, Engers R, et al. Diagnostic strategies in cervical carcinoma of an uknown primary (CUP). Eur Arch Otorhinolaryngol 2002; 259:325–33.

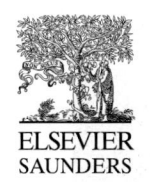

Congenital Neck Masses

Peter A. Rosa, DDS, MD[a,b],
David L. Hirsch, DDS, MD[a,b,*],
Eric J. Dierks, DMD, MD, FACS[c,d]

[a]Department of Oral and Maxillofacial Surgery,
New York University College of Dentistry, New York, NY, USA
[b]New York University School of Medicine, New York, NY, USA
[c]Oregon Health & Science University, Portland, OR, USA
[d]Legacy Emanuel Hospital, Portland, OR, USA

Congenital neck masses are subdivided based on their anatomic location in the neck. Midline neck masses include thyroglossal duct cyst (TDC), dermoid cyst, epidermoid cyst, ranula, thymic cyst, and teratoma. Lateral neck masses include branchial cleft cyst (BCC), laryngocele, lymphangioma, hemangioma, and fibromatosis coli. Although these lesions are congenital in nature, manifestations of these lesions may not occur until later in life. This may lead to a mistaken suspicion of acquired lesions of inflammatory or neoplastic origin. The appropriate diagnosis of these lesions is necessary to provide appropriate treatment and long-term follow up, because some of these lesions may undergo malignant transformation or be harbingers of malignant disease.

Midline congenital neck masses

Thyroglossal duct cyst

Epidemiology and etiology

Seven percent of the population has remnants of the thyroglossal duct. This lesion is the most common congenital anomaly of the neck. It represents 70% of congenital neck masses [1] and is the second most common neck mass after cervical adenopathy in the pediatric population.

TDC is diagnosed in 40% of childhood neck masses and has no gender predilection [2]. There is less than a 1% incidence of thyroid carcinoma or other malignancy within a TDC, 90% of which occur in adulthood [3].

The etiology of TDC is reflected by the embryology and formation of the thyroid gland (Fig. 1). The thyroid gland is the first endocrine gland formed in embryogenesis [1]. It begins in the third embryonic week as an endodermal thickening in the floor of the primitive pharynx-tuberculum impar. A downgrowth develops called the thyroid diverticulum (median thyroid anlage) [4]. This diverticulum opening, which is caudal to the median tongue bud, becomes the foramen cecum of the tongue. During elongation of the embryo, the diverticulum descends into the neck and becomes the thyroglossal duct [1]. The diverticulum descends and fuses with components of the fourth and fifth branchial pouches (lateral thyroid anlage). Because this occurs before the formation of the hyoid bone, remnants of the duct can become trapped within the hyoid bone during its formation. The pyramidal lobe of the thyroid gland, which is present in 30% of the population, may represent distal remnants of the TGD [2]. The proximal remnant becomes the foramen cecum. The duct usually obliterates between the fifth and eighth weeks. Failure of obliteration leads to formation of the TDC. The cyst is usually lined by respiratory epithelium, which can undergo squamous metaplasia with repeated superinfection. Thyroid tissue can be seen within the cyst in

* Corresponding author. 366 5th Avenue, Suite 709, New York, NY 10001
E-mail address: davidlhirsch@yahoo.com (D.L. Hirsch)

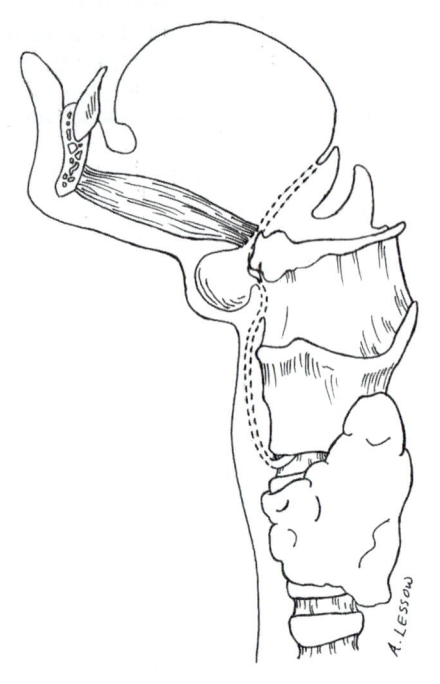

Fig. 1. TDCs can form anywhere along the embryologic path of descent of the thyroid gland. The dotted line indicates the path of thyroid descent. (*Courtesy of* Alexa Lessow, MD, New York, NY.)

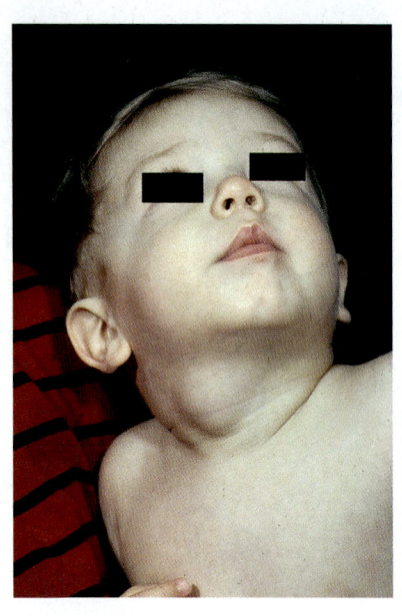

Fig. 2. TDC in a child. Note the midline position of the neck mass.

45% of cases. Infection with *Haemophilus* influenza, *Staphylococcus aureus*, and *Staphylococcus epidermidis* can occur [5].

Diagnosis

Most TDCs present in the first 5 years of life [6]. Two thirds are diagnosed within the first 3 decades. They are usually painless cystic masses in the midline of the neck, two thirds of which are adjacent to the hyoid (Fig. 2) [4]. They can, however, be located anywhere from the tongue to the pyramidal lobe of the thyroid. The cyst usually moves with deglutition and with protrusion of the tongue, unlike dermoid cysts. This finding can be helpful in the differential diagnosis. One third of these can present with concurrent or prior infection, which is the most common way they are diagnosed in the adult population [5]. Patients rarely present with a chief complaint of foul taste attributable to a draining fistula from the foramen cecum. Most present with an asymptomatic mass or infection. TDCs at the base of the tongue and large neck TDCs may lead to dyspnea because of airway obstruction.

An appropriate physical examination, medical history, and history of presenting illness are vital in narrowing down the differential diagnosis for this lesion. An imaging study, such as an ultrasound or CT scan, and a screening thyroid-stimulating hormone (TSH) level should initially be performed. If TSH levels are elevated or a solid mass is seen on ultrasound examination, a radionucleotide scan may be indicated to rule out median ectopic thyroid [4]. Some investigators advocate radionucleotide scans in all patients with TDC because median ectopic thyroid may be present in 1% to 2% of TDCs [4]. If the cyst is excised along with ectopic thyroid, replacement thyroid hormone therapy may be necessary if all functioning thyroid tissue is present within the ectopic specimen [4].

CT scans are not necessary for the diagnosis but aid in planning surgical excision. A TDC is seen as a hypodense lesion with variable rim enhancement with intravenous contrast. The lining of the cyst may be thickened secondary to repeated infection, chronic inflammatory reaction, or malignancy.

Treatment

The Sistrunk procedure is the classic procedure performed for the uncomplicated TDC. A transverse incision is made in the neck. The cyst and the distal portion of the tract are identified, and a wide-field dissection of the tract and adjacent tissues is continued from the thyroid gland, including the pyramidal lobe, if present, superiorly toward the hyoid bone. The central component of the hyoid bone associated with the TDC is excised. Further en bloc removal of the proximal tract contained within a cylinder of tongue musculature is performed up to the foramen cecum so that the entire tract is appropriately removed. If the pharynx is entered, the opening is suture ligated and the lesion is removed (Figs. 3 and 4) [6].

Surgical intervention during episodes of acute inflammation leads to high recurrence rates (40%) compared with treatment after inflammatory episodes have subsided (8%) [7]. It is preferable to wait to excise a recently infected TDC until at least 4 to 6 weeks after treatment with antibiotics. A more recent review, however, has shown that there may be no association between preoperative infection and increased recurrence rates [8].

In approximately 1% of all TDCs, excised carcinoma is detected incidentally. In such cases, 94% are thyroid in nature (mostly papillary thyroid carcinoma) and 6% are of squamous cell origin. If differentiated thyroid carcinoma within the cyst is diagnosed, it is appropriately managed within the normal treatment for TDC [9] (Sistrunk procedure). If invasive or extensive carcinoma is found, more extensive treatment is needed. This may require a total thyroidectomy with or without neck dissection in addition to the Sistrunk procedure, followed by radioactive iodine therapy and

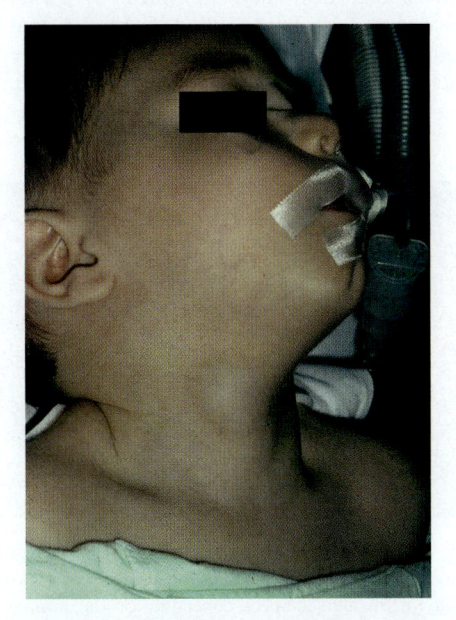

Fig. 3. Patient prepared for removal of a TDC.

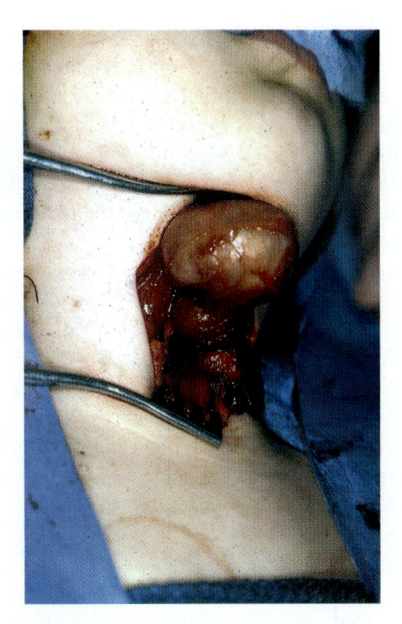

Fig. 4. Exposure and removal from a midline neck incision.

TSH suppression [9]. Portions of geniohyoid, mylohyoid, genioglossus, and hyoid may be removed with the TDC [10].

Recurrence of TDC can occur even with a properly performed Sistrunk operation. One possibility is that the original Sistrunk procedure performed on the patient did not include laterally directed or branching tracts [11]. Hewitt and colleagues [11] suggest dissecting a cuff of normal tissue with the specimen and removing granulation tissue because it may represent an inflammatory reaction to adjacent retained epithelium. Close dissection to the hypoglossal nerve (in some situations) may be necessary to prevent leaving residual TDC, in addition to taking intraoperative frozen sections of nearby tissue. Close follow-up is important because recurrences do occur, even with the most comprehensive treatment.

Dermoid cyst

Epidemiology and etiology

Dermoid cysts are germ cell tumors that are made up of ectodermal and mesodermal elements but have no endodermal elements. Hair follicles, smooth muscle, fibroadipose tissue, and sebaceous glands may be found within them. Several theories have been formulated as to their etiology. The first is that they are derived from anatomically isolated totipotential rests from the mesoderm and ectoderm that undergo disorganized growth. The acquired implantation theory postulates that the cysts come from germinal derivatives that were implanted into deeper tissue by a traumatic event. The third theory is congenital inclusion of germ layers into deeper tissues along embryonic fusion lines that have failed to close completely, thereby trapping epithelial debris [12].

Twenty percent of all head and neck dermoids are found in the cervical region, most often in the submental region. Seven percent of all dermoids occur in the head and neck [13]. Most often, dermoids present in the periorbital region (especially in children [14]), nasal region, or scalp. They rarely manifest in infants and usually manifest in childhood or later. They have no gender-related predilection [15].

Clinical presentation and evaluation

These lesions present as mobile midline neck masses that are soft, nontender, and filled with sebaceous debris (cheesy keratinous material). Some may manifest in the lateral neck submandibular triangle between the mylohyoid and hyoglossus. They usually do not move with protrusion of the tongue or swallowing; however, in some instances, they may have fibrous attachments to the hyoid, and thus may present similar to TDC. The usual clinical presentation is a lump or swelling under the tongue or submental region, which can measure up to 10 to 12 cm in diameter [15]. They are slow growing and become bothersome to the patient if they interfere with speech, mastication, or tongue mobility, but they rarely obstruct the airway. Dermoids in this area can become infected; in such cases, they become painful and erythematous and could present with a draining sinus tract. They can usually be diagnosed by CT or ultrasound imaging. A fine needle aspirate (FNA) biopsy can be used but is not always diagnostic and may not be necessary. Ultrasound can differentiate between simple cysts and dermoids based on echogenicity, but dermoids may be similar in echogenicity to lipomas [13].

Histologically, the presence of keratinizing stratified squamous epithelium, hair follicles, and sebaceous glands is characteristic of these cysts.

Treatment

Dermoid cysts are excised to prevent subsequent infection, to establish a diagnosis, and for cosmetic and functional purposes. Lesions located above the mylohyoid can be excised orally, whereas large neck lesions are excised transcervically (Fig. 5). Recurrence of these lesions is unusual with appropriate excision, and malignant transformation is rare [14].

Epidermoid cyst

Epidemiology and etiology

Epidermoid cysts are usually seen after puberty and are most common in the acne-prone areas of the face and neck. If seen before the onset of puberty, they may be associated with Gardner's syndrome. Younger people more commonly have these lesions on the face and neck, whereas older individuals are more prone to developing these lesions on the back. They occur more commonly in men and boys than in women and girls.

The epidermoid cyst is lined by stratified squamous epithelium, and sometimes ciliated epithelium, in addition to mucous-secreting cells. The epidermoid cysts in the submental region originate from epidermal cells that become trapped during closure of the first and second branchial arches during the third and fourth weeks of development [16]. They may arise after inflammation or infection of the hair follicle, which may be attributable to a postinflammatory nonneoplastic proliferation of the follicular epithelium. They may also sometimes arise from traumatic implantation much like dermoid cysts.

Clinical presentation and evaluation

Histologically, they are lined by stratified squamous epithelium with orthokeratin that is sloughed into the cystic lumen. The cyst may or may not have a granulomatous inflammatory reaction surrounding it in reaction to exposed

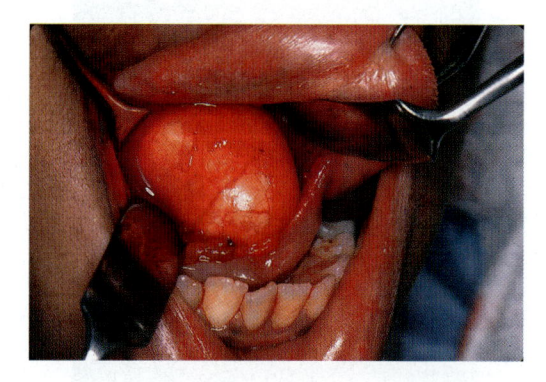

Fig. 5. Large dermoid cyst of the submental region. Large dermoids of the submental region can be removed orally or through the neck depending on the amount of exposure needed.

orthokeratin. These cysts are mobile and fluctuant to palpation.

Imaging studies

The same imaging modalities as those that aid in the diagnosis of dermoid cysts can be implemented to diagnose epidermoid cysts. Dermoids and epidermoids are differentiated histologically by content. Epidermoids contain one germ cell layer, whereas dermoids have derivatives of two germ cell layers.

Treatment

Simple excision is the treatment of choice. Recurrence is uncommon if epidermoid cysts are properly excised, and malignant transformation is rare [17].

Plunging ranula

Epidemiology and etiology

A ranula is a mucocele in the floor of mouth that can "plunge" into the neck. Its course splits the mylohyoid muscle, and the mass can be felt in the submental triangle. It is usually associated with the sublingual gland; however, it can be associated with the submandibular gland. Blockage of the gland ducts leads to a build-up of mucus material. This blockage can be attributable to direct trauma to the sublingual gland or to prior surgery to the floor of the mouth. The ranula does not possess a true cystic lining and forms a pseudocyst.

Simple ranulas do not penetrate through the mylohyoid muscle. The plunging ranula presents as a neck lesion by entering the fascial plane between the hyoglossus and mylohyoid, where the deep lobe of the submandibular gland is located. A defect in the mylohyoid muscle (mylohyoid boutonniere) that may be congenital in origin can predispose a simple ranula to conversion into a plunging ranula [18].

The presentation of a plunging ranula in the pediatric population is rare. Sixty-two percent of simple ranulas occur on the left side, and 58% of plunging ranulas occur on the right side [19].

Clinical presentation and evaluation

Ranulas appear as blue dome-shaped lesions in the floor of mouth, usually on either side of the midline. The extraoral appearance of a plunging ranula is seen as a submental mass extending along the inferior border of one side of the mandible, which may be quite large in size. They are filled with mucinous material. The spilled mucin from the ranula elicits a granulation tissue response that usually contains foamy histiocytes (Figs. 6–9).

Imaging studies

A combination of a CT scan or MRI along with FNA is effective in diagnosing the lesion. On FNA, saliva is aspirated from the lesion. The absence of keratin or epithelial or glandular elements further substantiates the diagnosis and differentiates between ranula and dermoid or epidermoid cyst.

Treatment

Surgical excision of the sublingual gland (the etiology in most cases) is the surgical procedure of choice. Marsupialization involves the removal of the roof of the lesion intraorally, thereby allowing the sublingual gland to communicate with the oral cavity. This allows it to drain intraorally. Marsupialization is noted to have a 67% recurrence rate, and transoral excision of the sublingual gland has the lowest possibility of ranula recurrence [20].

OK-432 (picibanil), which is a lyophilized mixture of low-virulence strain *Streptococcus pyogenes* incubated with zylpenicillin, has been successfully used as an intralesional sclerotherapy agent. This may serve as a potential treatment for plunging ranulas before considering surgery [21]. The surgical excision of plunging ranulas

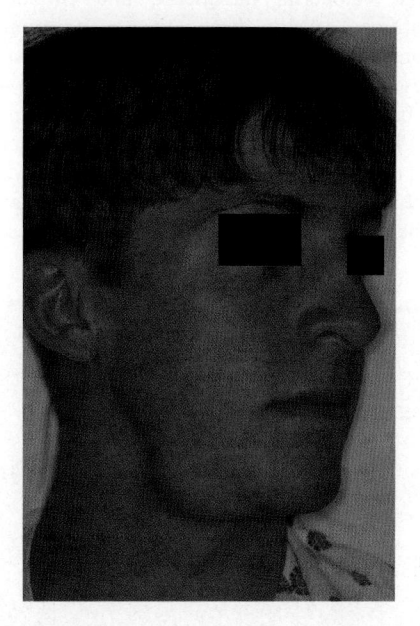

Fig. 6. Early plunging ranulas resolve with sublingual gland removal and decompression. Well-established or previously infected plunging ranulas may also require cervical exposure and excision.

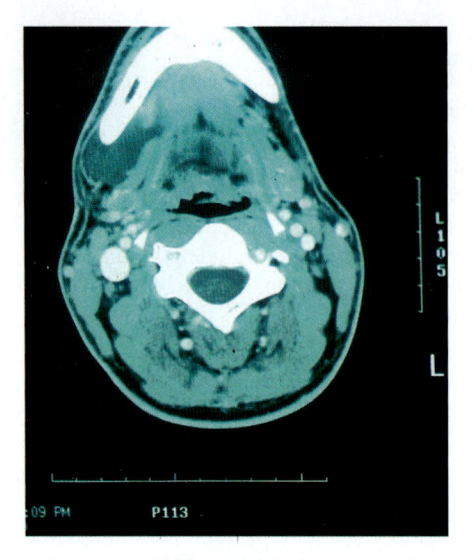

Fig. 7. Axial CT image of plunging ranula.

can be achieved orally; however, large plunging ranulas may need cervical excision for adequate access.

Teratoma

Epidemiology and etiology

A teratoma stems from all three germ cell layers (ectoderm, mesoderm, and endoderm). Teratomas develop during the second trimester of pregnancy and are seen as midline or sometimes lateral neck masses. They occur in 1 of 4000 live births [22] with a slight female predominance [23]. Ten percent of teratomas originate from the head and neck. The most common site of development is the neck, although they may also develop in the nasopharynx, oropharynx, and oral cavity.

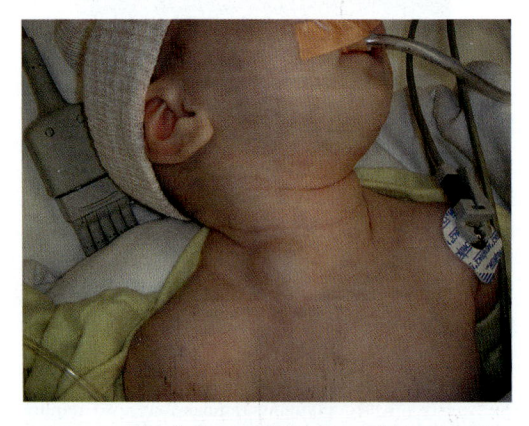

Fig. 8. Second BCC in a child.

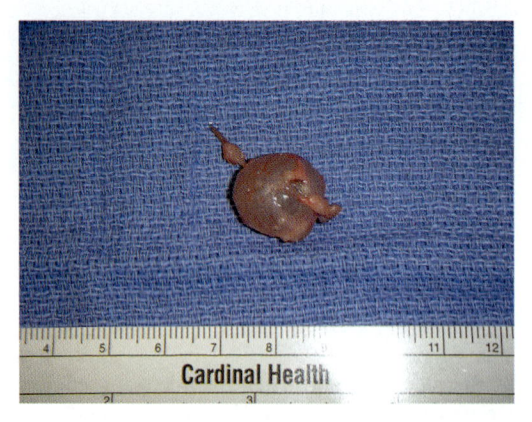

Fig. 9. Second BCC removed. Note that the tract of the lesion must be removed with the cyst.

There are four subdivisions of teratomas: the dermoid cyst or epithelium-lined cyst, which contains ectodermal and mesodermal elements (most common); the teratoid cyst, which contains poorly differentiated tissues from all three germ layers; the teratoma, which contains differentiated tissues from all three germ layers, and epignathi, which contain highly developed malformations resembling fetal organs [23].

The origin of teratomas is controversial. Some believe that they are derived from pluripotent stem cells sequestered during embryogenesis, emerging from an ectopic primitive streak. Another theory is that they arise from embryonic tissue that escaped the regional influences of the primary organizer [23].

Clinical presentation and evaluation

A teratoma may present in the neonatal period with airway obstruction. If they arise in the neck, these lesions can be fatal if untreated. They are frequently associated with polyhydramnios secondary to inhibition or obstruction to swallowing [23].

The diagnosis is usually made by prenatal ultrasonography. If seen on ultrasound, an ultrafast MRI scan can be obtained prenatally to determine the degree of tracheal compression and to differentiate this lesion from other lesions that it may mimic (ie, cystic hygroma) [24]. This allows better evaluation of the lesion without the use of radiation.

Treatment

Cesarean delivery can be considered for large congenital teratomas, and preparation for immediate surgical airway or intubation should be implemented. Excision is the treatment of choice. Malignancy has not been reported in pediatric cervical teratomas; therefore, critical structures should be spared during excision [4]. Malignancy has been documented among adults, and thus may require more aggressive management.

Lateral congenital neck masses

Thymic cyst

Epidemiology and etiology

The thymus is important for cell-mediated immunity during infancy. It grows to its maximum size at 2 to 4 years of age. It then involutes and becomes a fibrofatty remnant.

The thymus gland develops from the third and fourth pharyngeal pouches during the sixth week of development. By the eighth week, paired primordia fuse in the midline, attach to the pericardium, and begin their descent into the mediastinum [25]. As the superior attachment of the thymic primordium fails to regress at 8 weeks, solid or cystic ectopic tissue may be left behind along the path of migration [25].

Sixty seven percent of thymic cysts occur in the first decade of life [26]. They are present on the left side in 68% of cases, on the right side in 25%, and on the midline in 7% [26]. The gender distribution is reported to be equal or to have a 2:1 male predominance [27].

Clinical presentation and evaluation

Thymic cysts are usually located anterior or deep to the sternocleidomastoid muscle (SCM), and 50% extend into the mediastinum by direct extension or by connection to a vestigial remnant or as a solid cord [26]. They are exceedingly rare and are not reported because of the fact that they remain dormant, and thereby clinically insignificant. Eighty percent to 90% of cervical thymic cysts are asymptomatic [27]. They may enlarge because of hemorrhage or infection and then become symptomatic [27]. These can cause dysphagia, pain, dysphonia, and dyspnea based on mass effect on the neck. Thymic cysts are known to expand with the Valsalva maneuver.

These cysts can be congenital or acquired. The congenital type is usually unilobular and originates from persistent rudiments of the thymopharyngeal duct [27]. They sometimes have epithelium from the thyroid and parathyroid glands because of their close association during development. The acquired thymic cysts are multilobular and develop from degenerated Hassall's corpuscles (degenerated epithelial cells).

The cysts contain lymphocytes, along with multinucleated giant cells; macrophages; cholesterol clefts; and an epithelial lining that may be cuboidal, columnar, or stratified squamous [25]. The size of the cyst wall can vary from a few millimeters to as much as 1 cm [26].

Imaging studies

The study of choice, ultrasound examination, can demonstrate homogeneous and nonhomogeneous masses and a solid or cystic mass [26]. CT scans can guide surgical resection by giving more detail as to the location of the mass and its association with adjacent structures. MRI is excellent for soft tissue evaluation and can be a valuable tool to determine the location of the cyst and its mediastinal extension. FNA has little diagnostic value [25]. Chest radiography is important for the confirmation of normal thymic tissue in the mediastinum in children.

Treatment

The presence of a normal thymus is vital before excision of this lesion in children, because the thymus is important in their cell-mediated immunity. Therefore, removal of a thymic cyst in a child with an abnormal thymus may compromise that child's cell-mediated immunity. If normal thymic tissue is present, complete surgical excision that spares the surrounding vital structures is the treatment of choice [26].

There is a 2% recurrence rate of thymic cysts in adults, and no recurrences have been noted in children with complete excision [26]. In addition, there have been reports of rare malignant transformation of these cysts [28].

Branchial cleft cyst

Epidemiology and etiology

Branchial cleft anomalies arise from the branchial apparatus, which develops between the third and seventh weeks of embryologic growth. There are five branchial arches of mesodermal origin, each of which gives rise to specific bony, cartilaginous, muscular, and neurovascular structures in the head and neck (Table 1). Between each arch is a groove, or cleft, arising from ectoderm. The formation of a BCC is thought to be attributable to incomplete obliteration of the branchial tracts [29]. It is imperative that the surgeon be familiar with the structures associated with each arch,

Table 1
Branchial arch derivatives

	Nerve	Artery	Muscle	Cartilage/Bone
First arch	V_3	None	Tensor tympani, masticator mm Mylohyoid, anterior belly of digastric, tensor palatini	Malleus head and neck, incus body and short process, mandible, anterior malleal ligament, sphenomandibular ligament
Second arch	VII	Stapedial artery (degenerates)	Platysma, facial mm, stapedius, post belly of digastric, buccinator, styloid	Malleus manubrium, incus long process, hyoid lesser cornu and part of body, stapes, styloid process, stylohyoid ligament
Third arch	IX	Common carotid artery and internal carotid artery	Stylopharyngeus, superior and middle constrictors	Greater cornu of hyoid, rest of body of hyoid
Fourth arch	X Superior laryngeal	Aorta on left, proximal subclavian artery on right	Inferior pharyngeal constrictor, cricopharyngeus, cricothyroid mm	Thyroid cartilage, cuneiform cartilage
Fifth arch	X Recurrent laryngeal	Ductus arteriosis	Intrinsic laryngeal mm (except cricothyroid)	Cricoid, trachea, arytenoid cartilages, corniculate cartilage

Abbreviation: mm, muscle.

because the tracts of the cysts follow a pathway between the associated arch derivatives.

Clinical presentation

First branchial cleft cyst. Work [30] described first branchial cleft anomalies by dividing them into two types: type I, which arise from the cleft and are therefore ectodermal only, and type II, which have contributions from the first and second branchial arches as well, and therefore contain some mesodermal elements. Type I cysts typically course parallel to the external auditory canal (EAC), superior and lateral to the facial nerve, and may terminate in the bony-cartilaginous junction of the EAC or in the middle ear space They are considered to be duplications of the membranous EAC; if infected, they can drain as a fistula inferior to the lobule or in the preauricular or postauricular area. Type II cysts can contain cartilage and adnexal structures in addition to skin and are considered to be a duplication of the cartilaginous and bony EAC. The tract can lie medial or lateral to the facial nerve; if infected, it can present with drainage at the angle of the mandible [31] or internally, in the EAC, with otorrhea [32]. Type II cysts can present as cysts in the parotid gland [32] and can be confused with primary parotid lesions.

Second branchial cleft cyst. Second branchial cleft anomalies are the most common, representing up to 95% of all branchial anomalies [33]. Thirty-seven percent present as cysts alone, and 63% are also associated with fistulas or sinuses [34]. A complete fistula, with internal and external openings, is rare but has been reported [35]. The tract of a second BCC courses superficial to cranial nerves XII and IX; between the internal carotid artery and external carotid artery; and then pierces the middle constrictor, deep to the stylohyoid ligament, and opens into the tonsillar fossa. The cysts typically present as a mass along the anterior border of the SCM or near the angle of the mandible. They can present anywhere along the course of the tract, however, from the anterior border of the SCM to the tonsillar fossa. Unusual locations have been reported, including a cystic mass in the parapharyngeal space [34]. Three percent to 10% are bilateral [33] and can be associated with other congenital anomalies, such as branchiootorenal syndrome, which is associated with conductive hearing loss and renal abnormalities. They can be asymptomatic, or they can present with recurrent infection, sore throat, and dysphagia. Patients with a second BCC often present with a history of recurrent unilateral tonsillitis (Figs. 10 and 11). Note that in an adult with a cystic neck mass, it is imperative to rule out malignancy; most commonly, tonsillar and papillary thyroid carcinoma can present with a cystic metastatic lymph node (Figs. 12 and 13).

Third branchial cleft cyst. Third branchial cleft anomalies usually present anterior to the SCM near the superior pole of the thyroid lobe. The tract of the third branchial cleft anomaly courses from anterior to the SCM superficial to cranial nerve XII, deep to the carotid artery and cranial nerve IX, to pierce the thyrohyoid membrane above the internal branch of the superior laryngeal nerve and open into the pyriform fossa. Patients may present with what seems to be acute thyroiditis [36].

Fourth branchial cleft cyst. Fourth BCCs are rare, representing only 2% of all branchial anomalies [36,37]. The tract of the fourth branchial cleft anomaly is different on each side of the neck. On the right side, the tract traces from anterior to the SCM inferiorly to loop around the subclavian artery, deep to it and the carotid artery, lateral to cranial nerve XII, and inferior to the superior laryngeal nerve, to open into the pyriform fossa or the larynx. On the left side, which is the more common presentation, the course is lateral to cranial nerve XII, inferior to the superior laryngeal nerve, to open into the lower pyriform sinus or larynx. Only the relation of the tract to the superior laryngeal nerve distinguishes a third from a fourth branchial anomaly because they both open into the pyriform sinus. Because a fourth BCC usually presents as a neck mass near the inferior lobe of the thyroid gland, it can be confused with other entities, such as TDC, cystic hygroma, and thyroid cyst [36]. It should be high in the differential diagnosis when a patient presents with a neck mass that increases in size with crying or the Valsalva maneuver or with recurrent infections of the neck or thyroid gland. A neonate may present with a lateral neck mass and airway compromise [36].

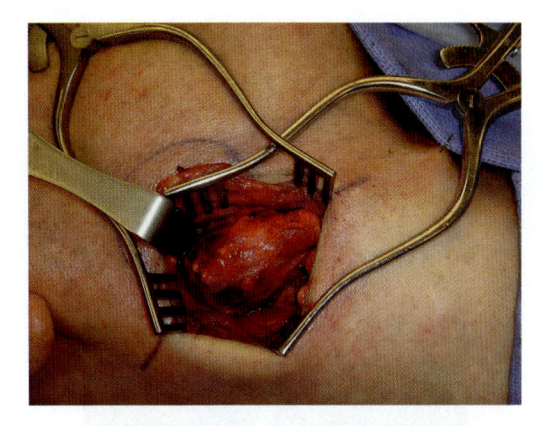

Fig. 11. Operative exposure of a right second BCC.

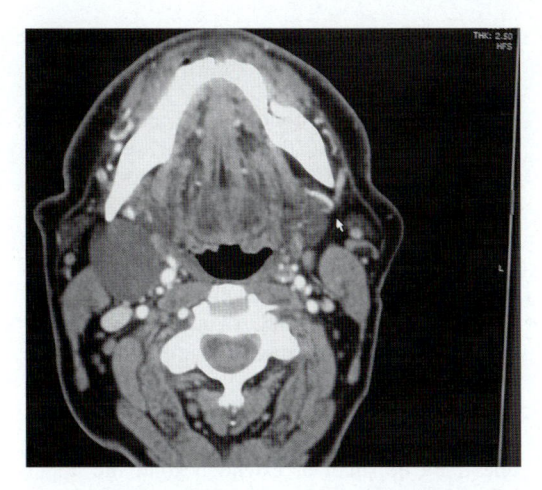

Fig. 10. Axial CT image of a left second BCC in an adult.

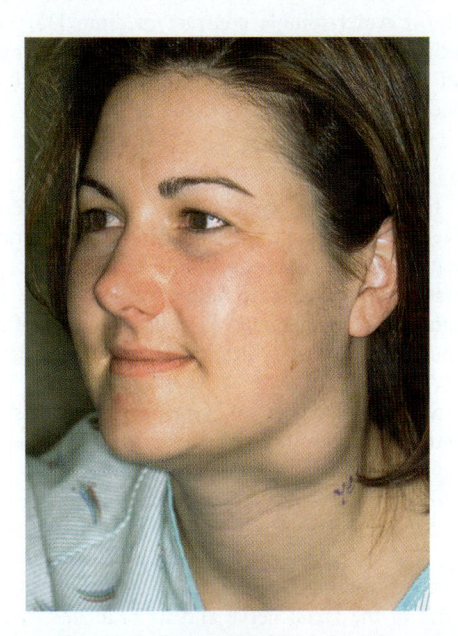

Fig. 12. Left second BCC in an adult.

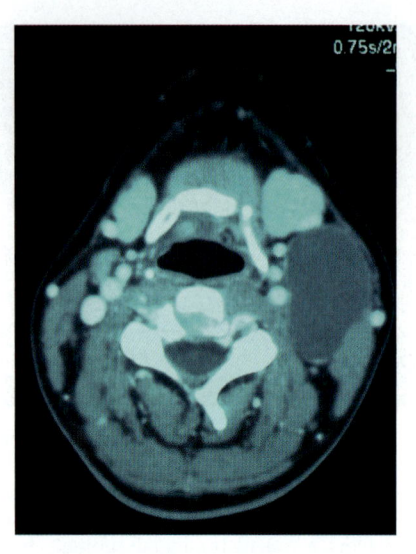

Fig. 13. CT appearance compatible with left second BCC. Final pathologic examination revealed a cystic metastatic lymph node from an unknown primary, which later proved to be the ipsilateral tonsil.

Imaging studies and diagnostic tests

CT of the neck with contrast shows the location of the cyst and the relation of the tract to the surrounding structures, aiding in the differential diagnosis. In the case of first branchial cleft anomalies, MRI shows the extent of the lesion in the parotid area and the location of the facial nerve in relation to the cyst tract. Injecting the tract with oily or water-soluble contrast medium [35] and taking radiographs can be diagnostic but may not show the whole extent of the tract if it is blocked by inflammatory tissue or secretions.

Treatment

If the cyst is infected, a course of antibiotics is given and preliminary incision and drainage may be unavoidable. Excision should be delayed for at least 4 to 6 weeks to allow resolution of inflammation and greater ease of dissection. Previous incision and drainage can make later excision more difficult.

Surgical excision of type I first BCCs is relatively straightforward; if there is a fistula, an ellipse of skin must be removed along with the epithelial tract and the opening into the EAC must be repaired. Excision of type II first BCCs can be more complicated, because the tract has an intimate although variable relation to the main trunk of the facial nerve and its branches within the parotid gland. Some advocate that it is not necessary to identify and dissect the facial nerve branches if electrophysiologic facial nerve localization is used throughout the case [31]. A superficial parotidectomy is often necessary to preserve the facial nerve. If a fistula ends in the EAC, a portion of skin and cartilage surrounding the fistula must be removed. There is a high rate of recurrence if the tract is not completely excised; in a review of 39 patients presenting with first BCCs, 50% of the cases had had a previous resection [32]. Injecting methylene blue dye into the fistula or inserting a lacrimal probe to cannulate the tract can aid in excision [33,36].

The second BCC is the most common brachial cyst to require excision. If there is a fistula, an ellipse of skin must be removed along with the epithelial tract and cyst. An isolated level II lymph node that contains a cystic metastasis from an occult primary squamous cell carcinoma, frequently from the tonsil, can present in the adult as a second BCC. Preoperative pharyngeal examination is appropriate for adult patients with an apparent second BCC. Should the final pathologic examination demonstrate a cystic metastasis rather than a second BCC, the patient should undergo an appropriate workup for an unknown primary. This can be done in one or two stages.

For third and fourth branchial cleft anomalies, direct laryngoscopy is used to explore the pyriform sinus for a tract to cannulate [36]. After dissection, the pharyngeal defect is closed with a purse-string suture. Endoscopic cauterization of fourth branchial cleft sinuses as an alternative to excision has been reported by Verret and colleagues [37] in a cohort of 10 patients.

Laryngocele

Epidemiology and etiology

Laryngoceles are abnormal saccular dilations of the appendix of the laryngeal ventricle of Morgagni [38]. The sac is lined by pseudostratified columnar ciliated epithelium and communicates with the ventricle by a narrow stalk. Development of the congenital laryngocele is contingent on the presence of a congenital saccular dilatation of the ventricular appendage [38]. An increase in intralaryngeal pressure may cause the sac to distend and sometimes to extend into the aryepiglottic fold.

There are three types of laryngoceles (internal, external, and combined type). Internal laryngoceles may be small or extend beyond the upper border of the thyroid cartilage. The external type forms when the dilated appendage penetrates the thyrohyoid membrane and extends into the subcutaneous tissues of the neck [38]. The combined type has components of the first two types. Laryngoceles are reported to be less common in women [38].

Clinical presentation and evaluation

Most laryngoceles are asymptomatic. There can be symptoms of hoarseness or cough. Dyspnea can be a symptom in children and infants because of obstruction. The laryngocele may be palpable as a soft reducible mass in the lateral cervical region that may be more pronounced during the Valsalva maneuver [38]. Laryngoceles are normally filled with air but may be filled with mucus or pus to form laryngomucoceles or mucopyoceles [39].

Evaluation involves CT or MRI, along with laryngoscopy. Ultrasound can also be a useful initial imaging modality. Localization of a mass dorsal to the hyoid bone and strap muscles and the depiction of a communication through the thyrohyoid membrane suggest the diagnosis of a laryngocele on ultrasound [40].

Treatment

Treatment is surgical. There are endoscopic microsurgical techniques that may be used in the removal of internal laryngoceles [41]. The external approaches begin with following the external portion of the laryngocele sac through the thyrohyoid membrane. The laryngocele is then transected close to the orifice of the saccule. Endoscopic marsupialization is another option that may be attempted instead of excision, but this technique has variable recurrence rates. Because symptomatic laryngoceles have an occult cancer rate of 4% [42], histopathologic evaluation of the lesion is vital.

Lymphangioma

Epidemiology and etiology

Approximately 50% to 65% of lymphangiomas are present at birth, with 90% presenting by 2 years of age [43] as compared with hemangiomas, which begin to involute at this age. The head and neck are the most frequent sites of presentation. Lymphangiomas are considered to be a subset of vascular malformations and are classified according to the size of the endothelially lined sinuses they contain:

1. Capillary lymphangioma (or lymphangioma simplex): small capillary-sized vessels
2. Cavernous lymphangioma: large dilated lymphatic vessels; violates tissue planes
3. Cystic lymphangioma (or cystic hygroma): large macrocystic cystic spaces

Smaller vessel lymphangiomas (capillary and cavernous) are typically found above the mylohyoid muscle in the lip, tongue, or oral cavity. They can be infiltrative and difficult to demarcate on CT. Cystic hygromas, the most common type of lymphangioma in the neck, are more sharply demarcated on CT and tend not to be as infiltrative.

Clinical presentation and evaluation

Cystic hygromas are painless and compressible, and they tend to enlarge gradually over time. The posterior triangle of the neck is the most common location (Figs. 14 and 15), with approximately 56% presenting in this location and approximately 44% presenting in the anterior triangle [43]. Occasionally, these lesions enlarge rapidly over days, which is thought to be attributable to concurrent upper respiratory infection; however, there have been reports of rapid enlargement, seemingly with no antecedent event [43]. Ultrasound, MRI, and CT are all useful adjuncts to diagnosis and surgical planning.

Treatment

Surgical resection is definitive therapy; however, the lesion can be difficult to resect depending

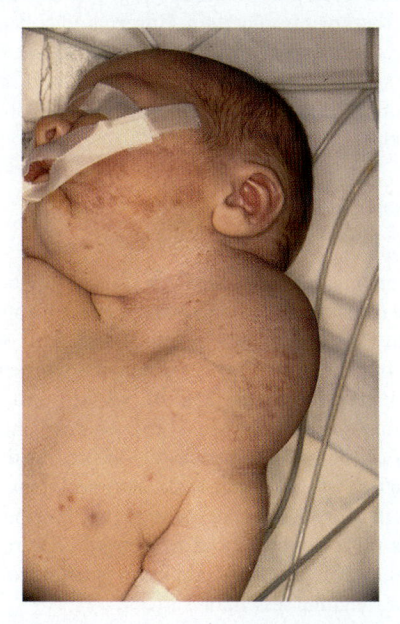

Fig. 14. Large supraclavicular lymphangioma in an infant.

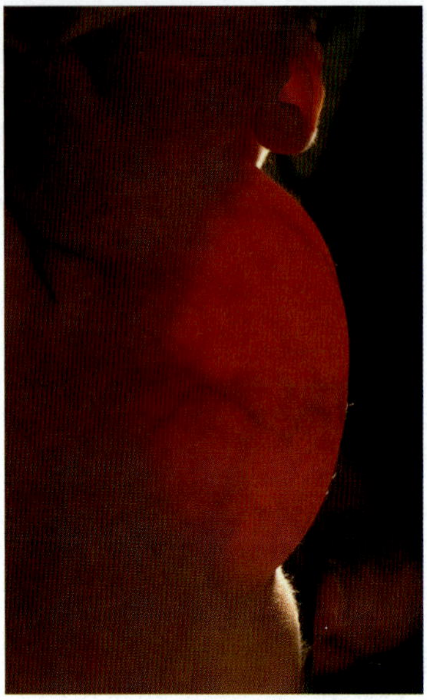

Fig. 15. Transillumination of lymphangioma.

on its proximity to vital structures and its tendency not to follow natural anatomic tissue planes. Recurrence rates can be high if the tumor is not excised completely. Alternative therapies include systemic and intralesional steroids, intralesional injections of sclerosing agents [44], intralesional injections of fibrin and bleomycin, and systemic cyclophosphamide [43]. The efficacy of these therapies is uncertain. Burezq and colleagues [45] recommend aspiration as conservative treatment, with excellent results in 14 cases of cystic hygromas that were diagnosed over a 30-year period.

Hemangioma

Epidemiology and etiology

Hemangiomas account for 7% of all benign neoplasms [46].Hemangiomas affect approximately 10% of infants in their first year of life [47]. Intramuscular hemangiomas can present in the masseter muscle (5% of all intramuscular hemangiomas) [48]. Most congenital hemangiomas of the head and neck region present during the first 6 weeks of life. Head and neck hemangiomas have a 3:1 female gender predilection and occur more commonly in whites [49]. There also seems to be a greater incidence in premature newborns weighing less than 1 kg.

Hemangiomas enter into the proliferative phase of their development in the first 8 months to 1 year of life and slowly regress for the next 5 or more years, which is known as the involuting phase. The involuting phase is completed in 70% of children by the age of 7 years [50]. During the first year, the lesion appears bright red, and as it involutes, it changes its color and begins to dull.

Historically, the terms *capillary hemangioma* and *cavernous hemangioma* are used for superficial and deep lesions, respectively. These terms are no longer clinically relevant, however, because, histologically, the endothelial pattern is similar throughout the depth of the lesion.

Hemangiomas are classified based on their rate of clinical regression: rapidly involuting congenital hemangiomas and noninvoluting congenital hemangiomas.

Clinical presentation and evaluation

Most of these lesions appear as isolated lesions that are firm to palpation and usually red in color. A thrill can sometimes be palpable over the lesion. Infants who present with these lesions in the lower face are more likely to have tracheal and laryngeal hemangiomas [51].Glut-1 is an important histochemical marker (erythrocyte-type glucose transporter protein) present in all stages of hemangioma development and involution, and it can help to differentiate hemangiomas from vascular malformations [47].

Ultrasound can be useful in differentiating these rapidly flowing vascular lesions from slower flowing venous malformations. Magnetic resonance angiography (MRA) can provide a great deal of information in terms of the vascular flow characteristics, which may indicate which phase the lesion is in. Three-dimensional CT angiography has been shown to differentiate hemangiomas from other vascular malformations [47].

Treatment

Intralesional and systemic steroids can reduce the size of these lesions. Vincristine has been successfully used in lesions unresponsive to steroids and has now replaced interferon-α as a medical treatment because of interferon's side effect of permanent spastic diplegia [47]. Becaplermin gel (recombinant human platelet-derived growth factor) is used to treat superficially ulcerated hemangiomas refractory to standard wound care [47].

Surgical resection can be considered in any phase of the hemangioma. Ulceration, bleeding, airway compromise, and extent of cosmetic defect must be accounted for as a risk for this decision.

Fibromatosis coli (congenital muscular torticollis)

Epidemiology and etiology

Congenital muscular torticollis, or "SCM tumor of infancy," is secondary to fibrosis of the SCM. It is the third most common pediatric orthopedic diagnosis in childhood [52]. There is a slight male predilection ($\sim$3:2) and an overall incidence of 1 in 250 live births [52].

Clinical presentation and evaluation

Children present with a stiff neck tilted to one side, most commonly to the right.

Imaging studies and diagnostic tests

Ultrasound shows a mass in the SCM. A biopsy confirms the diagnosis.

Treatment and prognosis

Physical therapy is the usual treatment of choice, with 50% to 70% of SCM tumors seen to resolve spontaneously during the first year of life. Surgical lengthening of the SCM is rarely performed.

Summary

Congenital neck lesions reflect abnormal embryogenesis in head and neck development. A thorough knowledge of embryology and anatomy is critical in the diagnosis and treatment of these lesions.

Acknowledgments

The authors thank Alexa Lessow, MD, for contributions to this article.

References

[1] Enepekides DJ. Management of congenital neck masses. Facial Plast Surg Clin North Am 2001; 9(1):131–45.

[2] Organ GM, Organ CH. Thyroid gland and surgery of the thyroglossal duct: exercise in applied embryology. World J Surg 2000;24:886–90.

[3] Roback SA, Telander RL. Thyroglossal duct cysts and branchial cleft anomalies. Semin Pediatr Surg 1994;3(3):42–6.

[4] Acierno SP, Waldhausen JHT. Congenital cervical cysts, sinuses, and fistulae. Otolaryngol Clin North Am 2007;40:161–76.

[5] Foley DS, Fallat ME. Thyroglossal duct and other congenital midline cervical anomalies. Semin Pediatr Surg 2006;15:70–5.

[6] Tracy TF, Muratore CS. Management of common head and neck masses. Semin Pediatr Surg 2007; 16:3–13.

[7] Ghaneim A, Atkins P. The management of thyroglossal duct cysts. Int J Clin Pract 1997;51(8):512–3.

[8] Ostlie DJ, Burjonrappa SC, Snyder CL, et al. Thyroglossal duct infections and surgical outcomes. J Pediatr Surg 2004;39(3):396–9.

[9] Motamed M, McGlashan JA. Thyroglossal duct carcinoma. Curr Opin Otolaryngol Head Neck Surg 2004;12(2):106–9.

[10] Sistrunk WE. Technique of removal of cysts and sinuses of the thyroglossal duct. Ann Surg 1920;71: 121–4.

[11] Hewitt k, Pysher T, Park A, et al. Management of thyroglossal duct cysts after failed Sistrunk procedure. Laryngoscope 2007;117(4):756–8.

[12] Rosen D, Wirtschafter A, Rao VM, et al. Dermoid cyst of the lateral neck: a case report and literature review. Ear Nose Throat J 1998;77(2):125–32.

[13] Yasumoto M, Shibuya H, Gomi N, et al. Ultrasonographic appearance of dermoid and epidermoid cysts in the head and neck. J Clin Ultrasound 1991;19(8):455–61.

[14] Pryor SG, Lewis JE, Weaver AL, et al. Pediatric dermoid cysts of the head and neck. Otolaryngol Head Neck Surg 2005;132(6):938–42.

[15] Leveque H, Saraceno CA, Tang CK, et al. Dermoid cysts of the floor of mouth and lateral neck. Laryngoscope 1979;89:296–305.

[16] Bataineh AB, Mansour MJ. Extraoral epidermoid cysts. Br J Oral Maxillofac Surg 1997;35:49–51.

[17] Lopez-Rios F, Rodriguez-Peralto JL, Castano E, et al. Squamous cell carcinoma arising in a cutaneous epidermal cyst. Am J Dermatopathol 1999;21: 174–7.

[18] Mahadevan M, Vasan N. Management of pediatric plunging ranula. Int J Pediatr Otorhinolaryngol 2006;70:1049–54.

[19] Zhao YF, Jia Y, Chen XM, et al. Clinical review of 580 ranulas, oral surgery, oral medicine, oral pathology. Oral Surg Oral Med Oral Pathol Oral Radiol Endod 2004;98(3):281–7.

[20] Zhao YF, Jia J, Jia Y, et al. Complications associated with surgical management of ranulas. J Oral Maxillofac Surg 2005;63(1):51–4.

[21] Rho MH, Kim DW, Kwon JS, et al. OK-432 sclerotherapy of plunging ranula in 21 patients: it can be a substitute for surgery. AJNR Am J Neuroradiol 2006;27:1090–5.

[22] Celik M, Akkaya H, Arda IS, et al. Congenital teratoma of the tongue: a case report and review of the literature. J Pediatr Surg 2006;41:E25–8.

[23] Kountakis SE, Minotti AM, Maillard A, et al. Teratomas of the head and neck. Am J Otolaryngol 1994;15(4):292–6.

[24] DeBacker A, Madern GC, Van de Ven CP , et al. Strategy for management of newborns with cervical teratoma. J Perinat Med 2004;32:500–8.
[25] Newman JG. Case report of an anterior neck thymic cyst. Otolaryngol Head Neck Surg 2001;125(6): 656–7.
[26] Delbrouck C, Choufani G, Fernandez-Aguilar S, et al. Cervical thymic cyst: a case report. Am J Otolaryngol 2002;23(4):256–61.
[27] Berenos-Riley L, Manni JJ, Coronel C, et al. Thymic cyst in the neck. Acta Otolaryngol 2005;125:108–12.
[28] Yamashita S, Yamazaki H, Kato T, et al. Thymic carcinoma which developed in a thymic cyst. Intern Med 1996;35:215–8.
[29] Girvigian MR, Rechdouni AK, Zeger GD, et al. Squamous cell carcinoma arising in a second branchial cleft cyst. Am J Clin Oncol 2004;27(1):96–100.
[30] Work WP. Newer concepts of first branchial cleft defects. Laryngoscope 1972;82:1581–93.
[31] Isaacson G, Martin W. First branchial cleft cyst excision with electrophysiological facial nerve localization. Arch Otolaryngol Head Neck Surg 2000; 126(4):513–6.
[32] Triglia JM, Nicollas R, Ducroz V, et al. First branchial cleft anomalies: a study of 39 cases and a review of the literature. Arch Otolaryngol Head Neck Surg 1998;124(3):291–5.
[33] Stone R, Devaiah A, Pistey RW. Pathology quiz case 2. Arch Otolaryngol Head Neck Surg 2004; 130(11):1137–9.
[34] Gadiparthi S, Lai S, Branstetter BF 4th, et al. Radiology quiz case 2. Arch Otolaryngol Head Neck Surg 2004;130(1121):1124–5.
[35] Ramirez-Camacho R, Garcia Berrocal JR, Borrego P. Radiology quiz 2. Arch Otolaryngol Head Neck Surg 2001;127(11):1395–6.
[36] Link TD, Bite U, Kasperbauer JL, et al. Fourth branchial pouch sinus: a diagnostic challenge. Plast Reconstr Surg 2001;108(3):695–711.
[37] Verret DJ, McClay J, Murray A, et al. Endoscopic cauterization of fourth branchial cleft sinus tracts. Arch Otolaryngol Head Neck Surg 2004;130:465–8.
[38] Lindell MM, Jing BS, Fischer EP, et al. Laryngocele. AJR Am J Roentgenol 1978;131:259–62.

[39] Harney M, Patil N, Walsh R, et al. Laryngocele and squamous cell carcinoma of the larynx. J Laryngol Otol 2001;115:590–2.
[40] VanVierzen PBJ, Joosten FB, Manni JJ. Sonographic, MR, and CT findings in a large laryngocele: a case report. Eur J Radiol 1994;18:45–7.
[41] Frederick FJ. Endoscopic microsurgical excision of internal laryngocele. J Otolaryngol 1985;14(3): 163–6.
[42] Canalis RJ. Observations on the simultaneous occurrence of laryngocele and cancer. J Otolaryngol 1976;5:207–12.
[43] Sherman BD, Kendall K. A unique case of the rapid onset of a large cystic hygroma in the adult. Am J Otolaryngol 2001;22(3):206–10.
[44] Greinwald J, Burke D, Sato Y, et al. Treatment of lymphangiomas in children: an update of picibanil (OK-432) sclerotherapy. Otolaryngol Head Neck Surg 1999;121(4):381–7.
[45] Burezq H, Williams B, Chitte S. Management of cystic hygromas: 30 year experience. J Craniofac Surg 2006;14(4):815–8.
[46] Sarteschi LM, Bonanomi G, Mosca F, et al. External jugular vein hemangioma occurring as a lateral neck mass. J Ultrasound Med 1999;18:719–21.
[47] MacArthur CJ. Head and neck hemangiomas of infancy. Curr Opin Otolaryngol Head Neck Surg 2006;14:397–405.
[48] Wolf GT, Daniel F, Krause CJ, et al. Intramuscular hemangioma of the head and neck. Laryngoscope 1985;95:210–3.
[49] Mulliken JB, Glowacki J. Hemangiomas and vascular malformations in infants and children: a classification based on endothelial characteristics. Plast Reconstr Surg 1982;69(3):412–22.
[50] Mulliken JB, Fishman SJ, Burrows PE. Vascular anomalies. Curr Probl Surg 2000;37(8):517–84.
[51] Berenguer B, Mulliken JB, Enjolras O, et al. Rapidly involuting congenital hemangioma: clinical and histopathologic features. Pediatr Dev Pathol 2003;6(6): 495–510.
[52] Do TT. Congenital muscular torticollis: current concepts and review of treatment. Curr Opin Pediatr 2006;18:26–9.

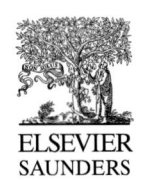

Deep Space Neck Infection: Principles of Surgical Management

Timothy M. Osborn, DDS, MD[a], Leon A. Assael, DMD[a,*], R. Bryan Bell, DDS, MD, FACS[a,b]

[a]*Department of Oral and Maxillofacial Surgery, Oregon Health & Science University, 611 SW Campus Drive, Mail Code SD 522, Portland, OR 97239, USA*
[b]*Oral and Maxillofacial Surgery Service, Legacy Emanuel Hospital and Health Center, 2801 N. Gantenbein Avenue, Portland, OR 97227, USA*

An intimate knowledge of the management of infections of the deep spaces of the neck is essential to the daily practice of oral and maxillofacial surgery. Decisions must be made in a timely fashion through the acute course of the disease. Interventions must be performed with the appropriate surgical and airway skill. The surgeon must decide on medical and surgical management, including

- Antibiotic selection
- How to employ supportive rescusitative care such as fluids and nutrition
- When to operate
- What procedures to perform
- How to secure the airway

To make these decisions the surgeon must understand the anatomy of the region, the etiology of infection, appropriate diagnostic workup, and medical and surgical management. This article provides a review of these pertinent topics.

Anatomy

Fascial layers

An understanding of the anatomy of the cervical fascia is critical in understanding the location of a deep neck infection, in predicting the extent of infection, and in choosing an approach for surgical drainage. The cervical fascia is the fibrous connective tissue that envelops and divides the structures of the neck and creates potential spaces (Fig. 1). The cervical fascia is divided into superficial and deep layers. The superficial fascia is immediately deep to the dermis and it ensheathes the platysma as well as the muscles of facial expression, the superficial musculoaponuerotic system (SMAS). It extends from the cranium down to the thorax and axilla. The deep layer is divided into superficial, middle, and deep layers.

The superficial layer of the deep cervical fascia (SLDCF) is an essential structure in understanding deep space infections of the neck. The SLDCF generally forms the outer margin of odontogenic deep space neck infections (DSNI). The tenacity of this fascia prevents the egress of pus toward the skin until neck infections are quite late. The result is that because of the barrier of the SLDCF, infections will expand to the point of descending toward the mediastinum, ascending to the lateral pharynx and masticator spaces, or will expand to the point of causing airway obstruction. Understanding the SLDCF is essential to understanding the pathway of infection.

The SLDCF begins posteriorly at the nuchal ridge and spreads laterally and anteriorly, splitting to envelop the trapezius and sternocleidomastoid (SCM). It attaches to the hyoid bone anteriorly. It envelops both the parotid and submandibular glands. It fuses with the fascia, covering the anterior bellies of the digastric and mylohyoid forming the inferior margin of the submandibular space. At the mandible, the fascia splits and the internal layer covers the medial surface of the pterygoid muscles up to the skull

*Corresponding author.
E-mail address: assaell@ohsu.edu (L.A. Assael).

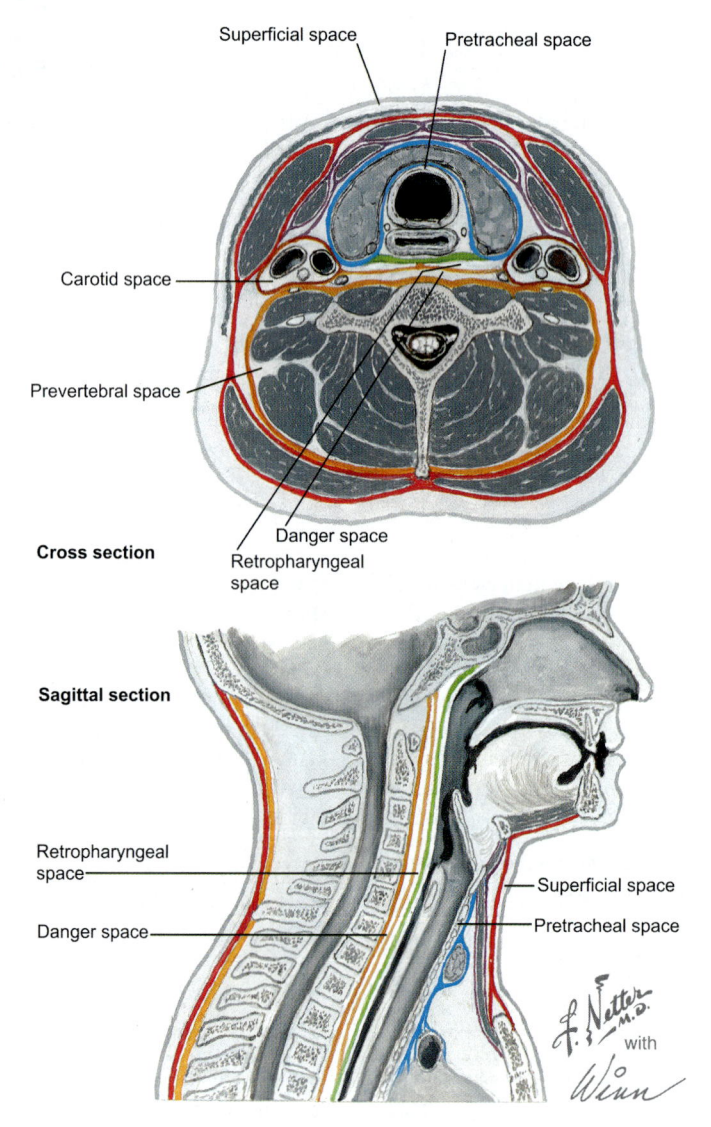

Fig. 1. Fascial spaces of the neck. (*Reprinted from* Netter anatomy illustration collection. Elsevier. All rights reserved; with permission.)

base. The external layer covers the masseter muscle and inserts into the zygomatic arch. Inferiorly, it inserts into the clavicles, sternum, and acromion of the scapula.

The middle layer of the deep cervical fascia (MLDCF) is also known as the pretracheal fascia. It often forms the base of deep space infections of the neck, thus creating a barrier to the extension of infection into the pulmonary, tracheobronchial tree, esophagus, and prevertebral space. It is separated into muscular and the visceral divisions. The muscular division surrounds the sternothyroid, sternohyoid, and thyrohyoid muscles. The muscular division does not offer important pathways for infection because the attachment is quite rigid, and no potential space is typically present except as it presents abutting the prevertebral fascia. Inferiorly this division also inserts into the clavicle and the sternum. Superiorly it inserts into the hyoid and thyroid cartilages. Posteriorly it fuses with the alar division of the deep layer of the deep cervical fascial at the level of T2 and forms the anterior wall of the retropharyngeal space.

The visceral layer of the MLDCF envelops the thyroid, trachea, and esophagus. It extends inferiorly into the upper mediastinum and joins the fibrous pericardium The middle layer also encloses the pharyngeal constrictors and the buccinator muscles. The visceral layer of the MLDCF is the pathway to mediastinitis in the deep space head and neck infection, forming the anterior barrier that must be traversed by advancing infection.. To descend, the infection will also disrupt the alar division of the DLDCF, described below.

The deep layer of the deep cervical fascia (DLDCF) separates into a posterior prevertebral division and an anterior alar division. The prevertebral division is adherent to the anterior aspect of the vertebral bodies from the base of the skull down the spine. It extends posteriorly around the spine and the muscles of the deep neck, the vertebral muscles, muscles of the posterior triangle, and the scalene muscles. It envelops the brachial plexus and subclavian vessels, extending laterally into the axillary sheath. The alar division is located between the visceral division of the middle layer and the prevertebral division of the deep layer. The deep layer corresponds to the posterior boundary of the retropharyngeal space, extending down to the level of T2, where it fuses with the visceral fascia. Thus the DLDCF is important in providing the posterior boundary for extension of infection to the mediastinum. The DLDCF is rarely perforated by infection, but when this occurs, it can result in cervical spine osteomyelitis or epidural abscess following head and neck infection.

Spaces

The spaces created by these fascial planes are potential spaces that are useful to consider in understanding the pathway of infection (Fig. 2). They include the lateral pharyngeal, retropharyngeal, submandibular, and pretracheal.

The floor of the mouth and mandible, the superficial layer of deep cervical fascia, and the lateral pharyngeal space bind the submandibular space. This space is divided by the mylohyoid muscle into sublingual and submandibular portions that are continuous posteriorly around the free margin of the muscle. The sublingual portion contains the submandibular duct, lingual nerve, and hypoglossal nerve, whereas the submandibular portion contains the anterior belly of the digastric. The lateral pharyngeal space is an inverted, cone-shaped potential space that extends from the skull base to the hyoid. The medial border is the buccopharyngeal fascia; the lateral border is the pterygoid muscles and mandible. Overlying the buccopharyngeal fascia is the superior pharyngeal constrictor muscle, which separates the peritonsillar "space" from the lateral pharyngeal space. The lateral pharyngeal space communicates anteriorly with the submandibular space and posteriorly with the retropharyngeal space. The styloid process and its attached structures divide the lateral pharyngeal space into two compartments; the anterior and posterior. The anterior compartment contains fat and connective tissue, whereas the posterior compartment contains cranial nerves IX, X, XII, the cervical sympathetic chain, the internal jugular vein, and the carotid artery. The retropharyngeal space lies between the middle and deep layers of cervical fascia, and extends from the skull base to the bifurcation of the trachea. There is a midline raphe that is formed by the attachment of the superior constrictor muscle to the alar layer of the deep cervical fascia. This midline raphe separates two chains of lymph nodes that lie within the space. The pretracheal space is located below the hyoid bone and extends inferiorly to the level of the fourth thoracic vertebrae along the arch of the aorta. The pretracheal space has the MLDCF as its anterior border, and is bounded posteriorly by the esophagus.

The infections in these spaces can be direct extensions from other spaces of the head and neck, or from the primary site. Extensions of infections can follow the fascial planes into the mediastinum or the axilla. Of special mention are the so-called "danger space" and the carotid sheath. The danger apace is the area between the alar and prevertebral fascia that extends from the skull base to the diaphragm. The carotid sheath forms a potential space that allows for infection to descend into the mediastinum, whereas infection that rests between the MLDCF and the DLDCF in the retropharyngeal region will create a retropharyngeal abscess that will end at about the tracheoesophageal junction.

Microbiology

The most common organism associated with deep neck infections was *Staphylococcus aureus* in the pre-antibiotic era. Drug resistance has, however, contributed to a change in the microbial flora associated with these serious infections, which are now most commonly associated with aerobic streptococcal species and nonstreptococcal anaerobes. [1,2]. The bacteria that commonly cause deep

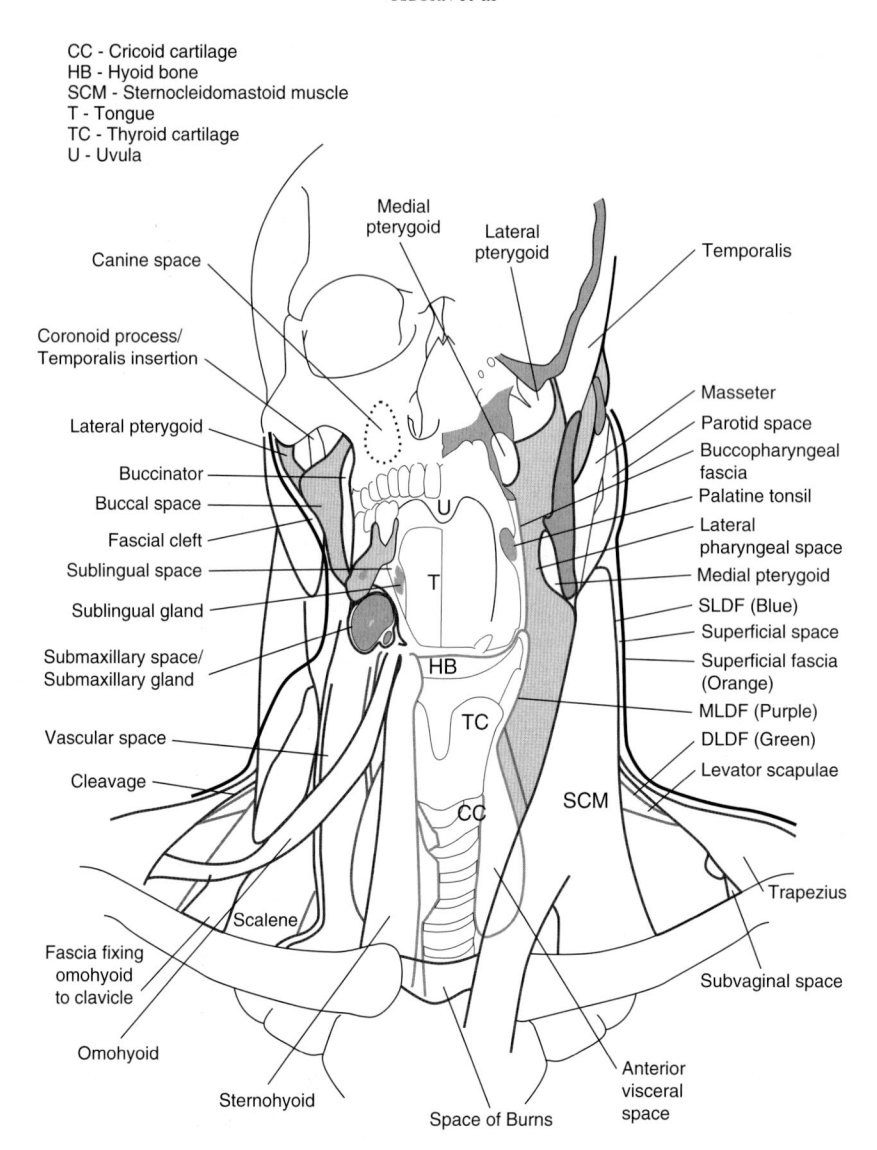

Fig. 2. Fascial spaces of the neck. (*Modified from* Janfaza P, Nadol JB, Galla RJ, et al. Surgical anatomy of the head and neck. Philadelphia: Lippincott Williams & Wilkins, 2000. p. 684; with permission.)

neck infections represent the normal oral flora that becomes pathogenic when normal host defenses are ineffective. Commonly cultured organisms include *Streptococcus viridans*, *Streptococcus milleri* group species, B-hemolytic streptococci, *Neisseria* species, *Peptostreptococcus*, coagulase-negative staphylococci and *Bacteroides* [2–4]. Other causes that should be considered but are uncommon are *Bartonella henselae* and *Mycobacterium tuberculosis* [5]. Anaerobic bacteria include *Prevotella* and *Porphyromonas* species, *Actinomyces* species, *Bacteroides* species, *Propionobacterium*, Hemophilus, and *Eikenella*. Anaerobic bacteria are found in more than half of severe odontogenic infections [6]. In diabetic patients, the microbial nature of DSNI shows a higher infection rate of *Klebsiella pneumoniae* when compared with those who do not have diabetes mellitus [4].

Diagnosis

When evaluating a patient in whom a deep neck infection is suspected, an orderly workup should be followed. As all evaluations should begin, a history and physical examination should be obtained, with focus on evaluation of the airway. Information on the time from initiation of symptoms to the present will give an understanding of the pace of advancement of the infection. Potential initiating factors such as dental problems, dental interventions, recent upper respiratory infection, recent surgery, or trauma need to be assessed. Any signs of impending airway obstruction should prompt immediate and necessary control of the airway. Patients who are deemed to have a stable airway may have a more leisurely history and physical examination performed. Physical examination should include intraoral evaluation with focus on the floor of mouth and dentition, oropharyngeal, and pharyngeal examination. Attention should also be directed behind the palatopharyngeal fold.

Understanding the common and uncommon presentation of DSNI is critical in the early recognition and management of these patients. Patients will often present with systemic signs and symptoms of disease, such as fever, chills, malaise, and loss of appetite. Because these are general symptoms, more localizing symptoms such as odynophagia, dysphagia, trismus, odontalgia, and dysphonia are often present. Mayor and colleagues [7] showed that the most common clinical presentation of DSNI was odynophagia in 84% of patients, followed by dysphagia (71%), fever (68%) neck pain (55%), neck swelling (45%), trismus (39%), and respiratory distress (10%). These symptoms have been shown to be similar in other series as well [8–10]. Signs include neck swelling, elevation of the floor of the mouth, drooling, diaphoresis, elevated temperature, and bulging of the pharyngeal wall or lingual aspect of the mandible. Classic description of pharyngeal wall bulging is midline bulging for prevertebral infections and unilateral for retropharyngeal space infections, because of the midline raphe formed by the superior constrictor muscle, which prevents space involvement crossing the midline [2].

There are a number of causes of deep neck infections. Determining the site of origin or cause of deep neck infections varies widely in the literature, ranging from 30% to 90% of cases having an identified source of infection [1,7]. The submandibular space is the most common site of deep neck infections and they are caused by odontogenic source in up to 85% of cases [11]. Other causes include laceration of the floor of the mouth, mandibular fracture, tumor, lymphadenitis, sialoadenitis, patient self-injection with intravenous drugs, systemic infection, and hematogenous spread of infection.

Infection of the lateral pharyngeal space is often caused by spread of tonsillar infection from the peritonsillar space through the superior pharyngeal constrictor muscle (Figs. 3 and 4). Other causes include posterior extension of infection from the submandibular space, anterior extension from the retropharyngeal space, and medial extenstion from a deep lobe parotid abscess or masticator space abscess. Common causes of retropharyngeal infection are from blunt or penetrating trauma, instrumentation (esophagoscopy, feeding tube placement, intubation), and suppurative lymphadenitis (rare after age 5). Spread of infection from the lateral pharyngeal space or prevertebral space can result in retropharyngeal space involvement (Fig. 5).

There are a number of imaging modalities that can be used once a history and physical have been performed. The potential for loss of airway during radiologic assessment should be considered in every case. Any patient who has airway compromise should have control of the airway ensured via intubation or tracheotomy before any imaging modalities are used. Clinicians can make use of plain radiographs (chest, lateral neck), ultrasonography, CT, MRI, and nuclear medicine scans. Inspiratory lateral cervical radiography has traditionally been used because it is simple, readily available, and applicable in cases of retropharyngeal and prevertebral space involvement. Increased thickness of the distance from the anterior aspect of the vertebral body to the air column in the posterior pharyngeal wall (>7 mm at C-2), loss of cervical lordosis, and presence of air in the soft tissues suggest space involvement [10,12]. In most institutions, this method is rarely used because of the 33% false-negative rate as well as the wide availability of CT scans.

CT scanning is the most widely used modality for diagnosing DSNI because it is less expensive, readily available, and can localize abscesses in the head and neck, as well as other structural abnormalities. The results of CT scans are easily interpreted by surgeons and allow for precise surgical planning. CT is not as effective as ultrasound in determining abscess from cellulitis. On CT, cellulitis appears as soft-tissue swelling, increased density of surrounding fat, enhancement of involved muscles, and obliteration of fat planes, whereas abscess is suspect when there is a low density area with a peripheral enhancement. With any radiologic evaluation, the findings must be correlated with clinical findings. A study by Miller and colleagues [13] found combination of

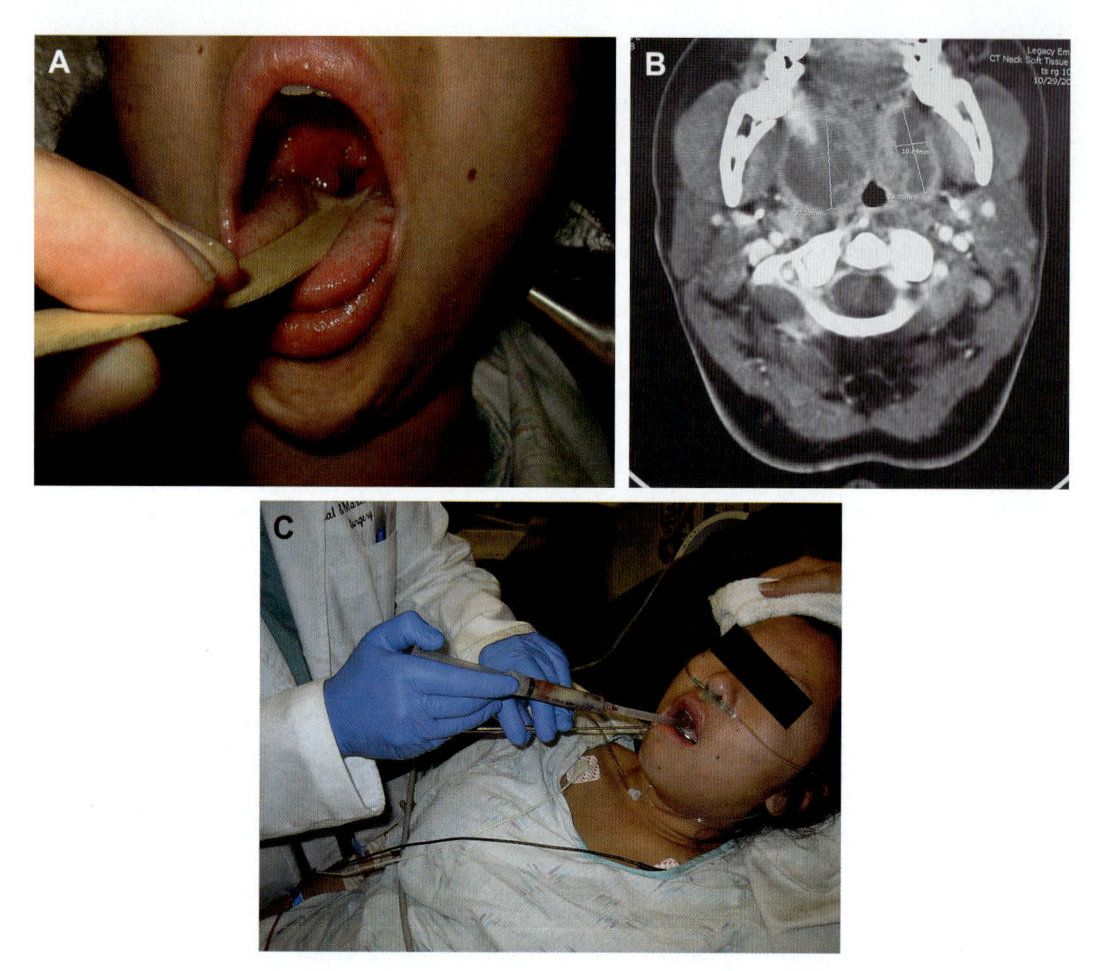

Fig. 3. Fourteen-year-old patient who has peritonsillar abscess (PTA). Note lack of trismus, differentiating this from a lateral pharyngeal space infection, which almost universally presents with trismus. PTAs can be safely managed by needle aspiration combined with appropriate antibiotic therapy, again differentiating them from lateral pharyngeal space infections, which generally require extraoral/transcervical drainage. (*A*) Clinical appearance. (*B*) CT scan of the same patient demonstrating peritonsillar fluid collections bilaterally. (*C*) Needle aspiration.

clinical evaluation and CT findings led to accuracy in identifying drainable collection of 89%, sensitivity of 95%, and specificity of 80%. In a series reported in one paper [8], CT scans were not readily available, and the lack of CT with contrast was an important contributing factor in all patient deaths.

Use of ultrasound gives reliable determination of abscess versus cellulitis. The advantages of ultrasound is that it is transportable to the patient, can be used to direct an aspirating needle, and involves no radiation [14]. Ultrasound is particularly useful in children and in peritonsillar-upper parapharyngeal infections, to avoid incision and drainage in cellulitis and to support medical treatment in those cases [15].

Use of MRI gives improved soft-tissue definition over CT without the use of radiation. MRI and magnetic resonance angiography (MRA) may also be more useful than CT technology in diagnosis of vascular complications of DSNI—internal jugular vein thrombosis (IJVT), carotid erosion or rupture [16,17]. MRI should also be used when central nervous system (CNS) involvement is suspected.

Patients with DSNI should undergo incision and drainage that includes a culture and sensitivity as a guide antimicrobial therapy. There is varying susceptibility of organisms in head and neck infections, and culture and sensitivity allows identification of resistant organisms [18]. Gram's stain is a quick and useful tool to assist in initial

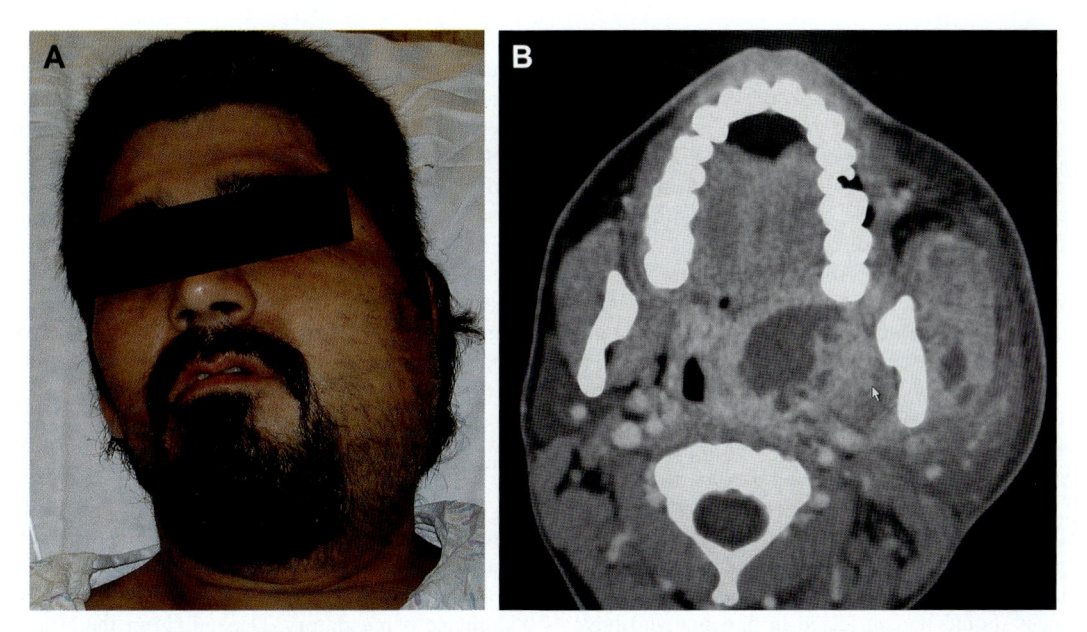

Fig. 4. Forty-five-year-old patient who has lateral pharyngeal space abscess with involvement of the masticator space. Note external swelling caused by the masticator space infection and severe trismus. (*A*) Clinical appearance. (*B*) CT scan demonstrating fluid collections involving the lateral pharyngeal space, submandibular space, and masticator space.

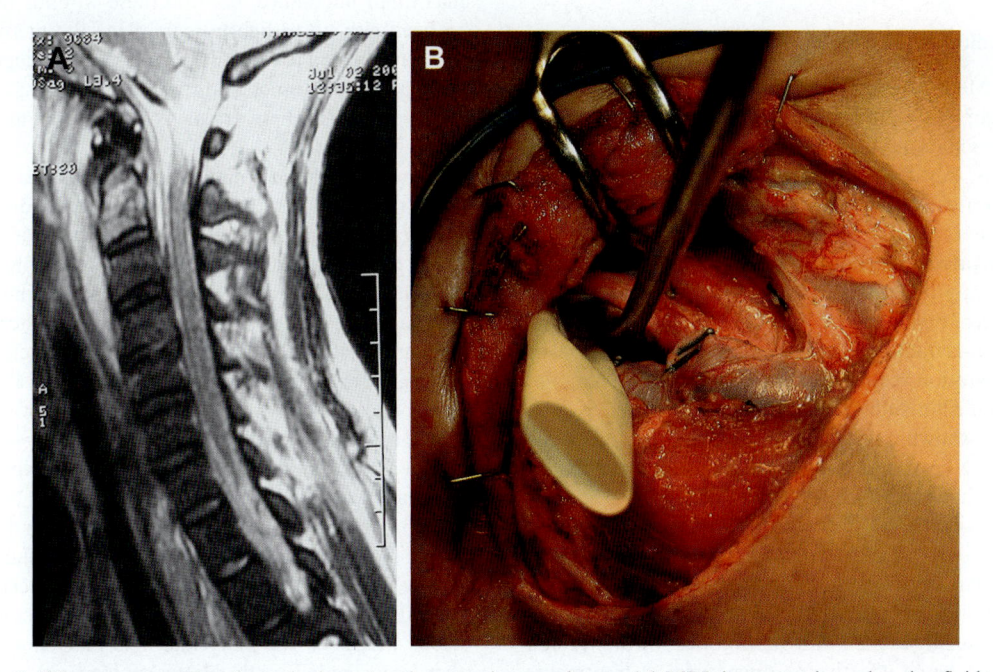

Fig. 5. Fifty-two-year-old patient who has retropharyngeal space abscess. (*A*) MRI demonstrating enhancing fluid collection in retropharyngeal space. (*B*) Clinical photograph demonstrating surgical approach to open drainage. Dissection begins at the anterior border of the sternocleidomastoid muscle; the internal jugular vein and carotid artery are identified and protected, and the retropharyngeal space is entered high in the neck. Note retraction of the internal carotid artery.

antibiotic choice, such as when Gram's stain may suggest staphylococcal infection versus streptococcal infection. Although there are improved techniques for isolating anaerobic bacteria, there is little use for anaerobic culture in DSNI. The majority of isolates in head and neck infections are aerobic in nature, particularly with use of the swab technique of collection [19].

Routine sampling of blood cultures is not widely practiced for patients in the absence of signs of systemic symptoms such as fever, chills, night sweats, or hypotension. Blood cultures are positive in 10% to 15% of patients who have systemic symptoms [4]. Patients who develop signs and symptoms of septicemia despite adequate medical or surgical treatment should have blood cultures.

An important consideration in people who have DSNI is that in one series, the cause in 6% of patients was malignant tumor [20]. Therefore the use of panendoscopy following acute phase treatment should be considered in patients who have no clear etiology of infection. One should also consider sampling of accessible lymph nodes if they are found enlarged or abnormal. It may also be prudent to take a biopsy specimen of the abscess wall to establish or exclude the diagnosis of malignancy [20].

Medical management

Medical management of these patients should begin promptly with intravenous access, fluid resuscitation, and administration of IV antibiotics. Antibiotic therapy should be administered empirically and tailored to culture and sensitivity results. Early intervention with a penicillin derivative and clindamycin is the key to successful therapy and avoidance of complications [21,22]. Other regimens include the use of penicillins with -lactamase inhibitor, second, third, or fourth generation cephalosporins, and metranidazole. Ampicillin/sulbactam and clindamycin have each been shown to be effective for anaerobic infections of the head and neck [18,23]. Pipercillin/tazobactam has shown efficacy in treating polymicrobial infections as a single agent [24]. Deep neck infections in the cellulitis stage can be successfully treated with antibiotic therapy alone [4,25]. Mayor and colleagues [7] showed that medical treatment alone with antibiotics and steroids could be as effective as open surgical treatment. The traditional approach is for open surgical drainage when the presence of purulence is suspect.

Comorbid medical conditions are found in many patients who have DSNI. Some of the more common are diabetes mellitus, chronic hepatitis, uremia or chronic renal failure, and relative immune-suppressed states such as HIV/AIDS or in patients on chemotherapy [4]. These conditions require thorough workup and monitoring because they can be exacerbated by the infection, and can also lead to more severe infections. Diabetes in particular requires strict management, and control of blood sugar below 200 mg/dL is imperative for good control of infection [26].

Surgical treatment

Many deep infections of the head and neck require surgical intervention in the form of incision and drainage. Many would argue that when there is an abscess in the deep neck, surgical drainage is mandatory. Depending on the series, surgical drainage is required in 10% to 83% of patients who present with deep neck space infections [7,20]. When surgical drainage is necessary, Topazian and Goldberg [27] recommend the following principles in their text: incise in healthy skin and mucosa when possible, not at the site of maximum fluctuance, because these wounds tend to heal with an unsightly scar; place the incision in a natural skin fold; place the incision in a dependent position; dissect bluntly; place a drain; and remove drains when drainage becomes minimal [27].

Drainage of the submandibular space can be by intraoral or extraoral incision. Intraoral drainage is via incision in the anterior aspect of the floor of the mouth, and is indicated only in uncomplicated infections limited to the sublingual compartment; otherwise an external approach is recommended [1]. The external approach is through an incision approximately 3 to 4 cm below the angle of the mandible and below the inferior extent of swelling. If the incision is placed in the area of swelling and erythema, the wound may heal with excessive scarring. The 2 to 3 cm incision should roughly parallel the inferior border of the mandible, but more importantly, should follow relaxed skin tension lines. The incision should be carried down through skin and subcutaneous tissues to the platysma. The platysma can then be divided with electrocautery or sharp dissection. The superficial layer of deep cervical fascia should then be incised parallel to the inferior border of the mandible. Blunt or finger dissection is then used in a superior-medial direction to enter the submandibular space. Care should be taken to dissect toward the lingual aspect of the mandible in the area of the posterior molars so as to avoid the facial vessels. It is often impossible to avoid penetration of the oral mucosa when teeth are extracted concomitantly, and in the authors' experience this has not led to orocutaneous fistula. Surgical drains should always be left in the space, or in multiple sites within the space. We often use red rubber catheters in addition to Penrose drains to irrigate the space.

Drainage of the lateral pharyngeal space is approached mainly through an external approach. An intraoral approach to the lateral pharyngeal space is discouraged because of the presence of the carotid sheath within the space [1]. In cases where no access to the carotid artery, internal jugular vein, or mediastinum are anticipated, an approach similar to that of the submandibular space can be used. As the authors have often seen, there is extension of submandibular space infections into the lateral pharyngeal space, and we approach both through the same incision. The only difference is that the superomedial vector of dissection is carried through aiming for the angle of the mandible and into the lateral pharyngeal space. Another approach is through the anterior SCM approach, which should be used if access to the carotid artery or internal jugular vein may be necessary. The incision is oriented vertically along the anterior border of the SCM beginning 3 to 4 fingerbreadths inferior to the auricle. The incision is carried down to the superficial layer of deep cervical fascia, and the carotid sheath is identified and opened. Dissection is carried superiorly along the vessels as indicated. Once near the angle of the mandible, blunt dissection can be used in a superior-medial direction to enter the space, as described before. If vascular complications are likely, proximal and distal closure should be achieved with loose ligature. In any case, drains should be left in the space. The authors routinely use two drains, one in the anterior and one in the posterior compartment.

Drainage of the retropharyngeal space can be accomplished through an intraoral or extraoral approach (see Fig. 5). When draining the space intraorally, it is wise to first aspirate the area of induration or fluctuance to confirm the presence of pus and not blood. If there is blood, one should suspect carotid artery erosion, which dictates an external approach. Once the presence of pus is confirmed, then a vertical incision can be made over the mass. Blunt dissection with hemostats should then be used to widely spread in the space. Copious irrigation should be used. The authors use an intraoral approach to this space with a clearly defined area of loculation, especially in children. Drains are not routinely used with an intraoral approach, but can be used if necessary, and sutured to the lateral pharyngeal wall and buccal mucosa. In adults and in people who have large retropharyngeal space abscesses, an external approach is used. The approach is through an anterior SCM approach as previously described. The carotid sheath is identified and mobilized medially. If there is sheath involvement, it can be opened. With the sheath and vessels mobilized medially, the prevertebral fascia will be encountered. Blunt dissection with hemostat or finger dissection is then used to enter the space. Drains are used, and again, the authors commonly use multiple drains in the space. Adequate drainage can be obtained without thoracotomy o the level of T-4 [1].

Although it is a rare phenomenon, Ludwig's angina deserves special mention (Fig. 6). It is defined as firm, acute, toxic cellulitis of the bilateral submandibular and sublingual spaces in addition to the submental space, most commonly secondary to dental infection. Ludwig's requires prompt diagnosis and surgical intervention. As with all infections if the head and neck, airway security is of prime concern. There is a higher incidence of upper airway obstruction in cases of Ludwig's as well as greater need for tracheostomy. Parhiscar and Har-El [28] noted that 16 of 36 patients underwent elective tracheostomy under local anesthesia without complication. In this series, when intubation was attempted, it failed in 55% of cases and emergent tracheostomy was necessary [28]. Therefore, with patients who have Ludwig's angina, or anyone who has similar risk of upper airway obstruction, the authors perform urgent elective tracheostomy under local anesthesia.

Airway management

Airway compromise is the most immediate and life-threatening of the complications encountered in management of deep neck infections. Proper management of the airway can be a lifesaving measure in certain patients and should be of primary focus. There are three options for airway management: close clinical observation,

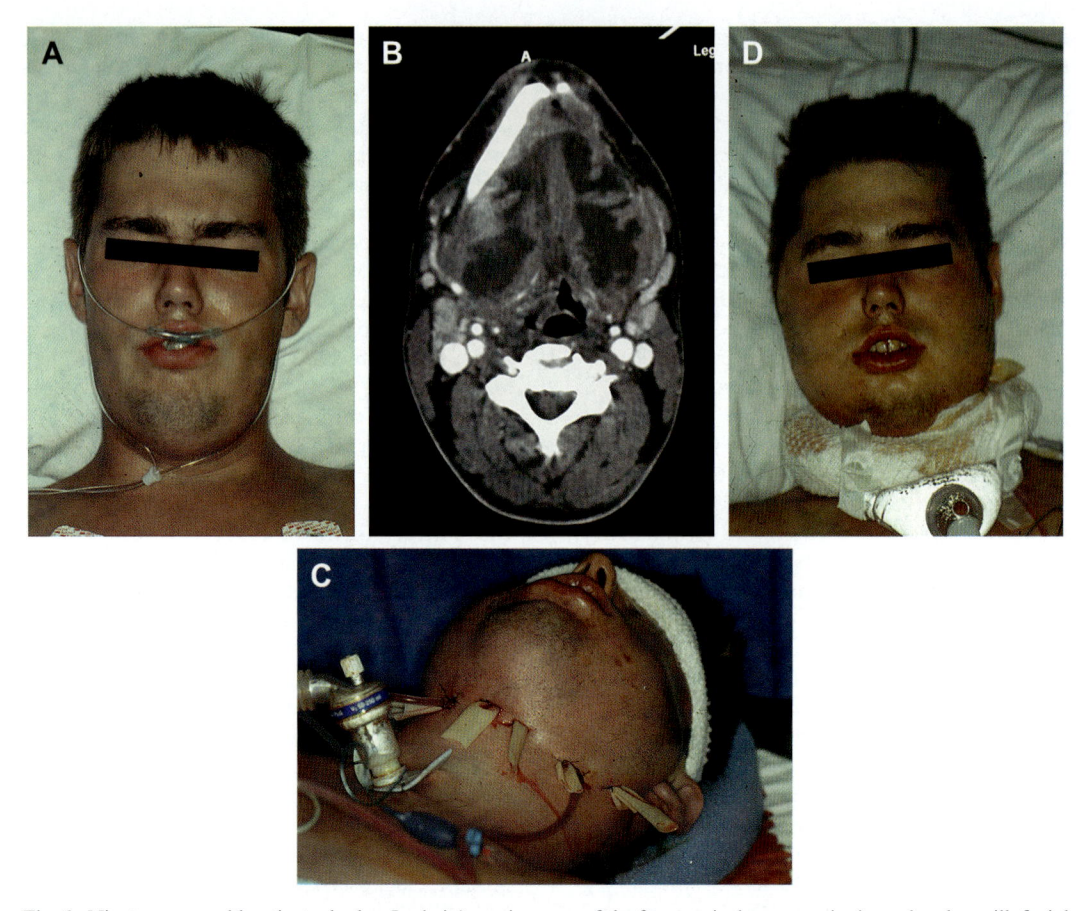

Fig. 6. Nineteen-year-old patient who has Ludwig's angina, one of the few surgical emergencies in oral and maxillofacial surgery. (*A*) Clinical appearance. Note: patient upright to maintain airway in preparation for awake tracheostomy. (*B*) CT scan demonstrating involvement of the submandibular and submental spaces bilaterally. (*C*) Incision and drainage with instrumentation of all involved spaces bilaterally (sublingual, submental, submandibular, and lateral pharyngeal). (*D*) Postoperative appearance 1 day following surgical drainage. Note: with early tracheostomy the patient requires no short- or long-term ventilatory assistance and is transferred out of the intensive care unit on postoperative day 1.

endotracheal intubation (fiberoptic or direct), or surgical airway. There are different advantages and disadvantages to each. Observation of the airway is adequate if initial evaluation reveals no impending airway compromise, but does require close evaluation. The main complications of observation without mechanical intervention are unrecognized impending airway loss, risk of oversedation with loss of airway, or extension of infection and edema leading to asphyxiation. The benefit is that there is no mechanical intervention, which carries inherent risk. The advantages of endotracheal intubation include the speed with which airway control can be achieved, and that it is a nonsurgical procedure. Disadvantages include the potential for failed intubation, inability to bypass upper airway obstruction, requirement for mechanical ventilation, and subglottic stenosis, and endotracheal tube (ETT) displacement/unintentional extubation. Tracheotomy, on the other hand, allows for the bypass of upper airway obstruction. It is a very secure airway, there is less need for sedation and mechanical ventilation, and it allows for earlier transfer out of critical care units [29]. Tracheotomy is a surgical procedure with inherent risks such as pneoumothorax, bleeding, subglottic stenosis, tracheoinnominate or tracheoesophageal fistula, as well as unsightly scar. Training and comfort with airway management procedures, as well as available hospital resources such as anesthesiology, fiberoptic equipment, and critical care resources, also have an impact [21,30]. The decision to observe the airway, perform

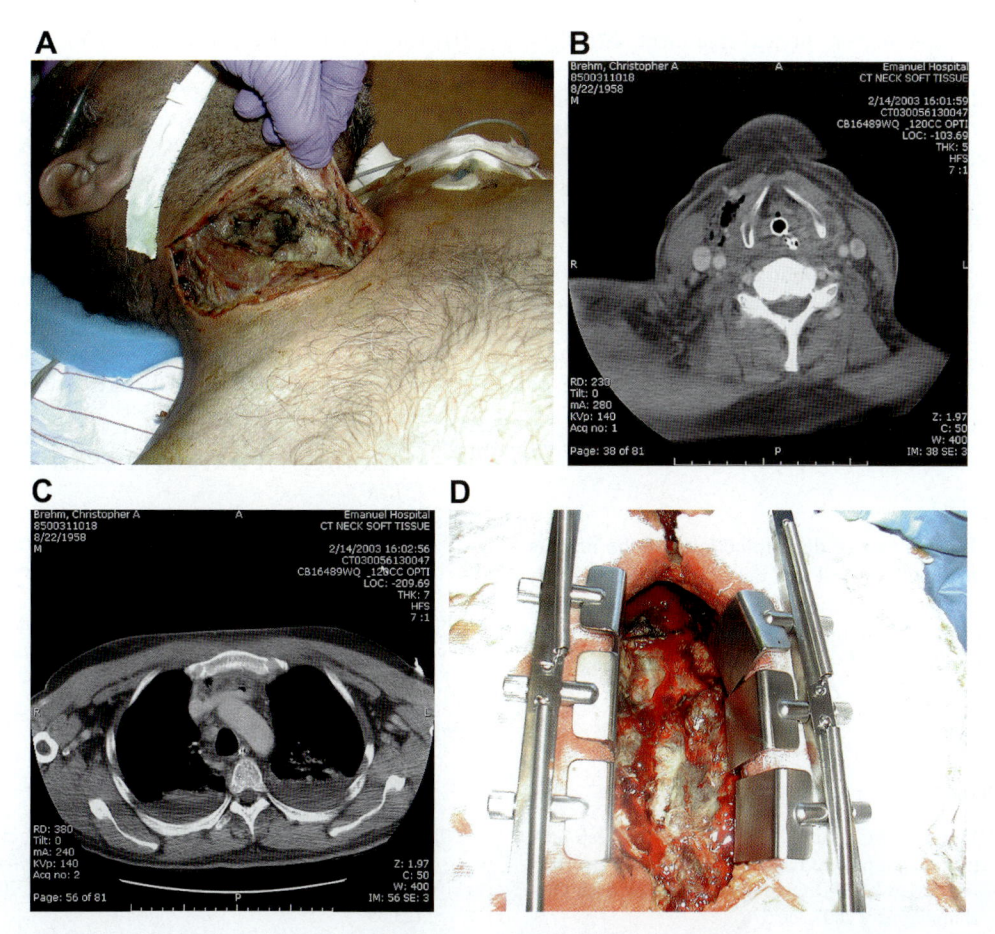

Fig. 7. Forty-nine-year-old patient who has cervical necrotizing fasciitis of odontogenic origin. Patient presented to emergency department in sepsis with mediastinal extension following inadequate drainage of a submandibular abscess at an outside office. (*A*) Intraoperative photograph at the time of initial neck exploration. Note necrotic tissue. (*B*) CT of the neck at presentation, demonstrating free air and inflammatory changes within the deep fascial spaces of the neck. (*C*) CT of the chest at presentation, demonstrating similar free air and inflammatory changes within the mediastinum in addition to pulmonary fluid collections. (*D*) Mediastinal exploration.

intubation, or tracheotomy must be made on an individual basis, considering the advantages and disadvantages of each.

Complications

Even in the advent of modern antibiotics, severe complications can occur in DSNI. These include airway compromise, jugular vein thrombosis, mediastinal involvement, pericarditis, pneumonia, emphysema, arterial erosion, meningitis, and extracranial or intracranial extension of infection if there is delay in diagnosis and treatment [8,31–33]. Carotid artery erosion is a devastating complication that can involve the common, internal, or external carotid branches. A bleed may be heralded by recurrent small hemorrhages, hematoma, bleeding, ipsilateral Horner's syndrome, unexplained cranial nerve IX to XII neuropathy, persistence of peritonsillar swelling, and blood clots on exploration or incision and drainage [34]. If carotid artery erosion is suspected, then aggressive treatment is warranted by gaining proximal and distal control with repair or ligation [10].

IJVT is the most common vascular complication. It is characterized by shaking chills, spiking fevers, tenderness, and swelling at the angle of the mandible or along the SCM [10]. IJVT may produce bacteremia, circulating septic thrombi with distant infection, or pulmonary embolism. Treatment is with medical management consisting of anticoagulation, or surgical treatment with ligation of the vein.

Mediastinitis is a rare complication of DSNI, and the descending necrotizing mediastinitis that results is one of the most serious and lethal forms (Fig. 7) [35]. The diagnosis of mediastinitis is based on clinical examination and cervicothoracic CT, which will show tracking of infection down the neck and signs of fluid collection or gas within the mediastinum. These patients are treated surgically through a cervical approach when there is no infiltration above the tracheal bifurcation or T4, and a combined cervical and thoracic approach in all other cases [36,37].

Summary

Management of deep infections of the neck is a critical skill of oral and maxillofacial surgery. It is a unique opportunity for the specialty to act as the primary managing team for these patients. A fundamental skill set is required for the diagnosis and management of these potentially life-threatening illnesses.

References

[1] Bottin R, Marioni G, Rinaldi R, et al. Deep neck infection: a present day complication. A retrospective review of 83 cases (1998–2001). Eur Arch Otorhinolaryngol 2003;260:576.
[2] Marra S, Hotaling AJ. Deep neck infections. Am J Otolaryngol 1996;17:287.
[3] Brook I. Microbiology and management of peritonsillar, retropharyngeal, and parapharyngeal abscesses. J Oral Maxillofac Surg 2004;62:1545.
[4] Huang TT, Lieu TC, Chen PR, et al. Deep neck infection: analysis of 185 cases. Head Neck 2004;26:854.
[5] Ridder GJ, Technau-Ihling K, Sander A, et al. Spectrum and management of deep neck space infections: an 8-year experience of 234 cases. Otolaryngol Head Neck Surg 2005;133:709.
[6] Flynn TR, Shanti RM, Levi MH, et al. Severe odontogenic infections, part 1: prospective report. J Oral Maxillofac Surg 2006;64:1093.
[7] Mayor GP, Milan JM, Martinez-Vidal A. Is conservative treatment of deep neck space infections appropriate? Head Neck 2001;23:126.
[8] Larawin V, Naipao J, Dubey SP. Head and neck pace infections. Otolaryngol Head Neck Surg 2006;135:889.
[9] Tom MB, Rice DH. Presentation and management of neck abscess: a retrospective analysis. Laryngoscope 1988;98:877.
[10] Gidley PW, Ghorayeb BY, Stiernberg CM. Contemporary management of deep neck space infections. Otolaryngol Head Neck Surg 1997;116:16.
[11] Patterson HC, Kelly JH, Stroone M. Ludwig's angina: an update. Laryngoscope 1982;92:370.
[12] Bank D, Krug S. New approaches to upper airway disease. Emerg Med Clin North Am 1995;13:473.
[13] Miller WD, Furst IM, Sandor GKB, et al. A prospective blinded comparison of clinical examination and computed tomography in deep neck infections. Laryngoscope 1999;109:1873.
[14] Baatenburg de Jong RJ, Rongen RJ, Lameris JS, et al. Ultrasound-guided percutaneous drainage of deep neck abscesses. Clin Otolaryngol 1990; 15:159.
[15] Quraishi MS, O'Halpin DR, Blayney AW. Ultrasonography in the evaluation of neck abscesses in children. Clin Otolaryngol 1997;22:30.
[16] Braun TF, Hoffman JC, Malko JA, et al. Jugular venous thrombosis: MRI imaging. Radiology 1985; 157:357.
[17] McArdle CB, Marfahraee M, Amparo EG, et al. MR imaging of transverse/sigmoid dural sinus and jugular vein thrombosis. J Comput Assist Tomogr 1987;11:831.
[18] Rega AJ, Aziz SR, Ziccardi VB. Microbiology and antibiotic sensitivies of head and neck space infections of odontogenic origin. J Oral Maxillofac Surg 2006;64:1377.
[19] Lewis MA, MacFarlane TW, McGowan DA. A microbiological and clinical review of the acute dentoalveolar abscess. Br J Oral Maxillofac Surg 1990;28:359.
[20] Ridder JG, Eglinger CF, Technau-Ihlinge K, et al. Deep neck abscess masquerading hypopharyngeal carcinoma. Otolaryngol Head Neck Surg 2000; 123:659.
[21] Har-El G, Aroesty JH, Shaha A, et al. Changing trends in deep neck abscess: a retrospective study of 110 patients. Oral Surg Oral Med Oral Pathol 1994;77:446.
[22] Stiernberg CM. Deep-neck space infection: diagnosis and management. Arch Otolaryngol Head Neck Surg 1986;112:1274.
[23] Retsema JA, English AR, Girard A, et al. Sulbactam/ampicillin: in vitro spectrum, potency, and activity in models of acute infection. Rev Infect Dis 1986;8(Suppl 5):S528.
[24] Gorbach SL. Pipercillin/tazobactam in the treatment of polymicrobial infections. Intensive Care Med 1994;20(Suppl 3):S27.
[25] Sakaguchi M, Sato S, Ishiyama T, et al. Characterization and management of deep neck infections. Int J Oral Maxillofac Surg 1997;26:131.
[26] Chen MK, Wen YS, Chang CC, et al. Deep neck infections in diabetic patients. Am J Otolaryngol 2000;105:169.
[27] Topazian RG, Goldberg MH. Odontogenic infections and deep fascial space infections of dental origin. In: Topazian RG, editor. Oral and maxillofacial infections. 4th edition. Philadelphia: WB Saunders Company; 2002.

[28] Parhiscar A, Har-El G. Deep neck abscess: a retrospective review of 210 cases. Ann Otol Rhinol Laryngol 2001;110:1051.
[29] Potter JK, Herford AS, Ellis E. Tracheotomy versus endotracheal intubation for airway management in deep neck space infections. J Oral Maxillofac Surg 2002;60:349.
[30] Peterson LJ. Contemporary management of deep infections of the neck. J Oral Maxillofac Surg 1993;51:226.
[31] Ruiz CC, Labajo AD, Vilas IY, et al. Thoracic complications of deeply situated serious neck infections. J Craniomaxillofac Surg 1993;21:76.
[32] Beck HJ, Salassa JR, McCaffrey TV, et al. Life-threatening soft tissue infections of the neck. Laryngoscope 1984;94:354.
[33] Chen MK, Wen YS, Chang CC, et al. Predisposing factors of life-threatening deep neck infection: logistic regression analysis of 214 cases. J Otolaryngol 1998;27:141.
[34] Blum DJ, McCaffrey TV. Septic necrosis of the internal carotid artery: a complication of peritonsillar abscess. Otolaryngol Head Neck Surg 1983;91:114.
[35] Roccia F, Pecorari GC, Oliaro A, et al. Ten years of descending necrotizing mediastinitis: management of 23 cases. J Oral Maxillofac Surg 2007;65:1716.
[36] Estrera AS, Lanay MJ, Grisham JM, et al. Descending necrotizing mediastinitis. Surg Gynecol Obstet 1983;157:545.
[37] Wheatley MJ, Stirling MC, Kirsh MM, et al. Descending necrotizing mediastinitis: transcervical drainage is not enough. Ann Thorac Surg 1990;49:780.

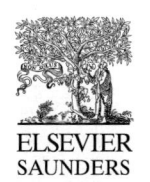

ORAL AND
MAXILLOFACIAL
SURGERY CLINICS
of North America

Deep Neck Infections: Clinical Considerations in Aggressive Disease

John F. Caccamese Jr., DMD, MD, FACS[a,b,*], Domenick P. Coletti, DDS, MD[a]

[a]Department of Oral and Maxillofacial Surgery, University of Maryland Medical System, 650 West Baltimore Street, Suite 1401, Baltimore, MD 21204, USA
[b]Department of Pediatrics, University of Maryland Medical System, 22 South Greene Street, Baltimore, MD 21204, USA

Deep neck infections (DNIs) are common and occur as a consequence of several etiologies. The result is either an abscess or cellulitis in the potential spaces of the neck. Countless reports exist in the literature detailing the management of infections arising from odontogenic sources, congenital lesions, cervical adenitis, malignancies, surgical treatment, upper respiratory infection, and penetrating trauma. Life-threatening complications that have been associated with DNI include airway obstruction, sepsis, septic emboli, Lemierre syndrome, descending mediastinitus, and pericarditis. Additionally, extremely aggressive forms of DNI exist, including necrotizing fasciitis (Fig. 1A, B and Fig. 2A, B, C).

Despite numerous reports, little information exists regarding the true incidence of these infections. As is true in many areas of medicine, limited prospective data are available to guide therapy. Treatment over the years has been based mostly on surgical principle, airway management, and an understanding of the microbiologic flora of these infections. Antibiotic therapy, interventional radiology, and patient support modalities have become more sophisticated, although surgery continues to be the mainstay of treatment for most patients. Today, neck infections are rarely life threatening when sound and timely management is applied.

Etiology

DNI can arise from many sources. Dental sources are widely held to be the most common in adults and give rise to some of the more aggressive infections [1–5]. Aside from odontogenic infections, the etiology varies significantly by report. In some of the larger series, upper respiratory tract infection, intravenous drug abuse, and penetrating neck trauma have all been major contributors to this disease process [1–5]; however, one should consider all possibilities when evaluating a patient for DNI. Branchial sinuses, thyroglossal duct cysts, and malignancies can all masquerade as infections or present secondarily infected [5–11]. A careful history, examination, and imaging will help to differentiate the causes (Fig. 3).

DNI in the pediatric patient can present more of a diagnostic dilemma. The origin of infection is more varied in the pediatric population, and the location and microbial flora can differ substantially as well. Although sinusitis, pharyngitis, and tonsillitis can all have important roles in pediatric DNI, patients and their families frequently present with no history of a precipitating event or illness. Even within the pediatric population, the age of the patient results in an altered distribution of the site and etiology of infection [12]. Several studies have noted a higher incidence of staphylococcal species in pediatric DNI, as well as

* Corresponding author. Department of Oral and Maxillofacial Surgery, University of Maryland Medical System, 650 West Baltimore Street, Suite 1401, Baltimore, MD 21204
E-mail address: jcaccamese@umm.edu (J.F. Caccamese).

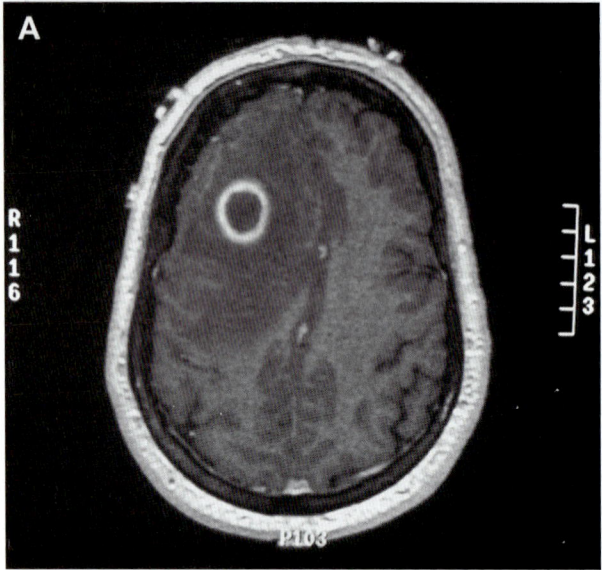

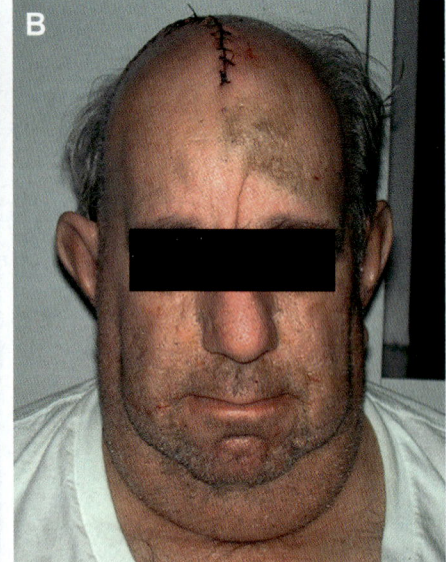

Fig. 1. (*A*) CT scan of an intraparenchymal abscess as a result of septic emboli from a dental source. (*B*) The patient following craniotomy for incision and drainage of the abscess.

a propensity for peritonsillar, retropharyngeal, and parapharyngeal space involvement [13–16]. History and physical examination can also present a challenge, making imaging more useful in the determination of etiology in this patient group.

The role of systemic disease

Systemic diseases, especially those that suppress the immune system, can make patients more susceptible to head and neck infections. Declining neutrophil function resulting in impaired phagocytosis and decreased bactericidal action have been demonstrated in the elderly, hemodialysis patients, and diabetic patients [17]. Other patients at risk are those who take immunosuppressive medications to treat chronic disease, such as cancer patients, patients with autoimmune disease, and transplant recipients.

Diabetic patients have long been known to have an increased susceptibility to infection, and DNI is no different in that regard [3,18]. In fact, studies suggest that diabetic patients not only become infected more frequency but also tend to be older, have a higher rate of complications, an increased severity of infection, prolonged hospitalization, and require more aggressive therapy [18,19]. Systemic hyperglycemia results in a derangement of the immune system involving neutrophil function, cellular immunity, and complement function; therefore, glycemic control is crucial in the management of diabetic infections. Additionally, diabetic infections might be populated with different bacterial flora, making culture and sensitivity data more important in their global management.

Microbiology

Most DNIs are polymicrobial, with only 5% identified as purely aerobic and 25% with isolated anaerobic species. Due to their fastidious nature, anaerobic organisms can be difficult to culture, and their exact role in disease is difficult to assess [20].

Neck infections commonly involve pathogens such as *Streptococcus viridans, Streptococcus milleri, Prevotella* spp, *Peptostreptococcus* spp, and *Klebsiella pneumoniae* [21–24]. Staphylococcal species are infrequently found in adult neck infections, many of which are coagulase negative and represent skin flora contamination. *Streptococcus viridans* is the predominant organism is adult neck infections (43.7%), but *Klebsiella pneumoniae* has been shown to be more common in diabetic patients (56.1%) [19]. Due to the predictable makeup of most polymicrobial head and neck infections, most patients can be treated empirically with regimens that include clindamycin or beta lactams alone or in combination with

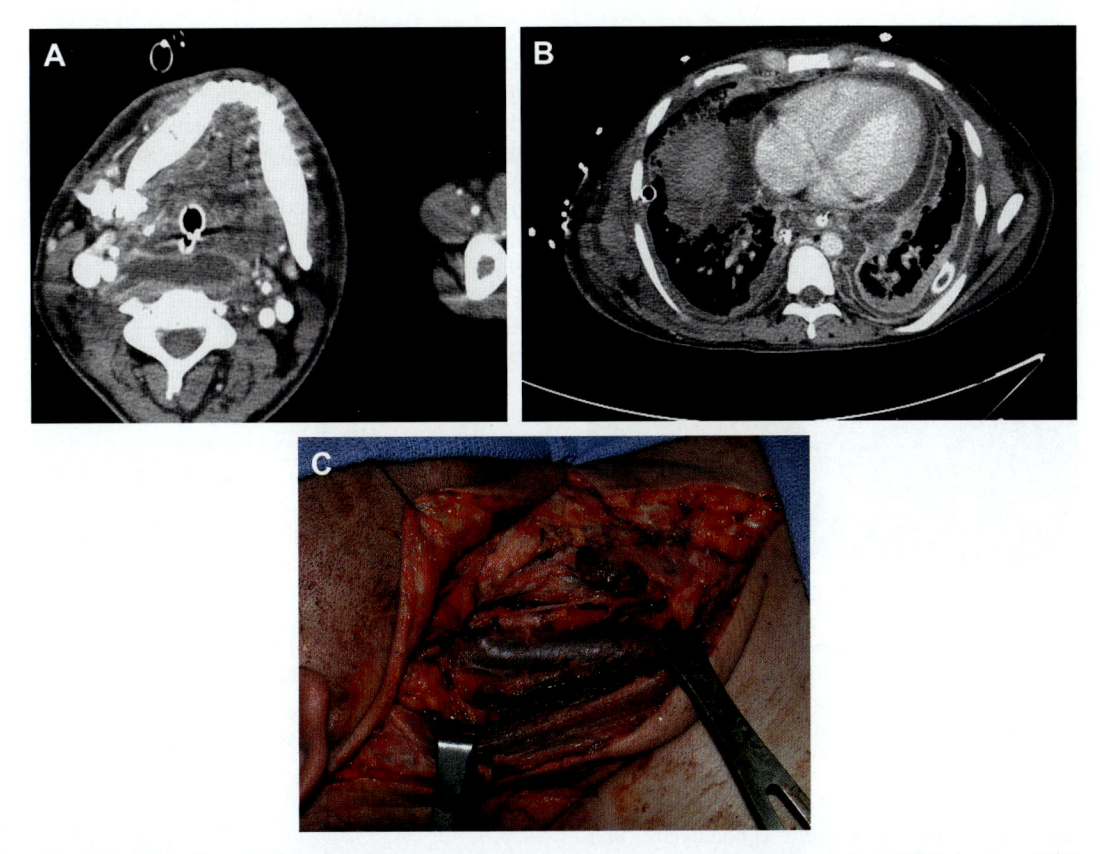

Fig. 2. (*A*) Retropharyngeal abscess from a dental source in an otherwise healthy young patient. (*B*) Extension of this abscess into the mediastinum and pericardium. The patient required thoracotomy. (*C*) An extended neck incision at the time of drainage. All neck spaces were drained.

metronidazole [25,26]. In a recent study of odontogenic infections by Flynn and colleagues [25], 19% of isolated species were found to be penicillin resistant, with only 4% of species with clindamycin resistance. These resistant strains accounted for 54% and 17% of cases with sensitivity data, respectively.

DNIs in children are also likely to be polymicrobial, with beta-lactamase producing organisms becoming more common. Group A streptococci represent the major pathogen, with *Prevotella* being the most common anaerobe; however, many studies have demonstrated an increased incidence of *Staphylococcus aureus* in pediatric neck infections [15,27–29]. This observation is most likely a result of fewer odontogenic infections in children and a higher rate of upper respiratory tract–related infections. Ever concerning is the increasing rate of methicillin-resistant *S aureus* (MRSA), which according to Ossowski and colleagues [29] has increased in their patient cohort of neck infections from 0% to 64% over 6 years.

The utility of cultures has been questioned, with some reports indicating that culture and sensitivity data do not lead to a change in antibiotic selection or treatment [26]. Others have recommended cultures for extensive or rapidly spreading infections, necrotizing and gas-forming infections, nosocomial or recurrent infections, and those that occur in an immunocompromised host [30]. Given the ever increasing possibility of drug-resistant organisms, perhaps this issue should be revisited.

In necrotizing fasciitis, the causative organisms are classically group A β-hemolytic streptococci and *Staphylococcus aureus*, alone or in synergism. Other aerobic and anaerobic pathogens can also be present, such as *Bacteroides, Clostridium, Peptostreptococcus, Proteus, Pseudomonas,* and *Klebsiella* [31]. Triple antibiotic therapy is usually instituted empirically, with regimens including

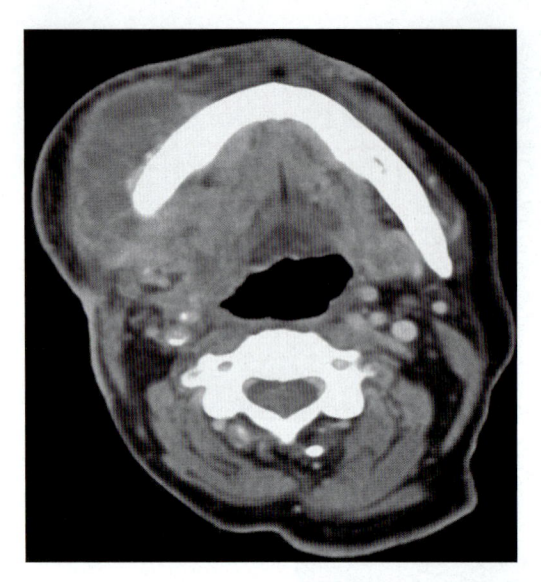

Fig. 3. CT scan of a neck "infection" referred for definitive treatment after several attempts at incision and drainage for presumed neck abscess at an outside institution. On further history, the patient described a recently excised squamous cell carcinoma of the ear. The mass was studied by biopsy rather than being re-drained and was found to be metastatic squamous cell carcinoma.

gentamicin, metronidazole, clindamycin and others to target these pathogens.

Pathogenesis of spread

Three patterns of spread are seen in severe head and neck infections—abscess formation, cellulitis, and necrotizing fasciitis. A variety of toxins, species, and strain-specific antigens are responsible for the infection's behavior. Classic teaching links abscess formation to staphylococcal species which produce coagulase, an enzyme that converts fibrinogen to fibrin. Fibrin-coated staphylococci resist phagocytosis, making the bacteria more virulent, and the bound coagulase induces the "clumping" of cells and the sequestration of bacteria and leukocytes. Streptococcal species give rise to cellulitis by producing invasins and protein toxins such as streptokinase and hyaluronidase that break down the ground substance and promote the spread of infection.

In necrotizing fasciitis, there is a rapid progressive liquefaction of subcutaneous fat and fascia, thrombosis of the subdermal veins, and decreased polymorphonuclear (PMN) leukocyte function promoted by hypoxic wound conditions.

Necrotizing fasciitis is associated with streptococcal pyrogenic exotoxins, thought to be responsible for toxic shock, and the enzyme cysteine protease that is involved in tissue destruction. Typically, the infection begins with an area of erythema that quickly spreads over a course of hours to days; as the skin's blood supply is lost, it necroses. The rate of necrosis is typically disproportionate to the clinical signs and symptoms (Fig. 4). Without prompt aggressive surgical drainage and debridement, secondary involvement of deeper muscle layers may occur, resulting in myositis or myonecrosis. The infection then progresses to systemic shock, organ failure, and death.

From a purely anatomic standpoint, DNIs usually follow the path of least resistance, penetrating the nearest and thinnest cortical bone and tracking along the fascial planes in the neck and face. Usually, infections spread from the primary fascial spaces (eg, sublingual, submandibular), extending by confluence to the secondary spaces of the retropharynx and prevertebral space as well as the carotid sheath, with eventual descent into the mediastinum, a possibility via the "danger space" or the anterior visceral space.

History

The diagnosis of severe aggressive odontogenic infection is initiated with a thorough history and physical examination. Important components of the history include the time course of the onset of

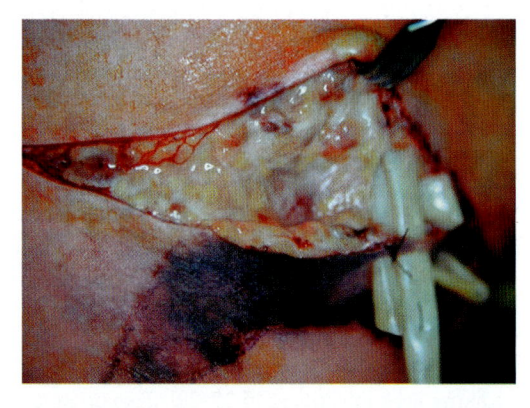

Fig. 4. Opening incision of necrotizing fasciitis infection. The infection developed in the patient after extraction of third molars at an outside institution. An attempt was made at conventional incision and drainage before transfer. Note the discoloration of the skin representing full-thickness necrosis as well as the necrotic appearance of the subcutaneous fat.

symptoms, fever, a history of a recent toothache or dental procedure, intravenous drug use, upper respiratory tract infection or tonsillitis, sinusitis, trauma, or skin abscess or infection. Exploring all potential etiologies in the history is important, and attention to specific symptoms suggestive of airway compromise is paramount. These symptoms include dysphagia, odynophagia, a muffled voice, inability to handle secretions, and, frequently, trismus as a result of inflammation adjacent to the muscles of mastication. Patients with the latter symptoms represent true surgical emergencies and can quickly progress to a life-threatening loss of airway.

A careful review of systems should focus on the presence of comorbid disease that might contribute to the infected state or complicate surgical management of the infection. Diabetes and other immunosuppressive diseases have been shown to contribute to infections in the head and neck and elsewhere. Additionally, immunosuppressive medications might necessitate modification of the surgical and anesthesia protocol as well as postoperative medical management.

Examination

A thorough head and neck examination must be performed efficiently following the basic principles of visualization, palpation, and percussion. A careful head and neck examination might obviate the need for adjunctive imaging in the acute setting, thereby decreasing the time until surgical management is initiated. The neck examination begins with a visual survey of the patient looking for swelling, erythema, pustules, or "pointing" of the infection (Fig. 5). Careful palpation of the anterior and posterior triangles should be performed. All fascial spaces of the oral cavity, face, and neck should be bimanually palpated to determine if the swelling is firm or fluctuant in nature. Draining sinus tracts and pits should be explored, and all carious teeth should be palpated and percussed to further elucidate the source of the infection. Crepitus can indicate gas-forming organisms and might also be a sign of a necrotizing infection. The palate, tonsils, and posterior pharynx should be examined for patency and symmetry. Nasal endoscopic examination is sometimes useful when trismus is severe. If trismus is present, the maximal interincisal opening should be measured because this can influence the anesthetic plan. A fetid odor is often detected in the oral cavity, indicating an infection of dental, salivary, sinus, or tonsillar origin.

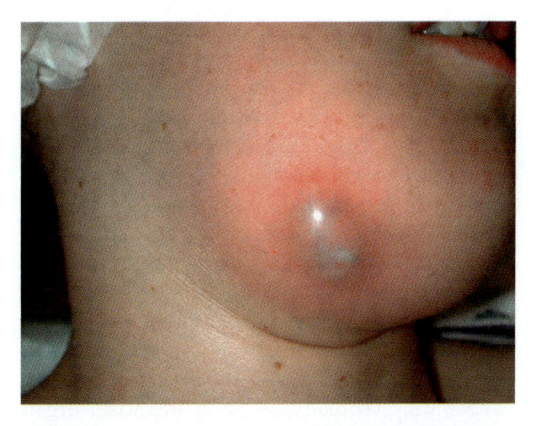

Fig. 5. This patient has an obvious right-sided neck swelling with erythema, ecchymosis, and a "pointing" infection.

A patient sitting postured in a sniffing position, drooling, and using their accessory muscles of respiration is an ominous sign of impending airway compromise (Fig. 6). Caution is advised at any attempt to lay the patient flat to obtain imaging or even intubate, because this may precipitate complete airway obstruction. Many of these patients have poor oral intake leading to dehydration, which, in addition to fever, will contribute to tachycardia. These acute infections can destabilize

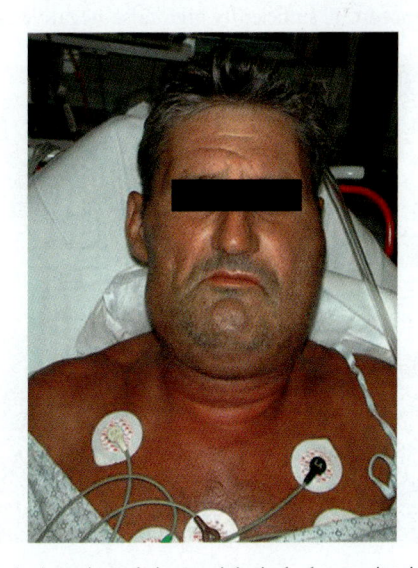

Fig. 6. A patient sitting upright in bed to maintain his airway. Note the appearance of distress and the fullness and erythema of the neck. This infection originated from an acute or chronic periodontal condition.

pre-existing diseases such as diabetes and cause hyperglycemia and ketosis.

Necrotizing fasciitis presents with an area of erythema that quickly spreads over a course of hours to days (Fig. 7). The margins of infection move out into normal skin without being raised or sharply demarcated. As the infection progresses, it gives way to a dusky or purplish discoloration of skin near the site of insult (Fig. 8). The patient usually appears moderately to severely toxic but, early on, may look deceptively well. The rate of necrosis is disproportional to the signs and symptoms of the infection, and the patient will eventually succumb to shock, organ failure, and death if early aggressive surgical management is not initiated. Fifty percent of patients with necrotizing infections present with hypotension; 10% to 30% have signs of acute renal failure, coagulopathy, abnormal liver function, acute respiratory distress syndrome, and hemolytic anemia [32].

Imaging

Plain radiographs such as a panoramic and periapical films are useful to identify an odontogenic source of infection. Soft tissue lateral views of the neck have been used to visualize increased prevertebral soft tissue thickening in retropharyngeal abscesses, but in the era of contrast-enhanced CT, sufficiently high false-negative rates have some centers abandoning their use [33,34]. CT scanning is now the imaging modality most used to assess severe neck infections (Fig. 9). Although CT scanning has an important role in diagnosing DNIs, it is not 100% predictive. Smith and colleagues [35] evaluated the positive predictive value of CT in DNIs. Seventy-five percent of the patients surgically drained had a discreet collection of pus correlating with CT findings; however, 25% did not. It was concluded that the decision for surgical drainage should be made

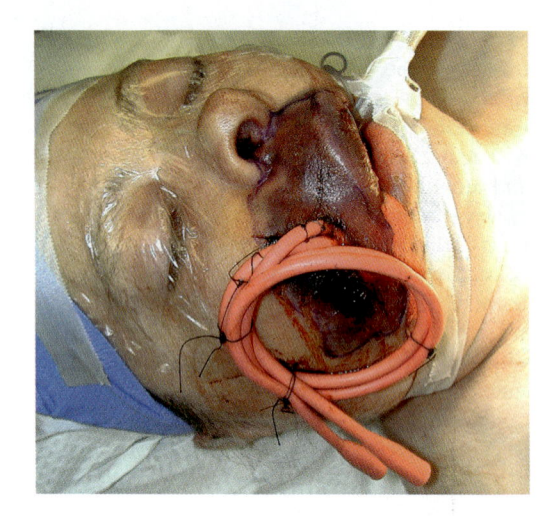

Fig. 8. This patient was transferred from an outside institution after multiple attempts at incision and drainage of the right side of the face. By history, the infection originated at the base of the nose. The infection progressed rapidly to a full-thickness necrosis, and the patient was diagnosed with necrotizing fasciitis at the time of definitive drainage and debridement. The organism was MRSA.

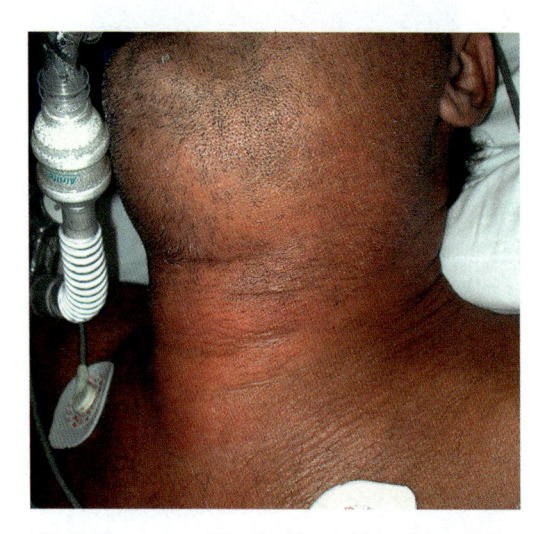

Fig. 7. The same patient in Fig. 6. Note the erythema and fullness of the submandibular region and the anterior neck. At the time of drainage and debridement, necrotizing fasciitis and myositis were observed.

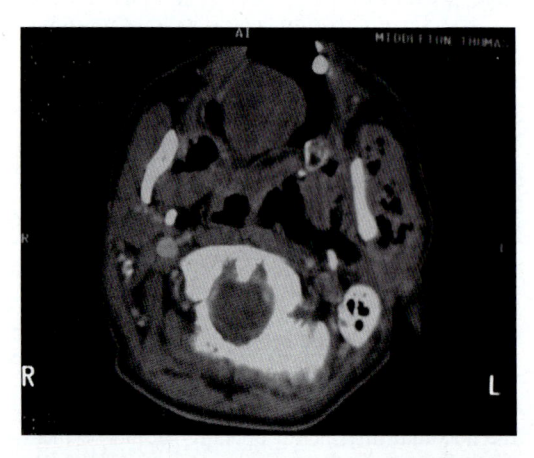

Fig. 9. CT scan of the neck demonstrating gas within the spaces of the neck indicating gas-forming organisms.

clinically, and that one should expect a 25% negative exploration rate. Lazor and colleagues [36] performed a 10-year retrospective review comparing preoperative CT with intraoperative findings. Similar to Smith and coworkers, they reported a positive correlation in 76.3% of patients. Both clinical examination and contrast-enhanced CT have been shown to be critical components in diagnosing DNIs. Miller and colleagues [37] performed a blinded prospective trial of 35 patients comparing the ability of clinical examination and contrast-enhanced CT to predict the presence of abscess formation in suspected DNIs. Twenty-two patients had drainable collections. Clinical examination was 63% accurate with 55% sensitivity and 73% specificity. CT was 77% accurate with 95% sensitivity and 53% specificity. If the two modalities were combined, the accuracy increased to 89%, with 95% sensitivity and 80% specificity. It was concluded that both clinical examination and contrast-enhanced CT were critical components in diagnosing these infections.

Munoz and colleagues [38] compared CT with MRI in the evaluation of head and neck infection. Although MRI was found to be superior in detecting abscess and defining spaces as well as lesion conspicuity and identification of source, CT depicted gas and calcification more accurately and was easier to interpret with regard to motion artifact. Overall, MRI was found to be superior for the initial evaluation of DNI; however, its utility is limited at the authors' center due primarily to the time involved in obtaining the study and the availability of MRI at all hours of the day.

Although CT scanning offers an advantage for the clinician by improving the identification of all involved spaces of the face, neck, brain, and mediastinum, patients with a compromised airway can be at risk for obstruction if placed supine for scanning. Despite the valuable information that can be gained from imaging, the clinician must weigh the risks and benefits of obtaining a scan. In situations in which airway loss is a real consideration and imaging is believed to be mandatory, the clinician should consider securing the airway (fiberoptic intubation, awake tracheotomy) before obtaining the study.

Airway

Potter and colleagues [39] reported that patients who had a neck infection and underwent tracheotomy had a shorter hospital and ICU stay when compared with those who were intubated. They concluded that tracheotomy provided better use of critical care resources with reduced cost.

In patients with a severe DNI, priority is given to securing the airway. This goal is facilitated by communication between the surgeon and anesthesiologist. Airway challenges specific to neck infections include trismus, neck swelling, mass effect, and edema of the tongue, pharynx, and larynx. If the vocal cords can be visualized with direct laryngoscopy, standard oral endotracheal intubation is safe. Recently, video-assisted direct laryngoscopy (GlideScope, Verathon, Bothell, Washington) has demonstrated value in management of the challenging airway, and this modality has been applied at the authors' institution [40]. The anesthesiologist should be informed of lateral pharyngeal, retropharyngeal, or peritonsillar collections of pus. Injudicious use of the laryngoscope could rupture an abscess in this location, resulting in aspiration of purulent material with subsequent pulmonary complications. If cord edema is present, excessive manipulation of the airway is ill advised, because this may cause further swelling, bleeding, or laryngospasm requiring an emergent surgical airway. In many severe DNIs, oral intubation is not possible. The recommended modality of airway management is an awake fiberoptic intubation or an awake tracheotomy. In emergent airway management, cricothyroidotomy is a quicker and safer choice, but swelling and edema may make palpation of the cricoid and thyroid cartilages difficult.

Potter and colleagues [39] reported that tracheotomy was the treatment of choice when severe DNIs were managed by otolaryngologists in a comparison with fiberoptic intubation managed by oral and maxillofacial surgeons. Ovassapian and colleagues [41] reported on 26 patients with deep DNI who underwent awake fiberoptic intubation. Three patients were intubated in the sitting position, two in Fowler's position, and 21 in the 10-to 15-degree supine position. Twenty-five of the intubations were successful; postoperatively seven patients were kept intubated and five underwent tracheotomy. Awake tracheotomy was recommended when fiberoptic intubation is not feasible or when intubation attempts fail. Awake fiberoptic intubation requires a skilled anesthesiologist facile with the technique. Tracheotomy also requires skill and experience in this patient population, because neck swelling may obscure the usual surgical landmarks and cause deviation of the trachea. There are risks and benefits associated with intubation and tracheotomy, and each case must be considered individually. The choice of procedure should be based on multiple issues, including the surgical plan, anticipated length of intubation, patient status at the time of drainage, and medical comorbidity. In Potter's series, 34 patients underwent tracheotomy and 51 were endotracheally intubated. One patient in the tracheotomy group had a cerebrovascular accident secondary to a ruptured carotid aneurysm. Two patients in the intubation group died, one from an unplanned extubation and the other from laryngeal edema post extubation with an inability to reintubate. According to their report, tracheotomy patients had a shorter hospital and ICU stay in comparison with intubated patients. It was concluded that tracheotomy provided better use of critical care resources with reduced cost [39]. In a review of retrospective data from a similar cohort of patients at the University of Maryland, only 2% of patients required tracheotomy, and a similar length of stay was observed [42].

In the setting of DNI, it is often difficult to assess when the patient is suitable for extubation despite the presence of inspiratory and expiratory cuff leaks and meeting appropriate ventilatory weaning parameters. Extubation of these patients has the potential of being disastrous, and it is recommended to err on the side of caution if any doubt exists, or to perform a tracheotomy.

Laboratory investigations

A complete blood count can show leukocytosis with an increased percentage of PMN leukocytes and a left shift; however, in isolated space abscesses, the white cell count might be normal. Many patients, especially those with necrotizing infections, have a metabolic acidosis as demonstrated by their basic metabolic panel and arterial blood gas. In cases of septic shock, lactate, blood urea nitrogen, creatinine, potassium, and glucose can all be elevated.

Surgical management

Medical therapy is primarily supportive in nature, because DNIs are primarily a surgical disease. For any patient demonstrating surgical urgency, the ABCs of basic life support are initiated. In deep neck and necrotizing infections in which patients are exhibiting signs of dehydration, fever, or shock, aggressive fluid resuscitation is initiated. Employment of vasopressors might be necessary for patients in septic shock once volume has been restored. The mainstay of therapy for DNI is prompt surgical drainage and removal of the source of infection when relevant, even in cases of cellulitis involving important fascial spaces. Aggressive incision and drainage will lead to earlier resolution by changing the local environment to one more favorable for antibiotic delivery and for the activity of host defense mechanisms. The authors' preference when dealing with infections that have progressed to the neck is to create an incision large enough to allow digital palpation of the involved drained spaces and bimanual inspection when anatomically possible. This inspection helps to ensure adequate drainage of all loculations and facilitates irrigation of the wound (Fig. 10).

Whether a role exists for nonsurgical management or minimally invasive intervention (eg, radiologically guided aspiration and drainage) is the subject of debate in the literature. Medical therapy alone seems to have a role in isolated space infections in the pediatric patient [28,43,44]; however, it has also been suggested that parapharyngeal abscesses could be treated medically with intravenous antibiotics alone or with needle aspiration. Oh and colleagues [45] performed an 8-year prospective study of 34 patients with CT-proven parapharyngeal abscesses. Nineteen of these patients were treated conservatively with antibiotics only or needle aspiration, and 15 were treated surgically with incision and drainage.

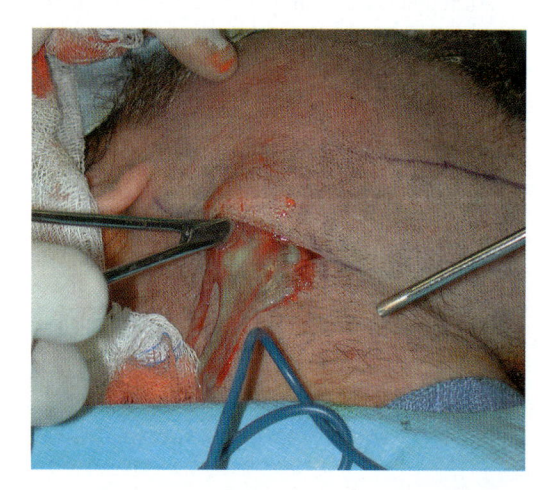

Fig. 10. At a minimum, access to the neck should be adequate to allow digital exploration of the involved spaces.

Patients with airway compromise had tracheotomies performed (n = 5). The length of hospital stay was 8.2 days in the conservative group and 11.6 days in the surgical group. One patient in the conservative group developed mediastinitis. It was concluded localized parapharyngeal abscesses may in some cases respond to antibiotics alone. Sichel and colleagues [46] performed a nonrandomized prospective study of infections limited to the parapharyngeal space without airway compromise or signs of shock. Twelve patients presented with this diagnosis; however, five were excluded due to extension into other spaces. Six of the seven cases were pediatric patients, and all were treated with a 9- to 14-day course of intravenous amoxicillin with clavulanic acid. All of the patients were cured without the need for drainage [46].

In peritonsillar abscesses, catheter or needle drainage has been recommended with the addition of ancillary steroids, and image-guided aspiration using either CT or ultrasound has been applied to DNIs [47]. Poe and colleagues [48] reported the use of CT-guided aspiration in a small series of four cases without complications. Yeow's group prospectively reviewed 15 cases of unilocular neck abscesses that failed antibiotic therapy alone. Thirteen patients were successfully treated with needle or catheter aspiration and two required re-aspiration. Two patients failed this therapy and required traditional surgical drainage [49]. Chang and colleagues [50] performed a prospective controlled study of 14 patients with well-defined unilocular abscesses. All of the patients were successfully treated by ultrasound-guided drainage, and eight patients had an indwelling catheter placed. It was concluded that ultrasound-guided percutaneous drainage was an effective treatment for well-defined unilocular abscesses in the head and neck.

Few trials have examined percutaneous methods for space infections from odontogenic sources. Additionally, many infections occupy more than one space or present with an indistinct cellulitic process. In these situations, aggressive surgical drainage is recommended with the employment of generous incisions. Adequate access allows an exploration of all involved spaces with digital palpation and manipulation to breakdown loculations, perform washout of necrotic debris, and place drains, all of which alter the wound environment to one more favorable for cure. Incisions should be placed to allow dependant drainage when possible and to avoid important anatomic structures (ie, facial nerve). Penrose drains are placed to keep the wound open for drainage and to allow for daily bedside irrigation as needed. Thorough digital exploration of these spaces using known anatomic landmarks will reduce the likelihood of missing loculations or involved spaces, thereby reducing the need for reoperation and decreasing hospital stays. Bross-Soriano and colleagues [51] conducted a retrospective review of 113 patients with Ludwig's angina treated with small incisions. Sixty-two patients had extension into the parapharyngeal space, and 32 had retropharyngeal involvement. Forty-six were diabetic, and 34 required tracheotomy. More than half of the patients were hospitalized for 6 or fewer days. In this series, 33 patients had major complications such as mediastinitis, sepsis, or death. Nevertheless, it was concluded that drainage using small incisions was safe and effective in patients with Ludwig's angina.

In necrotizing fasciitis, aggressive surgical debridement is crucial, and any delay in treatment can result in mortality. When the skin is incised, little to no bleeding is observed due to small vessel thrombosis. The underlying fascia is necrotic, and thin turbid "dish water" pus is classically seen. The skin and underlying fascia must be radically and aggressively excised until bleeding skin edges are achieved. In these circumstances, the authors have noted hesitation or avoidance by the inexperienced surgeon to perform such excision, because significant esthetic and functional deformities result from the debridement (Fig. 11A, B). It must be understood that this wide excision of affected tissue is a life-saving procedure, and that any hesitation to treat the disease aggressively will result in further tissue loss and possibly death. When underlying muscle is involved, it must also be excised. The wound is then packed open and irrigated with hydrogen peroxide and saline solution with frequent dressing changes. Daily washouts and wound inspections with further debridement are performed until the extent of the infection declares itself (Fig. 12A, B). Before considering reconstruction, it is usually recommended to wait at least 2 weeks or until a healthy bed of granulation tissue has developed and the patient is systemically stable. If available, hyperbaric oxygen may be helpful in the treatment of necrotizing fasciitis, although its role is controversial in the literature. Jallali and colleagues [52] performed a review of the English literature to review current practice and the evidence for the use of hyperbaric oxygen as adjunctive

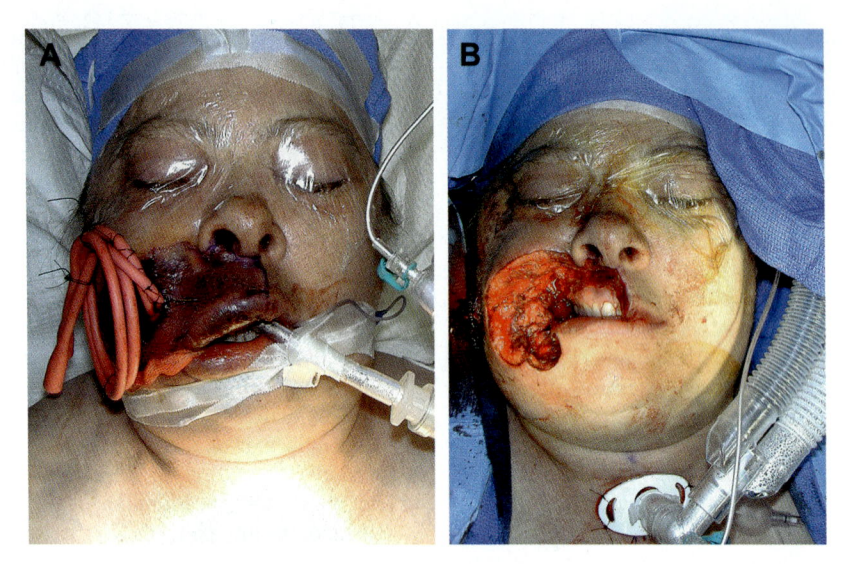

Fig. 11. (A) The patient shown in Fig. 8 with staphylococcal necrotizing fasciitis of the right side of the face. (B) The same patient after first stage drainage and debridement. She was eventually reconstructed with a radial forearm free flap.

therapy in necrotizing fasciitis. They concluded that the results are currently inconsistent, and that more robust evidence by way of prospective randomized trials is necessary before routine use of hyperbaric oxygen for necrotizing fasciitis can be recommended.

Reconstruction is not considered until after the wounds are stabilized with signs of a healthy granulation tissue bed (Fig. 13A, B, C). Furthermore, these patients are often profoundly catabolic as a result of sepsis and poor nutrition and have a diminished immunologic response.

Sequencing reconstructive strategies for patients with necrotizing fasciitis can be a monumental challenge. Extensive tissue loss following aggressive debridement may require composite (eg, skin, muscle, bone) tissue replacement. The challenges of reconstruction for these destructive head and neck infections are similar to those in oncologic head and neck surgery. They include a compromised airway, impaired sensory and motor function, esthetic facial deformity, an inability to control secretions, and impaired speech. The goals of reconstruction are the restoration of

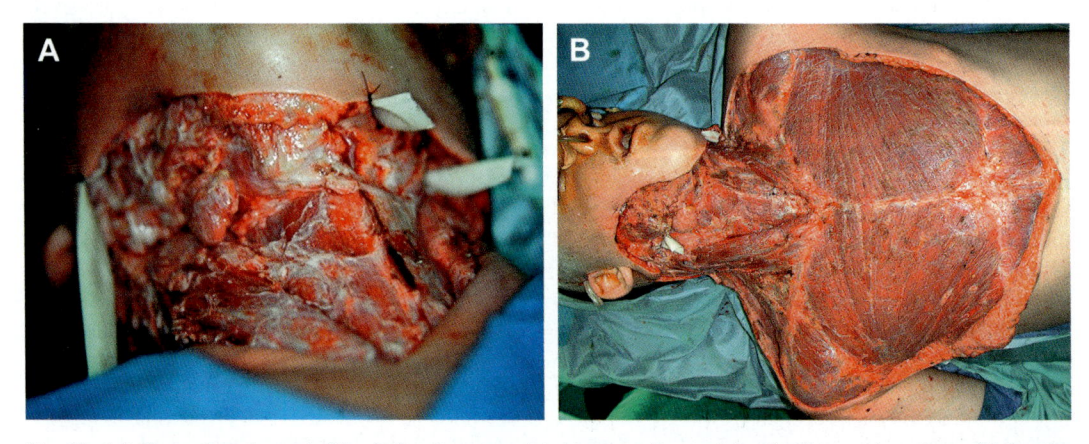

Fig. 12. (A) The patient shown in Fig. 4 after first stage debridement of necrotizing fasciitis resultant from third molar extraction. (B) The same patient at the time of final debridement once the infection had declared itself completely. Rapid spread along the relatively avascular fascial planes took this infection down onto the chest wall. The patient was eventually skin grafted and is alive and well.

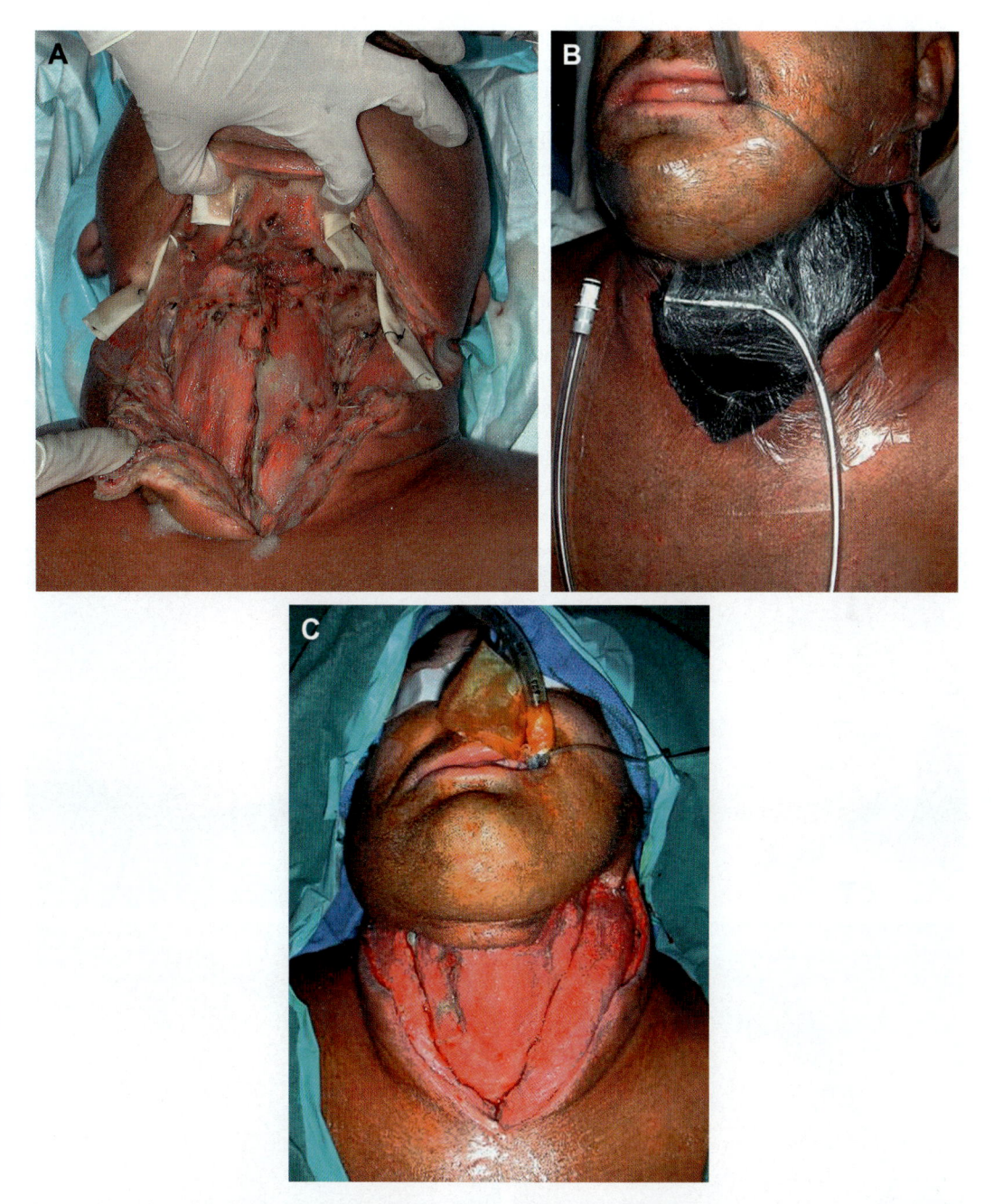

Fig. 13. (*A*) This patient had a necrotizing infection of the neck requiring debridement of skin, muscle, nerve, vascular structures, and the submandibular glands, leaving him with significant deficits and a soft tissue defect. He underwent serial debridements and meticulous wound management. (*B*) The same patient after stabilization of the wound size during a period of management that included frequent dressing changes and a vacuum-assisted closure device to facilitate a clean wound and encourage granulation tissue. (*C*) The same patient before definitive reconstruction. Note the healthy appearance of the wound.

function and form. To achieve these goals, the surgeon must understand the advantages and disadvantages of each rung of the reconstructive ladder. Local flaps have limited use with composite defects due to the limited volume of tissue, the limited versatility with composite defects, the typically modest vascular supply, the inability to transfer bone, and the possible need for a multistage approach (ie, walking tube flaps). Regional flaps are more versatile with defects related to necrotizing fasciitis. Advantages include (Fig. 14A–D) a reliable vascular supply and the presence of adequate soft tissue volume. Disadvantages are the pedicle base, which limits the arch of rotation; the many involved functional muscle units, which make the donor site a concern; and the negligible ability to transfer bone (a multistaged procedure with bone grafts).

The advantage of a free tissue transfer is its ability to simultaneously restore the multidimensional tissue loss in a single operative visit. It is more reliable in hostile environments when compared with local or regional flaps with bone grafting. Additionally, free tissue transfer is more versatile in reconstructing larger continuity defects, although necrotizing infections infrequently involve the resection of bone. When osseous reconstruction is required, there is greater success with placement of endosseous implants and decreased time to complete the oral rehabilitation. One important consideration in the use of free tissue is the recipient site vessels, especially in this environment of infection and inflammation. Frequently, target vessels have been debrided in the process of disease control. Additional imaging may be required to find suitable inflow and outflow for the flap.

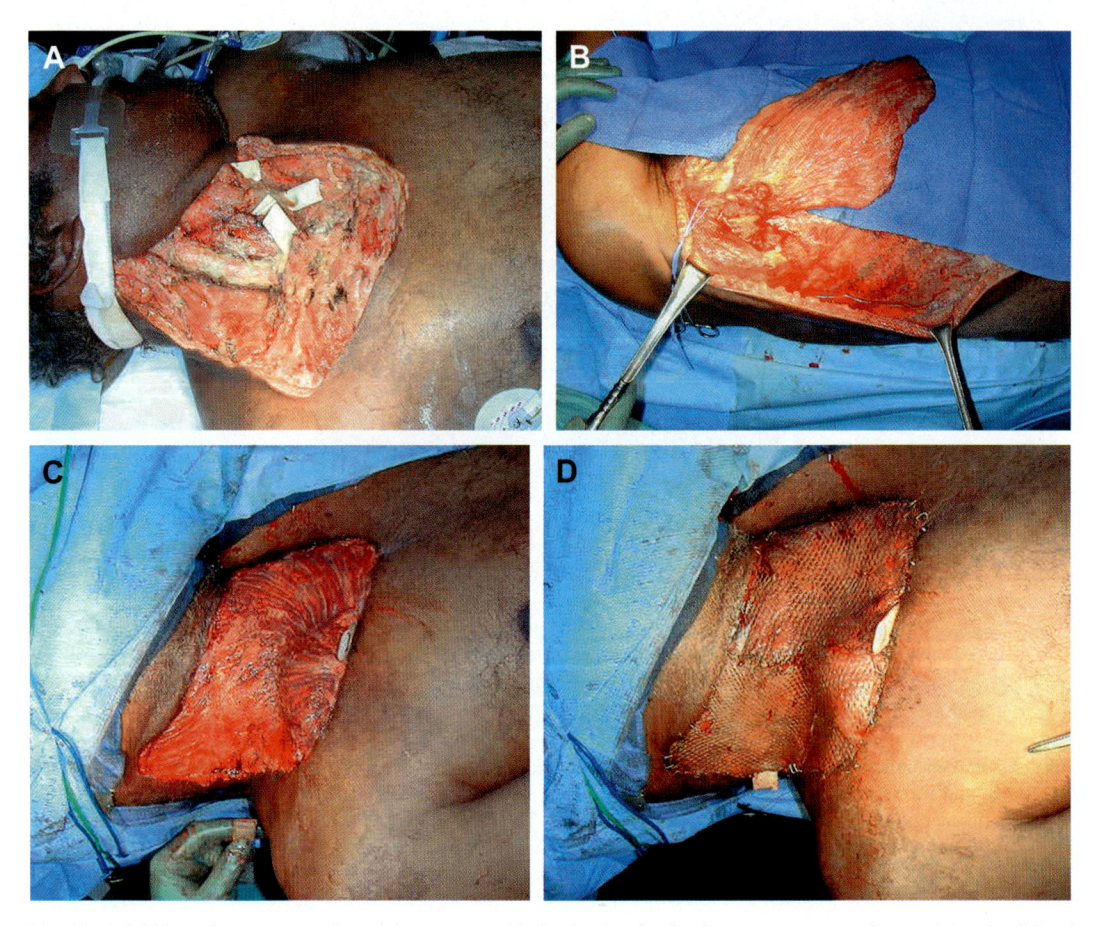

Fig. 14. (*A*) This patient was transferred from an outside institution for further management of necrotizing fasciitis of the right side of the neck. The exposed carotid sheath can clearly be visualized in the wound. The infection had entered the superior mediastinum. (*B*) The wound was reconstructed with a pedicled latissimus dorsi muscle flap. Photograph shows the flap at the time of elevation. (*C*) The flap at inset. (*D*) The flap after split-thickness skin grafting.

A true comprehension of the architectural hard and soft tissue defects facilitates a strategic approach to these difficult reconstructions. The initial sequencing of reconstruction is focused on restoring oral lining, followed by soft tissue coverage of the face and vital structures and then skeletal support. Before implementing any of the reconstructive options available, the patient should be medically stabilized, and all necrotic and infected tissue must be debrided with no signs of progression. Because necrotizing fasciitis can result in massive surface area skin loss beyond the limits of coverage that a single (or multiple) regional or free flaps can provide, the defects are reconstructed analogous to a burn patient with multiple skin grafting procedures, with flaps reserved for large areas of composite tissue loss. A population of patients is unsuitable for free flap surgery due to medical comorbidities; these patients are more suitable for regional flaps. Because each option has its own inherent advantages and disadvantages, the surgeon can employ a combination of each to achieve the best reconstruction possible.

Summary

The management of neck infections can be challenging. Careful attention to the source of infection and airway requirements yields the best medical and surgical results when it comes to treatment. Although there might be a role for carefully observed inpatient medical management in single space infections of non-odontogenic origin and in pediatric neck infections, it is the authors' opinion and that of the literature that neck infections are usually best managed with prompt surgical treatment and supportive medical care. When these methods are employed, complications are rarely encountered.

References

[1] Huang TT, Liu TC, Chen PR, et al. Deep neck infection: analysis of 185 cases. Head Neck 2004;26(10): 854–60.
[2] Har-El G, Aroesty JH, Shaha A, et al. Changing trends in deep neck abscess: a retrospective study of 110 patients. Oral Surg Oral Med Oral Pathol 1994;77(5):446–50.
[3] Parhiscar A, Har-El G. Deep neck abscess: a retrospective review of 210 cases. Ann Otol Rhinol Laryngol 2001;110(11):1051–4.
[4] Sethi DS, Stanley RE. Deep neck abscesses–changing trends. J Laryngol Otol 1994;108(2):138–43.
[5] Lee JK, Kim HD, Lim SC. Predisposing factors of complicated deep neck infection: an analysis of 158 cases. Yonsei Med J 2007;48(1):55–62.
[6] Brook I. Microbiology and management of peritonsillar, retropharyngeal, and parapharyngeal abscesses. J Oral Maxillofac Surg 2004;62(12): 1545–50.
[7] Brook I. Microbiology and management of infected solid tumours. Eur J Cancer Care (Engl) 2007;16(1): 12–6.
[8] Nusbaum AO, Som PM, Rothschild MA, et al. Recurrence of a deep neck infection: a clinical indication of an underlying congenital lesion. Arch Otolaryngol Head Neck Surg 1999;125(12):1379–82.
[9] Ostlie DJ, Burjonrappa SC, Snyder CL, et al. Thyroglossal duct infections and surgical outcomes. J Pediatr Surg 2004;39(3):396–9 [discussion: 396–9].
[10] Park SW, Han MH, Sung MH, et al. Neck infection associated with pyriform sinus fistula: imaging findings. AJNR Am J Neuroradiol 2000;21(5):817–22.
[11] Wang CP, Ko JY, Lou PJ. Deep neck infection as the main initial presentation of primary head and neck cancer. J Laryngol Otol 2006;120(4):305–9.
[12] Schweinfurth JM. Demographics of pediatric head and neck infections in a tertiary care hospital. Laryngoscope 2006;116(6):887–9.
[13] Choi SS, Vezina LG, Grundfast KM. Relative incidence and alternative approaches for surgical drainage of different types of deep neck abscesses in children. Arch Otolaryngol Head Neck Surg 1997;123(12):1271–5.
[14] Coticchia JM, Getnick GS, Yun RD, et al. Age-, site-, and time-specific differences in pediatric deep neck abscesses. Arch Otolaryngol Head Neck Surg 2004;130(2):201–7.
[15] Tan PT, Chang LY, Huang YC, et al. Deep neck infections in children. J Microbiol Immunol Infect 2001;34(4):287–92.
[16] Ungkanont K, Yellon RF, Weissman JL, et al. Head and neck space infections in infants and children. Otolaryngol Head Neck Surg 1995;112(3):375–82.
[17] Marioni G, Castegnaro E, Staffieri C, et al. Deep neck infection in elderly patients: a single institution experience (2000–2004). Aging Clin Exp Res 2006;18(2): 127–32.
[18] Chen MK, Wen YS, Chang CC, et al. Deep neck infections in diabetic patients. Am J Otolaryngol 2000; 21(3):169–73.
[19] Huang TT, Tseng FY, Liu TC, et al. Deep neck infection in diabetic patients: comparison of clinical picture and outcomes with nondiabetic patients. Otolaryngol Head Neck Surg 2005;132(6):943–7.
[20] Brook I. Microbiology and principles of antimicrobial therapy for head and neck infections. Infect Dis Clin North Am 2007;21(2):355–91.
[21] Flynn TR, Shanti RM, Levi MH, et al. Severe odontogenic infections. Part 1. Prospective report. J Oral Maxillofac Surg 2006;64(7):1093–103.

[22] Kuriyama T, Karasawa T, Nakagawa K, et al. Bacteriologic features and antimicrobial susceptibility in isolates from orofacial odontogenic infections. Oral Surg Oral Med Oral Pathol Oral Radiol Endod 2000;90(5):600–8.

[23] Sakamoto H, Kato H, Sato T, et al. Semiquantitative bacteriology of closed odontogenic abscesses. Bull Tokyo Dent Coll 1998;39(2):103–7.

[24] Stefanopoulos PK, Kolokotronis AE. The clinical significance of anaerobic bacteria in acute orofacial odontogenic infections. Oral Surg Oral Med Oral Pathol Oral Radiol Endod 2004;98(4):398–408.

[25] Flynn TR, Shanti RM, Hayes C. Severe odontogenic infections. Part 2. Prospective outcomes study. J Oral Maxillofac Surg 2006;64(7):1104–13.

[26] Wang J, Ahani A, Pogrel MA. A five-year retrospective study of odontogenic maxillofacial infections in a large urban public hospital. Int J Oral Maxillofac Surg 2005;34(6):646–9.

[27] Cabrera CE, Deutsch ES, Eppes S, et al. Increased incidence of head and neck abscesses in children. Otolaryngol Head Neck Surg 2007;136(2):176–81.

[28] Craig FW, Schunk JE. Retropharyngeal abscess in children: clinical presentation, utility of imaging, and current management. Pediatrics 2003;111(6 Pt 1): 1394–8.

[29] Ossowski K, Chun RH, Suskind D, et al. Increased isolation of methicillin-resistant *Staphylococcus aureus* in pediatric head and neck abscesses. Arch Otolaryngol Head Neck Surg 2006;132(11):1176–81.

[30] Jones JL, Candelaria LM. Head and neck infections. In: Fonseca RJ, Williams TP, Stewart JCB, editors. Oral and maxillofacial surgery, vol. 5. Philadelphia: WB Saunders; 2000. p. 77–117.

[31] Brook I, Frazier EH. Clinical and microbiological features of necrotizing fasciitis. J Clin Microbiol 1995;33(9):2382–7.

[32] McGurk M. Diagnosis and treatment of necrotizing fasciitis in the head and neck region. Oral Maxillofac Surg Clin North Am 2003;15(1):59–67.

[33] Nagy M, Backstrom J. Comparison of the sensitivity of lateral neck radiographs and computed tomography scanning in pediatric deep neck infections. Laryngoscope 1999;109(5):775–9.

[34] Haug RH, Wible RT, Lieberman J. Measurement standards for the prevertebral region in the lateral soft-tissue radiograph of the neck. J Oral Maxillofac Surg 1991;49(11):1149–51.

[35] Smith JL II, Hsu JM, Chang J. Predicting deep neck space abscess using computed tomography. Am J Otolaryngol 2006;27(4):244–7.

[36] Lazor JB, Cunningham MJ, Eavey RD, et al. Comparison of computed tomography and surgical findings in deep neck infections. Otolaryngol Head Neck Surg 1994;111(6):746–50.

[37] Miller WD, Furst IM, Sandor GK, et al. A prospective, blinded comparison of clinical examination and computed tomography in deep neck infections. Laryngoscope 1999;109(11):1873–9.

[38] Munoz A, Castillo M, Meichor MA, et al. Acute neck infections: prospective comparison between CT and MRI in 47 patients. J Comput Assist Tomogr 2001;25(5):733–41.

[39] Potter JK, Herford AS, Ellis E III. Tracheotomy versus endotracheal intubation for airway management in deep neck space infections. J Oral Maxillofac Surg 2002;60(4):349–54 [discussion: 354–5].

[40] Marrel J, Blanc C, Frascarolo P, et al. Videolaryngoscopy improves intubation condition in morbidly obese patients. Eur J Anaesthesiol 2007;24(12): 1045–9.

[41] Ovassapian A, Tuncbilek M, Weitzel EK, et al. Airway management in adult patients with deep neck infections: a case series and review of the literature. Anesth Analg 2005;100(2):585–9.

[42] Coletti DP, Caccamese JF, Hartman MJ, et al. The impact of substance abuse on the occurrence and outcome of odontogenic deep space infections. In: Proceedings of the Annual Scientific Meeting, British Association of Oral and Maxillofacial Surgeons. Eastbourne (U.K.): Elsevier; June 28-30, 2006.

[43] Al-Sabah B, Bin Salleen H, Hagr A, et al. Retropharyngeal abscess in children: 10-year study. J Otolaryngol 2004;33(6):352–5.

[44] McClay JE, Murray AD, Booth T. Intravenous antibiotic therapy for deep neck abscesses defined by computed tomography. Arch Otolaryngol Head Neck Surg 2003;129(11):1207–12.

[45] Oh JH, Kim Y, KY, Kim CH. Parapharyngeal abscess: comprehensive management protocol. ORL J Otorhinolaryngol Relat Spec 2007;69(1):37–42.

[46] Sichel JY, Dano I, Hocwald E, et al. Nonsurgical management of parapharyngeal space infections: a prospective study. Laryngoscope 2002;112(5): 906–10.

[47] Herzon FS, Martin AD. Medical and surgical treatment of peritonsillar, retropharyngeal, and parapharyngeal abscesses. Curr Infect Dis Rep 2006;8(3):196–202.

[48] Poe LB, Petro GR, Matta I. Percutaneous CT-guided aspiration of deep neck abscesses. AJNR Am J Neuroradiol 1996;17(7):1359–63.

[49] Yeow KM, Liao CT, Hao SP. US-guided needle aspiration and catheter drainage as an alternative to open surgical drainage for uniloculated neck abscesses. J Vasc Interv Radiol 2001; 12(5):589–94.

[50] Chang KP, Chen YL, Hao SP, et al. Ultrasound-guided closed drainage for abscesses of the head and neck. Otolaryngol Head Neck Surg 2005; 132(1):119–24.

[51] Bross-Soriano D, Arrieta-Gomez JR, Prado-Calleros H, et al. Management of Ludwig's angina with small neck incisions: 18 years experience. Otolaryngol Head Neck Surg 2004;130(6):712–7.

[52] Jallali N, Withey S, Butler PE. Hyperbaric oxygen as adjuvant therapy in the management of necrotizing fasciitis. Am J Surg 2005;189(4):462–6.

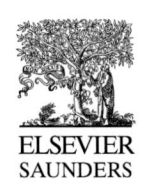

Cervical Spine Injuries

Jeff W. Chen, MD, PhD, FACS

Legacy Emanuel Hospital, Portland, OR, USA

Cervical spine injuries involve both fractures and spinal cord injuries. The fractures may be detected radiographically whereas the detection of spinal cord injuries may require both clinical and radiographic data. Spinal cord injuries may occur in the absence of a fracture if there is a herniated disc, spinal cord contusion, or ligamentous injury. The social impact of a cervical spinal injury is tremendous and carries both emotional and economic implications for the patient and the patient's family. Recognition of a cervical spine injury is important to avoid further neurologic compromise.

Facial or skull fractures are frequently associated with cervical spine fractures or spinal cord injury. The incidence of cervical spine injuries in trauma patients has been reported to range from 0% to 8%. This depends upon the mechanism of injury and the age and gender of the patient [1–4]. In a postmortem study of trauma patients, it has been estimated that approximately 24% of the patients examined had spinal injuries [1]. In a recent study of 3356 patients with craniomaxillofacial fractures, Elahi and colleagues [4] identified 124 cases of cervical spine injury for an incidence of 3.69%. The vast majority of the injuries occurred with motor vehicle accidents. They found that there were two main clusterings for the injuries: the C1 to C2 area and the C6 to C7 area. They also found an increased incidence with decreasing Glasgow Coma Score. This makes sense intuitively because more severe traumatic brain injuries are more likely to be associated with increased forces of injury [4].

This article briefly discusses the anatomy of the cervical spine and the most common types of fractures associated with the cervical spine. Cervical spinal cord syndromes are also reviewed because such syndromes, discovered during the neurologic examination, frequently provide the first clue that there is an underlying spinal cord injury. Because the majority of the associated maxillofacial and spinal injuries occur in the setting of motor vehicle accidents, it is particularly important for the maxillofacial surgeon to be cognizant of the injuries, particularly in the context of the need for facial/cranial surgery. Appropriate measures are necessary to immobilize or fixate the spine before surgery to avoid exacerbating the spinal injury.

Cervical spine anatomy

The occipital condyles

The occipital condyles are paired semilunar points of articulation that project off of the inferior surface of the skull. These lie along the anterior and lateral parts of the foramen magnum. They extend medially. The occipital condyles articulate with the superior concavities of the lateral masses of the atlas. The slope of the condyles matches the slope of the lateral masses of the atlas so that the condyle lies somewhat within the atlas (Fig. 1). This relationship is not as well developed in the pediatric population. This may explain the higher incidence of atlanto-occipital injuries in these patients [5].

Anatomy of the atlas (C1)

The term atlas is derived from Greek mythology after the god whose task it was to bear the heavens on his shoulders. The atlas is a ringlike structure with two lateral masses with smooth articulating surfaces superiorly and inferiorly (see Fig. 1). Above the atlas are the occipital condyles, which are below the superior articulating surfaces of the axis (C2). The anterior arch includes the anterior tubercle in the midline, while the posterior

E-mail address: jchen@lhs.org

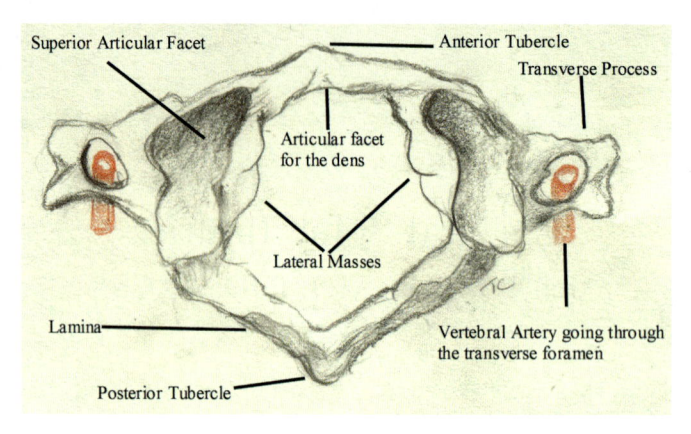

Fig. 1. The atlas (C1) from above. Note the lateral masses and the sites of articulation superiorly with the occipital condyles. The vertebral arteries are depicted in red.

arch includes the posterior tubercle in the midline. The anterior arch is about half the length of the posterior arch. The anterior tubercle is attached to the anterior longitudinal ligament and the longus coli muscles. The posterior tubercle is attached to the ligamentum nuchae. The transverse foramen are lateral to the lateral masses. The vertebral artery passes through the transverse foramen before turning medially and posteriorly to go behind the superior articular process [6]. A series of ligaments attach the atlas to the axis and the skull.

Anatomy of the axis (C2)

The axis has a vertebral body from which the toothlike dens or odontoid extends upward. The anterior articular surface of the dens articulates with the posterior surface of C1 (the articular facet for the dens). A series of ligaments connect the dens with the ring of C1 and the occiput. The lamina join posteriorly in a bifid spinous process. The axis has well-defined pedicles (Fig. 2). The transverse processes extend laterally and have foramen to accommodate the vertebral artery [6]. The C1–C2 junction is composed of the atlantoaxial joints on both sides with their lateral mass biconvex articulations, which have loosely associated joint capsules.

Occiput–C1–C2 relationships

The ligaments between the occiput, C1, and C2 are critical for the maintenance of stability in this region (Fig. 3). The primary motion at the occiput–C1 junction is in the sagittal plane [7]. Anteriorly, flexion is limited when the tip of the dens abuts the anterior margin of the foramen magnum. Posteriorly, the tectorial membrane is a continuation of the posterior longitudinal ligament as it passes from the body of C2 to the anterior rim of the foramen magnum. This limits extension. The alar ligaments extend from the tip of the dens to the medial aspects of the occipital condyles. These ligaments are primarily responsible for restraining lateral and rotational motion at the occiput–C1 junction [8].

The transverse ligament lies posterior to the dens and goes between the lateral masses of C1. This restrains the dens and prevents anterior translation. The apical ligament goes between the tip of the dens and the basion (anterior rim of the foramen magnum). This further restricts anterior translation. The anterior atlantodental ligament is a small ligament between the anterior part of the dens and posterior aspect of the anterior tubercle of C1. A great deal of rotation occurs at the atlantoaxial joint. Studies have demonstrated normal values of unilateral rotation that range from 34° to 47° [9,10].

Anatomy of the subaxial spine (C3–C7)

The lower cervical vertebrae have vertebral bodies that increase in size from a cranial to caudal direction. They are broader in the transverse dimension compared with the anteroposterior direction. Each intervertebral disc has an external annulus fibrosus that surrounds the nucleus pulposus. These discs act as cushions between the vertebral bodies and give the spine the ability to flex and extend. The vertebral bodies are joined anteriorly by the anterior longitudinal ligament, and posteriorly by the posterior longitudinal ligament.

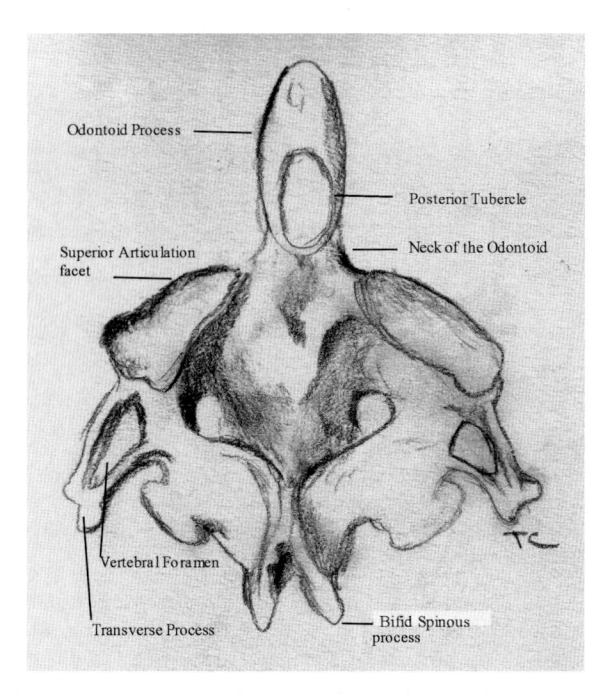

Fig. 2. The axis (C2) in an anterior-posterior view. Note the odontoid process and foramen for the vertebral arteries.

The pedicles extend posterolaterally from the vertebral body joining with the lamina that join posteriorly in the midline (Fig. 4). The processes of the articular pillars project laterally from the junction of the pedicles and lamina and support the superior and inferior articular facets. The transverse processes project laterally off of the vertebral bodies and house the transverse foramen, through which the vertebral artery passes.

Vascular anatomy

The paired vertebral arteries are the main vessels associated with the cervical spine. Typically the vertebral arteries arise off of the left and right subclavian arteries. They enter the transverse foramina between C6 and C7 and travel in a cephalad direction through the transverse foramen of C6 up to the transverse foramen of C1, where they exit and pass posteriorly behind the articular process of C1 (Fig. 5). The vertebral arteries join intracranially at the level of the pons to form the basilar artery. Before this junction, branches descend from the vertebral arteries and join, forming the anterior spinal artery, which courses along the length of the anterior spinal cord. There are contributions throughout its course from 6 to 10 anterior radicular arteries that arise from the vertebral arteries or the intercostals arteries [6].

Spinal cord

The spinal cord lies within the spinal or vertebral canal and extends from the foramen magnum down to the conus (approximately T12–L1). There is variability in the width of the spinal cord that corresponds to areas of increased innervation. The spinal cord demonstrates enlargement between C2 and C6 with a maximal transverse diameter of 13 to 14 mm [6]. The spinal nerve roots exit the neural foramina laterally. The cross-sectional anatomy of the spinal cord demonstrates topographic organization of the fiber tracts. The location of the fracture or compression relative to the different fiber tracts explains many of the clinical spinal cord injury syndromes.

Cervical spine fractures and dislocations

Occiput–C1 articulation

The occipital–cervical articulation is highly mobile. The stability in this region is largely provided by the series of ligaments discussed earlier. The occipital condyles are well visualized by CT scanning at the base of the skull and are classified according to CT scan findings. A type I fracture is a comminuted fracture of the occipital condyle or condyles that occurs as a result of a direct impact to the top of the head (axial loading). Thus, the

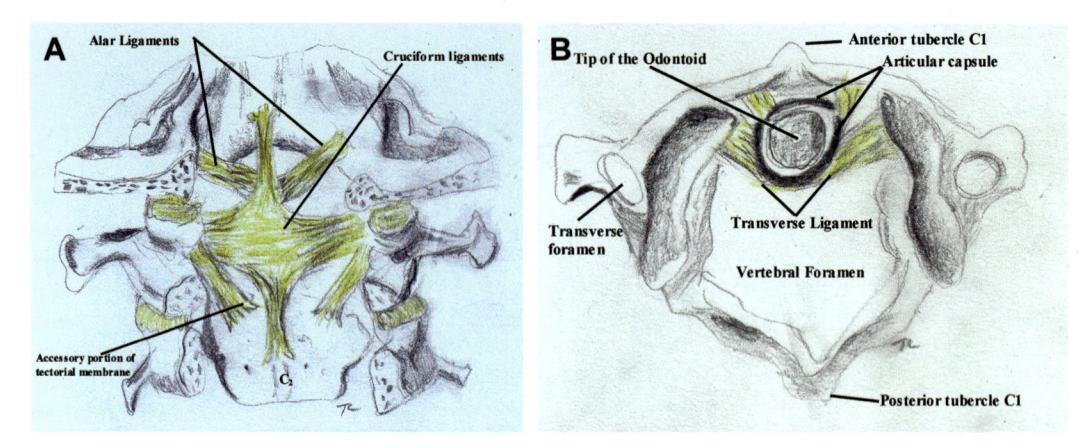

Fig. 3. Occipital–C1–C2 junction. The key ligaments holding this region together include the alar, the apical, and the transverse ligaments. (*A*) Posterior view with the removal of posterior elements and spinal cord. This demonstrates the alar and cruciform ligaments holding the odontoid process posteriorly. (*B*) Cross-sectional view from above showing the Odontoid being held forward by the transverse ligament.

occipital condyles impact upon the lateral masses of C1. A type II fracture involves a fracture of the occipital condyle with extension upwards to include the skull base. A type III fracture involves medial displacement of the bone fragments off of the occipital condyle. There is disruption of the attachment sites of the alar ligaments. These are frequently bilateral and occur in 30% to 50% of atlanto-occipital dislocations [11,12].

Type I and II fractures tend to be stable fractures and may be treated with cervical braces for 6 weeks. Type III fractures with minimal displacement are usually treated with a halo vest. Type III fractures that demonstrate instability are treated with posterior cervical fusion between the occiput, C1, and C2.

Traditionally, occipitalcervical dislocation injuries were fatal with few survivors. Forensic studies have demonstrated an up to 10% incidence of occipitalcervical dislocation injuries in fatal motor vehicle accidents [1,13]. Improved resuscitation techniques and triaging have resulted in more survivors with this dislocation. Many of these patients have a significant traumatic brain injury,

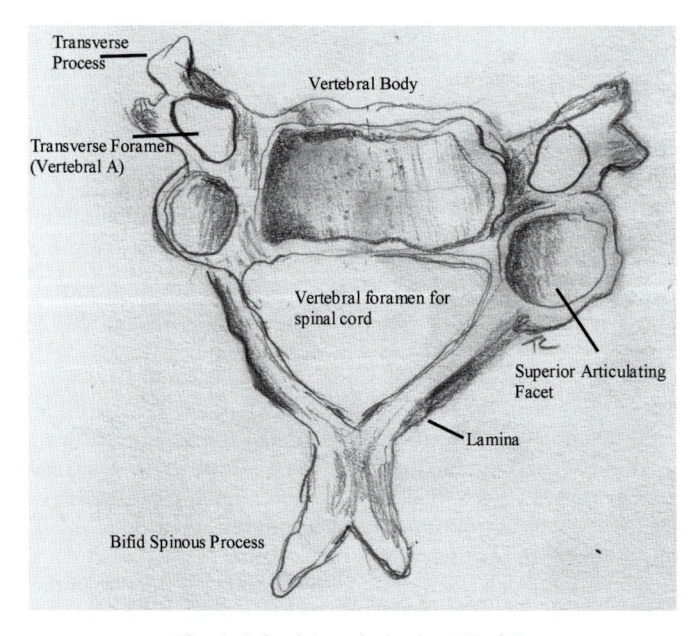

Fig. 4. Subaxial cervical spine (C3–C7).

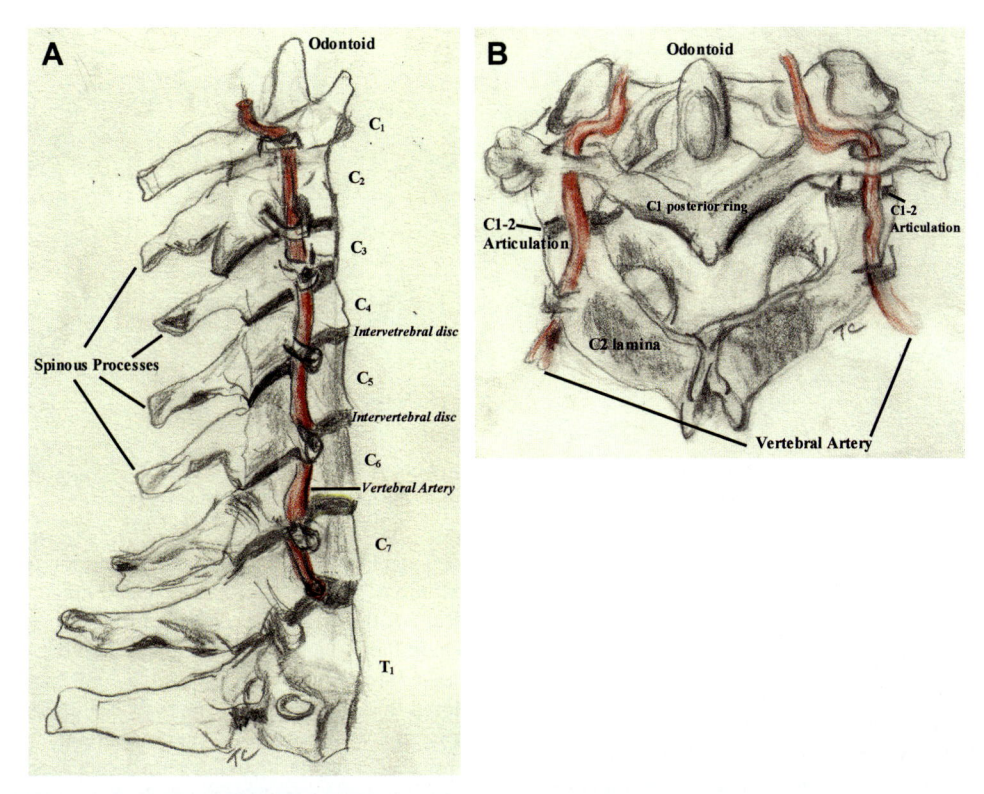

Fig. 5. Key arteries (*red*) of the cervical spine. The cervical spine's relationship with the course of the paired vertebral arteries is delineated. The vertebral arteries traverse the vertebral foramen before going medially at the level of C1. (*A*) Lateral view of the cervical spine. (*B*) Posterior view from above focusing on the C1-2 junction.

and this dislocation may not be recognized initially. Some of the clinical findings include brainstem injury with cardiopulmonary arrest; cranial nerve findings (VI, XI, and XII most frequently); Brown-Sequard syndrome, or central cord syndrome, or both; and subarachnoid hemorrhage. These occipitalcervical dislocations are highly unstable. The goal is to stabilize the spine to prevent further injury to the underlying neural tissue. These dislocations are treated with an occipital–C1–C2 fusion using posterior rods and screws [5,12,13].

Atlas fractures

Fractures of the atlas make up about 10% of all acute cervical spine injuries [11]. The most common type of C1 fracture involves the posterior arch bilaterally at the junction of the posterior arch and the lateral masses. The mechanism of this injury is hyperextension of the cervical spine, which leads to compression of the posterior arch of C1 between the occiput and the spinous process of C2. The second most common atlas fracture is the Jefferson fracture. This typically occurs by axial loading and is a burst fracture that results in three to four fractures that involve both the posterior and anterior arches of C1 (Fig. 6). For this fracture to occur, the axial load needs to be distributed fairly evenly [12]. The third type of C1 fracture is that which usually involves one lateral mass. This occurs if the head is deviated from the true saggital plane at the time of impact [11]. These fractures are described in isolation, but are frequently associated with fractures of the second cervical vertebra.

These atlas fractures are generally treated nonoperatively. This depends largely upon the amount of lateral displacement of the lateral masses. For those with a larger amount of displacement, thus suggesting more disruption of the ligaments, a halo brace with traction is used for 6 to 12 weeks. For the patient with isolated posterior arch fractures or Jefferson fractures with less than 2 mm of lateral displacement of the lateral masses, treatment is with a rigid orthotic brace for 10 to 12 weeks [11,12].

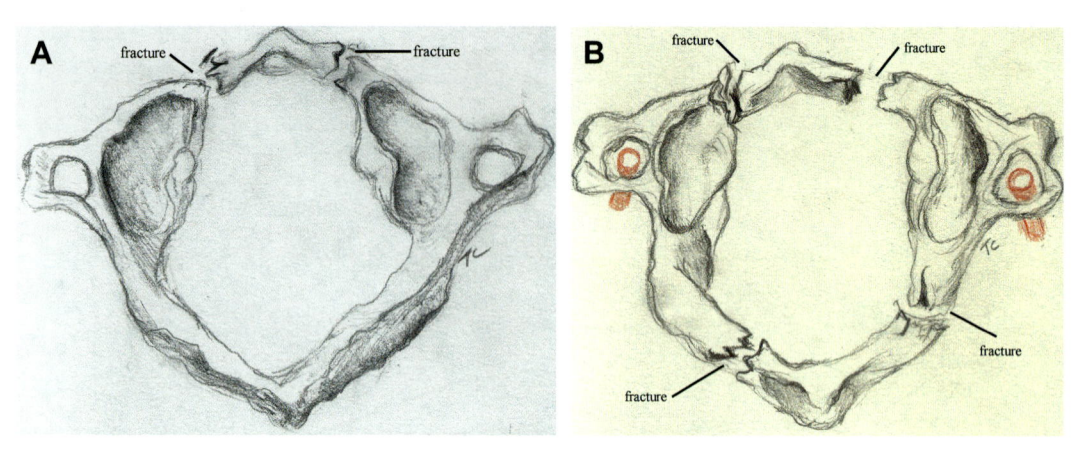

Fig. 6. C1 fractures. (*A*) Anterior ring fractures that may occur with axial loading with flexion. (*B*) Typical fracture pattern seen with the Jefferson fracture, where there are fractures in the anterior and posterior rings.

Axis fractures

Odontoid fractures

The prevalence of dens fractures in patients with cervical spine injuries that survive the initial injury ranges from 10% to 15% [14–16]. The classification scheme of Anderson and D'Alonzo [17] is the most widely adopted for odontoid fractures (Fig. 7). Type I fractures involve an oblique fracture off of the tip of the dens. These are rare fractures and are usually treated nonoperatively using a rigid brace.

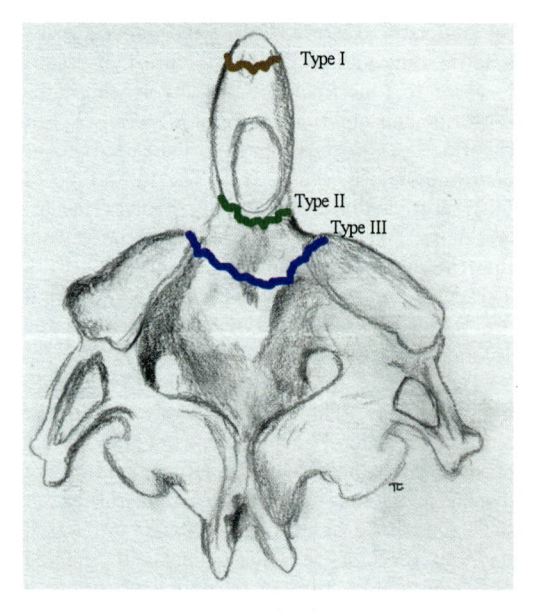

Fig. 7. Typical locations of the type I, II, and III odontoid fractures in the anterior-posterior view, according to the classification scheme of Anderson and D'Alonzo.

Type II fractures are the most common type of odontoid fracture and occur at the junction (or neck) of the odontoid process and vertebral body. These have the highest rates of nonunion, which range from 5% to 63% [18]. It has long been proposed that the reason for the poor healing rates at this site was because of poor vascular supply. However, further studies have demonstrated a rich vascular supply to the neck of the odontoid. It is currently believed that the poor rate of union is the result of the inability of the ligaments to stabilize this region when a break exists [18,19]. Therefore, it is not surprising that several different methods for stabilizing this fracture have evolved over the years.

Odontoid fractures as a proportion of all cervical fractures occur more frequently in the pediatric population than in the adult population. However, given that pediatric injuries are less common than adult injuries, this overall number is relatively low [18]. The adult population may be divided into those less than and those greater than 65 years of age. Odontoid fractures in those less than 65 years usually occur as a result of significant force, such as in a motor vehicle crash. In those over 65, ground level falls account for the majority of these fractures [20,21]. We have found that the elderly patients frequently have osteoporosis, which leads to a weakened neck of the odontoid.

Clinically, many of the younger patients are unconscious from concomitant traumatic brain injury and are unable to be examined. Elderly patients typically have severe pain at the base of the skull with increased pain upon movement. We have found that, in many of these patients, the odontoid fracture may not be recognized initially because the patient may not seek help right away. CT scanning through this region with coronal and saggital reconstructions provides the best means to visualize these fractures. Plain films with lateral and open-mouth odontoid views have been the traditional way to view this area. However, it is frequently difficult to visualize this region because of the osteopenia of the odontoid or obscuration by the surrounding teeth.

There are a several ways to treat these fractures. As mentioned above, the type II odontoid fractures have a poor rate of union without some type of immobilization. External immobilization using a halo apparatus has been used for many years. Nonunion rates in adults have been reported to range from 6% to 64% [22]. The alignment of the fracture is a key factor in the rate of fusion with an 88% nonunion rate reported if there is more than 4 mm of odontoid displacement. Similarly, age over 40 has been associated with a nonunion rate of 67% [18,22].

Although the halo has the advantage of a nonoperative approach, it does impede mobility and respiratory function. It is best suited for young, mobile patients. Elderly patients do not fare as well with halo immobilization [20,23]. Facial lacerations and facial fractures may also make it difficult to fixate the halo ring to the head. Typically, patients are treated in a halo for approximately 12 weeks. If there is still nonunion at 4 months, most advocate an operative stabilization.

Posterior cervical fusion of C1–C2 using a Gallie-type wiring technique has achieved excellent results with fusion rates in excess of 90%. Wires are placed in a sublaminar fashion between

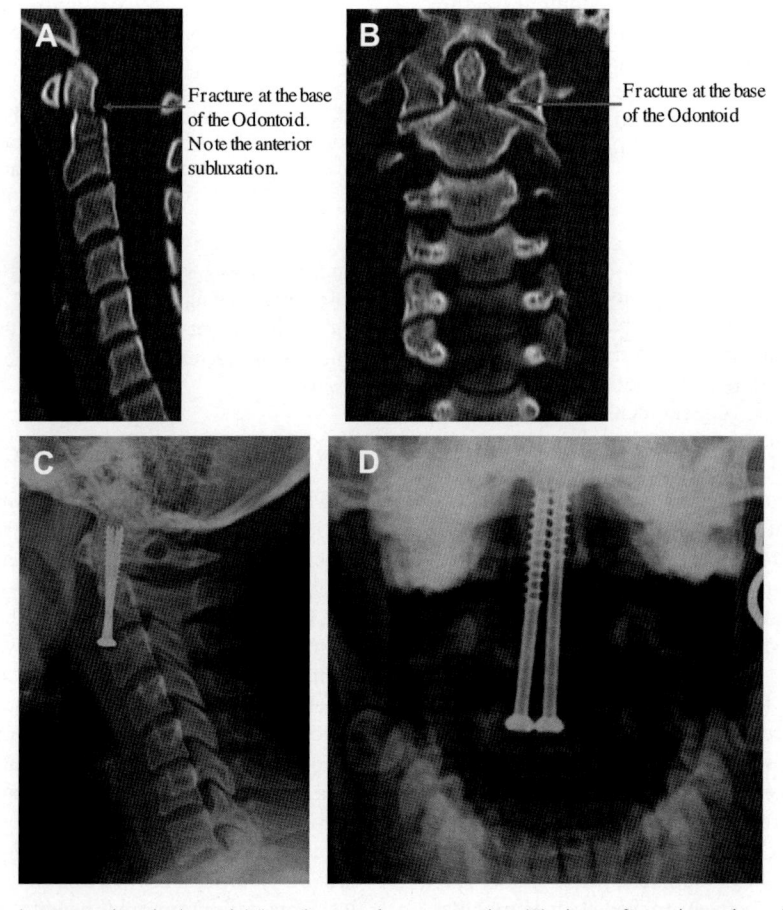

Fig. 8. CT scan demonstrating the lateral (*A*) and coronal reconstruction (*B*) views of a patient who suffered an odontoid fracture. This patient is an 18-year-old female who was in a high-speed rollover motor vehicle accident. She was neurologically intact with severe neck pain. Postoperative plain lateral (*C*) and open-mouth odontoid views (*D*) demonstrating the placement of two odontoid screws.

C1 and C2 with interposed bone graft [5,18]. There are variations on this procedure, depending on the location of the wires and the bone. Recently, advances in the use of polyaxial pedicle screws have allowed fixation using a rod and screw construct [24]. While posterior fusion procedures provide a firm fixation and a high rate of union, they also result in the loss of mobility at the C1–C2 junction [18].

Anterior odontoid screw fixation achieves a high rate of union and preserves the mobility of the patient at the C1–C2 level. One or two screws are placed along the axis of the odontoid, across the fracture line, and to the tip of the odontoid. This allows "lagging" of the fracture pieces together [25]. This technique is very dependent upon an ability to align the fracture and trajectory of the screw in the operating theater. We typically use orthogonally placed C-arm fluoroscopy to achieve fixation of the odontoid fracture.

Type III odontoid fractures extend into the base (vertebral body) of C2 (see Fig. 7; Fig. 8). These fractures typically have a large cancellous surface area that allows good approximation of the fragments. These have a high fusion rate using rigid bracing [18].

Traumatic spondylolisthesis of C2

These fractures involve bilateral pedicles of the axis (Fig. 9) and have been given various names, including hangman's fracture, fractures of the neural arch, fractures of the ring of the axis, and traumatic spondylolisthesis of the axis [26]. This fracture received a great deal of attention and notoriety in the last century as anatomic studies were done on criminals who died from judicial hanging. The submental placement of the knot was important in achieving the hyperextension that resulted in the posterior arch of C2 snapping off and adhering to C3 while the ends and anterior arch of C1 remained fixed to the skull. This led to instantaneous severing of the spinal cord [26,27].

In current times, these types of fractures are usually the result of motor vehicle accidents (Fig. 10). These fractures are subcategorized according to the amount of displacement of the body of C2 relative to C3. Generally, patients with traumatic spondylolisthesis of C2 have no neurologic findings but have neck pain. These fractures are effectively treated with immobilization in a halo brace for approximately 12 weeks. Surgically, these may be addressed with disc excision at C2–C3 with placement of a bone graft and anterior plating system. These may also be fused posteriorly using pedicle screws into the C2 body. This surgery is difficult because of the proximity of the vertebral arteries to the course of the screws.

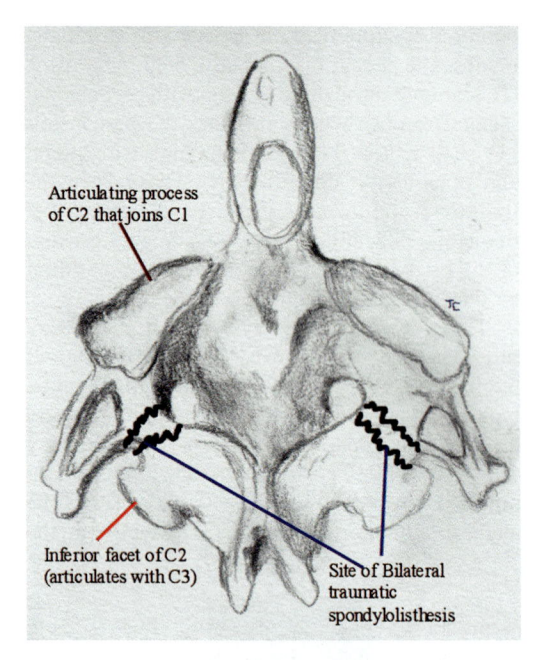

Fig. 9. Traumatic spondylolisthesis of C2 (hangman's fracture). The fracture occurs bilaterally along the pars articularis of C2 as indicated. A "disconnect" occurs between the junction of C2 and C3 and the articulation of C1 and C2. C2 may thus slip forward relative to C3.

Injuries of the subaxial spine (C3–C7)

The lower cervical spine from C3 to C7 accounts for most of the flexion and extension of the neck. The anterior and posterior longitudinal ligaments span the length of the cervical spine. The fact joint capsules, as well as the interspinous ligaments, give additional stability at each segment. The stability of the lower cervical spine depends on the integrity of the ligamentous structures. The forces of injury may lead to abnormal movement from ligamentous damage. This may occur in the absence of a fracture.

Subaxial spine injuries may be broadly categorized according to the mechanism of injury. Flexion injuries may occur in motor vehicle accidents, falls from great heights, and dives into shallow water. Evaluation includes plain radiographs, cervical CT scans and MRI scans. The "teardrop" fracture is an example of a flexion

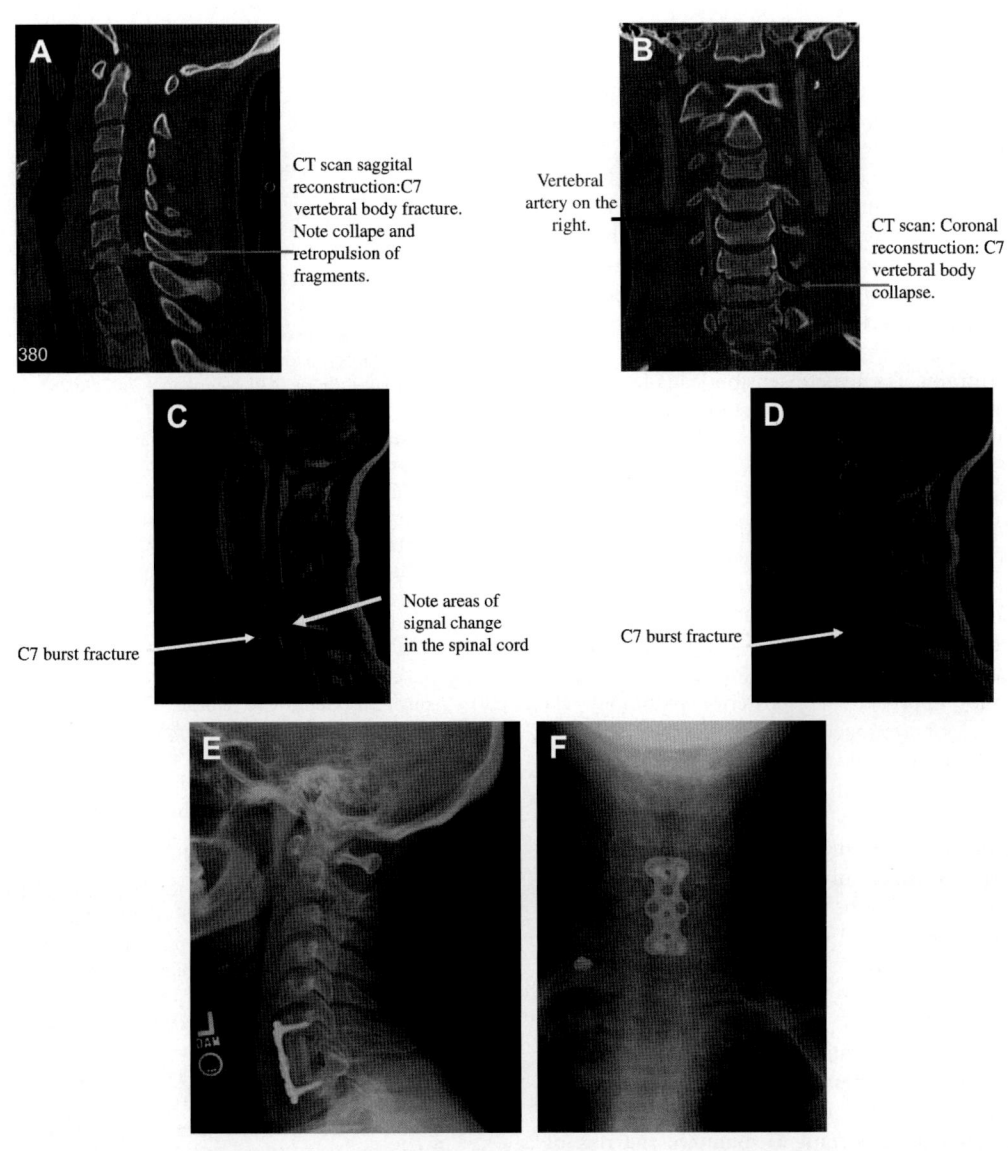

Fig. 10. CT scans demonstrating a C7 burst fracture and subluxation in a 23-year-old female involved in a motor vehicle accident. (*A*) Lateral reconstruction view. Note collapse and retropulsion of fragments (*arrow*). (*B*) Coronal reconstruction view. Black arrow indicates vertebral artery on the right. Blue arrow shows C7 vertebral body collapse. (*C*) MRI demonstrating signal change in the spinal cord. Left arrow indicates C7 burst fracture. Right arrow notes areas of signal change in the spinal cord. (*D*) T1 MRI demonstrating the fracture (*arrow*). (*E, F*) Stabilization after corpectomy is achieved with an anterior plating system.

injury and is characterized by complete ligamentous and disc disruption at the level of the injury with disruption of the facet joints posteriorly. The characteristic large triangular anterior bone fragment is the result of the superior vertebra being severely flexed on the inferior vertebra [28,29].

Axial loading injuries may lead to burst fractures of the cervical vertebrae. In combination with flexion forces, this may result in posterior disruption of the posterior elements and joints. This is a very unstable condition and is frequently associated with neurologic deficits [25].

Extension injuries may result in disruption of the anterior longitudinal ligament and disruption of the lamina and spinous processes. Fractures of the facets may also occur leading to potential instability. Hyperextension injuries frequently occur without fractures. However, such injuries often result in a central cord syndrome with profound neurologic deficits. Central cord syndrome is characterized by weakness that is greater distally than proximally. Patients frequently have weakness and numbness in the hands and fingers. The upper extremities are affected more than the lower extremities. This is believed to occur because of the topographic distribution of the nerve tracts in the cervical spine such that the representation of the hands and fingers is placed medially or centrally. The hyperextension leads to anterior compression of the blood vessels that supply the central spinal cord [30].

Subaxial spine fractures are treated with immobilization. Malalignment, for example, with jumped or locked facets is treated initially with cervical traction to restore the normal configuration to the spinal cord. Stabilization may be achieved by anterior or posterior fusions. This depends on the location of the disruption. As a general rule, anterior pathology is treated via an anterior approach and posterior pathology via a posterior approach. The development of new instrumentation and fusion techniques has greatly facilitated our ability to achieve solid constructs (see Fig. 10). Early stabilization allows for the aggressive treatment of injuries to other organ systems. Furthermore, this allows for early mobilization and thus decreased morbidity from pulmonary issues.

Summary

Cervical spine injuries occur frequently with traumatic brain injury and facial fractures. Care to immobilize the cervical spine in the early evaluation is important to minimize the risk of additional neurologic injury. Frequently, these patients are comatose and are not able to undergo neurologic examination. Thus, their neurologic status may be unknown. Comatose patients should be treated as though the cervical spine is unstable until proven otherwise. Even radiographic examinations with radiographs and CT scans may miss a ligamentous injury. The upper cervical spine and the lower cervical spine each have unique and different potential fracture patterns. Different techniques of arthodesis and instrumentation have been developed and tailored for each of these regions. These have greatly aided our ability to stabilize these fractures and provide for early mobilization.

Acknowledgment

All original art courtesy of Therese L. Chen, Portland, Oregon.

References

[1] Bucholz RW, Burkhead WZ, Graham W, et al. Occult cervical spine injury in fatal traffic accidents. J Trauma 1979;19:768–71.

[2] Holly LT, Kelly DF, Counelis GJ, et al. Cervical spine trauma associated with moderate and severe head injury: incidence, risk factors, and injury characteristics (Spine 3). J Neurosurg 2002;96:285–91.

[3] Luce EA, Tubb TD, Moore AM. Review of 1,000 major facial fractures and associated injuries. Plast Reconstr Surg 1979;63(1):26–30.

[4] Elahi MM, Brar MS, Ahmed N, et al. Cervical spine injury in association with cranial maxillofacial fractures. Plast Reconstr Surg 2008;121(1):201–8.

[5] Anderson PA. Injuries to the occipital cervical articulation. In: Clark CR, editor. The cervical spine. 3rd edition. Philadelphia: Lippincott-Raven; 1998. p. 387–99.

[6] Heller JG, Pedlow FX. Anatomy of the cervical spine. In: Clark CR, editor. The cervical spine. 3rd edition. Philadelphia: Lippincott-Raven; 1998. p. 3–36.

[7] Alund M, Larsson S. Three-dimensional analysis of neck motion: a clinical method. Spine 1990;15:87–91.

[8] Dvorak J, Panjabi MM. Functional anatomy of the alar ligaments. Spine 1987;12:183–9.

[9] Dvorak J, Hayek J, Zehinder R. CT-functional diagnostics of the rotatory instability of the upper cervical spine. Part two. Evaluation on healthy adults and patients with suspected instability. Spine 1987;12(8):726–31.

[10] Dvorak J, Panjabi MM, Gerber M, et al. CT-functional diagnostics of the rotatory instability of the upper cervical spine; an experimental study in cadavers. Spine 1987;12(3):197–205.

[11] Levine A, Edwards C. Treatment of injuries in the C1-C2 complex. Orthop Clin North Am 1986;17:31–44.

[12] Kurz LT. Fractures of the first cervical vertebra. In: Clark CR, editor. The cervical spine. 3rd edition. Philadelphia: Lippincott-Raven; 1998. p. 409–13.

[13] Davis D, Bohlman H, Walder AE, et al. The pathological findings in fatal craniospinal injuries. J Neurosurg 1971;34:603–13.

[14] Sherk HH. Fractures of the atlas and odontoid process. Orthop Clin North Am 1978;9:973–83.

[15] Wang GJ, Mabie KN, Whitehill R, et al. The nonsurgical management of odontoid fractures in adults. Spine 1984;9:229–30.

[16] Lipson SJ. Fractures of the atlas associated with fractures of the odontoid process and transverse ligament ruptures. J Bone Joint Surg Am 1977;59:940–3.

[17] Anderson LD, D'Alonzo RT. Fractures of the odontoid process of the axis. J Bone Joint Surg Am 1974; 56:1663–74.

[18] Ballard WT, Clark CR. Fractures of the dens. In: Clark CR, editor. The cervical spine. 3rd edition. Philadelphia: Lippincott-Raven; 1998. p. 409–13.

[19] Schatzker J, Rorabeck CH, Waddell JP. Fractures of the dens (odontoid process): an analysis of thirty-seven cases. J Bone Joint Surg Br 1971;53:392–404.

[20] Majercik S, Tashjian RZ, Biffl WL, et al. Halo vest immobilization in the elderly: a death sentence? J Trauma 2005;59:350–7.

[21] Sokolowski MJ, Jackson AP, Haak MH, et al. Acute outcomes of cervical spine injuries in the elderly: atlantaxial vs subaxial injuries. J Spinal Cord Med 2007;30:238–42.

[22] Apuzzo MLJ, Heiden JS, Weiss MH, et al. Acute fractures of the odontoid process. J Neurosurg 1978;48:85–91.

[23] Jackson AP, Haak MH, Khan N, et al. Cervical spine injuries in the elderly: acute postoperative mortality. Spine 2005;30:1524–7.

[24] Harms J, Melcher RP. Posterior C1-C2 fusion with polyaxial screw and rod fixation. Spine 2001;26: 2461–71.

[25] Aebi M, Benzel EC. Cervical spine burst fractures. In: Clark CR, editor. The cervical spine. 3rd edition. Philadelphia: Lippincott-Raven; 1998. p. 465–73.

[26] Levine AM. Traumatic spondylolisthesis of the axis. In: Clark CR, editor. The cervical spine. 3rd edition. Philadelphia: Lippincott-Raven; 1998. p. 429–48.

[27] Wood-Jones F. The ideal lesion produced by judicial hanging. Lancet January 4, 1913;53.

[28] Schneider RC, Kahn EA. Chronic neurological sequelae of acute trauma to the spine and spinal cord. Part I: the significance of the acute flexion or "teardrop" fracture-dislocation of the cervical spine. J Bone Joint Surg Am 1956;38:985–97.

[29] Harris JH, Edeiken-Monroe B, Kopaniky DR. A practical classification of acute cervical spine injuries. Orthop Clin North Am 1986;17:15–30.

[30] Schneider RC, Thompson JM, Rebin J. The syndrome of acute central cervical spinal cord injury. J Neurol Neurosurg Psychiatry 1958;21:216–27.

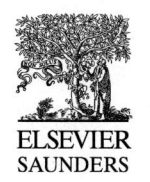

Penetrating Neck Injuries

Shahrokh C. Bagheri, DMD, MD[a,b,c], H. Ali Khan, DMD, MD[c], R. Bryan Bell, DDS, MD, FACS[d,e,f,]*

[a]Oral and Maxillofacial Surgery, Northside Hospital, Atlanta, GA, USA
[b]Division of Oral and Maxillofacial Surgery, Emory University School of Medicine, Atlanta, GA, USA
[c]Atlanta Oral and Facial Surgery, Atlanta, GA, USA
[d]Oral and Maxillofacial Surgery Service, Legacy Emanuel Hospital and Health Center, Portland, OR, USA
[e]Oregon Health & Science University, Portland, OR, USA
[f]Head & Neck Surgical Associates, Portland, OR, USA

The modern approach to patients presenting with penetrating injuries to the neck requires the cautious integration of clinical findings and appropriate imaging studies for formulation of an effective, safe, and minimally invasive modality of treatment. The optimal management of these injuries has undergone considerable debate regarding surgical versus nonsurgical treatment approaches. More recent advances in imaging technology continue to evolve, providing more accurate and timely information for the management of these patients. In this article the authors review both historic and recent articles that have formulated the current management of penetrating injuries to the neck.

The formidable anatomy of the neck demands carefully designed treatment planning when afflicted with penetrating injuries. Seven major body systems are confined within this relatively concentrated region of the body: (1) the vascular system, compromising the common, internal, and external carotid arteries, the highly variable jugular venous system, and the vertebral vessels; (2) the gastrointestinal system, including the oropharynx and esophagus; (3) the respiratory system, including the laryngo-tracheal structures; (4) the endocrine system, including the thyroid and parathyroid glands; (5) the lymphatic system; (6) skeletal structures, including the vertebral column, mandible, and hyoid bone; and (7) the nervous system, which includes several cranial nerves and the spinal cord.

It is clear that patients who present hemodynamically unstable, with severe hemorrhage, or with an expanding hematoma should undergo immediate surgical exploration. In patients who have no hard signs of vascular injury, however, it can be difficult to predict the presence of occult injury based on clinical examination alone. Surgical exploration of all penetrating neck injuries, although feasible, will result in a significant number of unnecessary operations. Monson and colleagues [1] attempted to reduce the number of negative neck explorations by describing three zones of injury, based upon their anatomic location and accessibility to surgical intervention. Traditionally, zone I and zone III injuries were managed selectively because of the difficulties associated with surgical access, and zone II injuries were routinely explored. This resulted in overtreatment of a significant number of zone II injuries (negative neck explorations) and undertreatment of zone I and III injuries (missed injuries). Today, there has been a shift toward selective intervention for injuries involving all three zones when "hard signs" of vascular injury are absent, and this has somewhat diminished the importance of the three zones of the neck. The current indications for immediate surgical intervention include an expanding hematoma, exsanguinating hemorrhage, shock, airway compromise, and massive subcutaneous emphysema [2]. Injury from a single projectile, regardless of velocity, may result in life-threatening penetration of the trachea or larynx, the esophagus, major blood vessels, or cervical nerve roots, cranial

* Corresponding author.
 E-mail address: bellb@hnsa1.com (R.B. Bell)

nerves, or the spinal cord. Surgeons managing these injuries must be familiar with the complex anatomic structures of the head, neck, and maxillofacial region to provide safe, rapid, and predictable therapy.

Historical perspective

Historic articles make reference to complications related to penetrating neck injuries over 5000 years ago [3]. According to Homer's *Iliad* (Chapter XXII, Verses 322–329), Hector, while fighting his last duel, was almost entirely protected by bronze armor except for a small area "where the clavicle marks the boundary between the neck and the thorax." The area above the suprasternal notch was described by Homer as "the shorter way to death," and it is in this area that Achilles delivered a fatal blow by thrusting his lance into Hector's neck (Fig. 1). Long after the collapse of the ancient civilizations of Greece, literary reports of wounds of the neck continue to be derived from surgery of warfare. The first documented case of the treatment of a cervical vascular injury is attributed to the great French surgeon Ambrose Pare (1510–1590), who ligated the carotid artery and jugular vein of a soldier who had a bayonet wound [4]. The patient survived but developed profound aphasia and left-sided hemiplegia. The first reported uncomplicated surgical procedure was done by Fleming [5] in 1803, in which he ligated the lacerated common carotid artery of a sailor. Several years later, in 1811, Abernathy reported a patient who was gored by a bull and was managed in similar fashion by ligation of the lacerated left common and internal carotid arteries. The patient developed a profound hemiplegia and subsequently died [6]. Since Abernathy, the outcome of patients who have penetrating neck injuries has made modest improvement, based upon the concomitant refinement of the instruments of warfare and the instruments of healing.

Experience during wartime has significantly contributed to the evolution of the current management protocols. During the period from the American Civil War to World War I, the reported mortality from penetrating neck injuries raged from 11% to 18% [7,8]. In this time period, the majority of the injuries where treated by expectant or nonsurgical management. In 1944, Bailey [9] proposed early exploration of all cervical hematomas on the basis of his wartime experience. By the end of World War II, an unacceptably high rate of initially unrecognized neurovascular injuries resulting from expectant treatment prompted most military surgeons to explore any injury that penetrated the platysma [9–19]. This practice was further popularized in the civilian sector by Fogelman and Stewart [15] in 1956, who reported a series of 100 patients treated at Parkland Memorial Hospital in Dallas, Texas, where patients underwent either early or delayed neck exploration following penetrating injuries to the neck. The study authors retrospectively reported a significantly lower mortality rate for patients receiving immediate/early treatment (6% versus 35%). Subsequently, mandatory early exploration of any neck injury violating the platysma muscle became the standard approach to diagnosis by the majority of trauma surgeons the United States.

The Korean War introduced two important logistic innovations that made invaluable contributions to decreasing overall mortality—the Mobile Army Surgical Hospital (MASH) and the concept of early evacuation by helicopter. Rapid evacuation of the severely injured patients, such as those who had penetrating neck injuries, reduced the overall mortality rate from wounds from 4.5% experienced during World War II to 2.5% in Korea [20]. Reports of mortality from penetrating neck injuries during the Korea

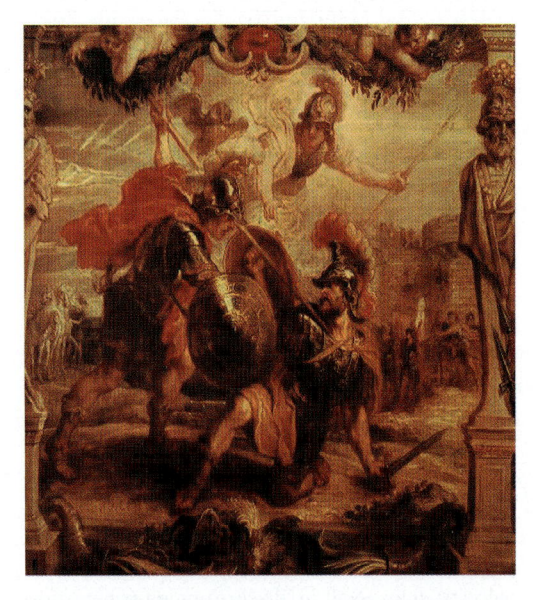

Fig. 1. "Achilles Kills Hector," c. 1631. A painting by Peter Paul Rubens depicting the death of Hector as Achilles thrusts his lance through Hector's neck—"the shorter way to death".

(2.5%) and Vietnam war (15%) demonstrate significantly different survival rates [21,22]. The development of high-velocity weapons (ballistic speeds of over 2000 m/second) used by the military in the Vietnam conflict contributed to the higher mortality of penetrating injuries. Table 1 illustrates the mortality rates of military and civilian neck wounds reported during recent military conflicts, and also civilian experience [21,23]. Fig. 2 outlines the balance between mortality and medical and surgical advances that have influenced the outcome of neck trauma.

As conflicts in the Balkans, the Middle East, and North Africa began during the later part of the twentieth century and the beginning of the twenty-first century, mortality rates from civilian penetrating neck injuries were generally accepted to be from 2% to 11% [23–43]. It is difficult, however, to compare the civilian data to the military experience: most civilian reports do not distinguish between gunshot wounds and stab wounds when reporting mortality. More importantly, most civilian injuries are the result of low-velocity weapons such as handguns, which is not the case in a war zone. Prgomet and colleagues [44] reported a 2.1% mortality for 187 patients who had war-related neck injuries occurring during the war in Croatia from 1991 to 1992 that were treated with selective neck exploration based in large part on physical examination. Although the experience from the Gulf Wars is still being accrued, there are data based on the Kosovo experience that the incidence of head and neck injuries in modern warfare is more than twice that of

Table 1
Mortality rates of military and civilian neck wounds

War	No. of cases reported	Mortality
American Civil War	4114	15
Spanish-American War	188	18
World War I	594	11
World War II	851	7
Korea	?	2.5
Vietnam	?	15
Croatia	187	2.1
Gulf War I & II	?	12
Civilian experience	4193	3.7–5.9

Data from Asensio JA, Valenziano CP, Falcone RE, et al. Management of penetrating neck injuries. The controversy surrounding zone II injuries. Surg Clin North Am 1991;71(2):267–96, and Chipps JE, Canham RG, Makel HP. Intermediate treatment of maxillofacial injuries. U S Armed Forces Med J 1953;4:951.

Mortality (200 years)=2-18%

- Bronze and iron
- Steel
- Gunpowder
- Modern ballistics

- Surgical technique and instrumentation
- Anesthesia
- Antibiotics
- Imaging

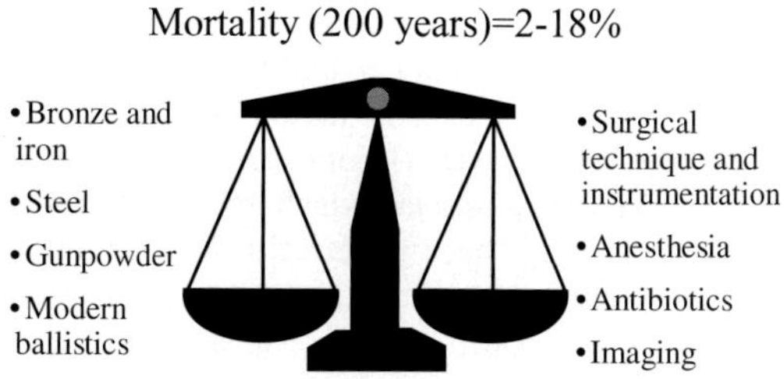

Fig. 2. Mortality and medical and surgical advances that have influenced the outcome of neck trauma.

previous major conflicts [45]. A recent analysis of battlefield injuries from the second Gulf War in Iraq and Afghanistan found that, excluding intracranial and ophthalmic injuries, 21% of all patients will present with at least one injury involving the head and neck region [46]. Data from Operation Iraqi Freedom II suggests that roughly 10% of all combat casualties will have neck injuries, and that mortality approaches 12% [47].

The incidence and significance of head and neck injuries appears to be increasing with changes in mechanisms of injury. A recent study evaluated 10 retrospective studies selected from the period 1982 to 2005 that reviewed war injuries from Vietnam, Lebanon, Slovenia, Croatia, Iraq, Somalia, and Afghanistan [48]. Injuries from fragments (improvised explosive devices, IEDs) were more common during the 90s than during the Vietnam War, when shooting injuries predominated. Injuries to the trunk were reduced in conflicts from 1991 onwards as military personal armor systems including protective vests were used; however, the mortality of wounded soldiers in all conflicts was consistently between 10% and 14%. There was a high incidence of injuries to the head and neck (up to 40%), though they affected only 12% of the body surface area. Though the data from the different military conflicts are not always comparable, there are trends in the type of injuries and mortality, which may lead to changes in existing systems of medical care.

Anatomic considerations

Key to understanding the physical signs and symptoms of penetrating neck injuries is appreciating anatomy and the fascial envelope that surrounds the various anatomic structures. The neck is invested by two fascial layers: the superficial fascia, which encompasses the platysma and is part of the superficial musculoaponeurotic system (SMAS) in the face; and the deep cervical fascia, which comprises the investing, pretracheal, and prevertebral layers. Injuries that are confined to the superficial fascia, which means that the platysma has not been penetrated, are not lethal because there are no vital structures superficial to the platysma. Deep to the superficial fascia, however, lies a network of interconnected connective tissue layers that split to surround muscles and other vital structures and then unite on the other side. Below the hyoid bone the superficial layer of the deep cervical fascia encircles the entire neck deep to the superficial fascia. The prevertebral (deep) fascia encloses the vertebral column and its associated muscles, thus forming the vertebral compartment. Condensations of connective tissue stretch anteriorly to surround the great vessels and vagus nerve, forming the carotid sheath. It is this tight fascial compartmentalization of the vital neck structures that limits external bleeding from vascular injuries, thus minimizing the chance of exsanguination. The pretracheal layer (middle) makes up the anterior compartment of the neck, is bounded by the carotid sheaths laterally, and the prevertebral fascia posteriorly, and forms the visceral compartment containing the trachea, esophagus, and associated structures. A comprehensive review of head and neck anatomy is beyond the scope of this article.

Monson and colleagues [1] described the most widely accepted anatomic classification with regard to penetrating neck injuries by dividing the neck into three anatomic zones anterior to the sternocleidomastoid muscle (Fig. 3). Zone I extends from the level of the clavicles and sternal notch at the thoracic inlet to the cricoid cartilage. The important structures in zone I include the arch of the aorta, proximal carotid arteries, vertebral arteries, subclavian vessels, innominate vessels, apices of the lungs, esophagus, trachea, brachial plexus, and thoracic duct (Fig. 4). Patients often present with exsanguinating hemorrhage that may require transthoracic as well as transcervical approaches to affect repair. Zone II is the largest and most exposed area, and extends from the level of the cricoid cartilage to the angle of the mandible (Fig. 5). The important structures in zone II include the common, internal, and external carotid arteries, the jugular veins, various cranial nerves, the larynx, hypopharynx, and proximal esophagus. Bleeding is often tamponaded by the fascial layers of the neck. Proximal and distal control of the bleeding vessels is readily achieved through various standard neck incisions (Fig. 6). Zone III extends from the level of the angle of the mandible to the base of the skull.

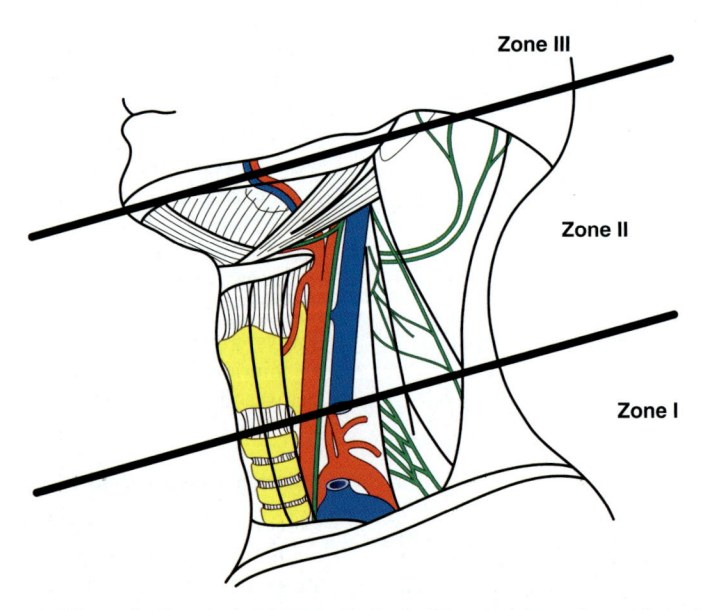

Fig. 3. Anatomic zones of the neck. Zone 1 extends from the level of the clavicles and sternal notch at the thoracic inlet to the cricoid cartilage. Zone II extends from the level of the cricoid cartilage to the angle of the mandible. Zone III extends from the angle of the mandible to the base of the skull.

1. Brachial plexus
2. Subclavian vein
3. First rib
4. Anterior scalene muscle
5. Suprascapular artery and vein
6. Omohyoid muscle (cut)
7. Scapular vein
8. Middle scalene muscle
9. Posterior scalene muscle
10. Sternocleidomastoid muscle (cut)
11. Internal jugular vein
12. Transverse cerviacl vein
13. Omohyoid muscle (cut)
14. Inferior thyroid vein and artery
15. Common carotid
16. Thyrocervical trunk
17. Phrenic nerve
18. Sternocleidomastoid muscle
19. Pectoralis muscle
20. Subclavian artery

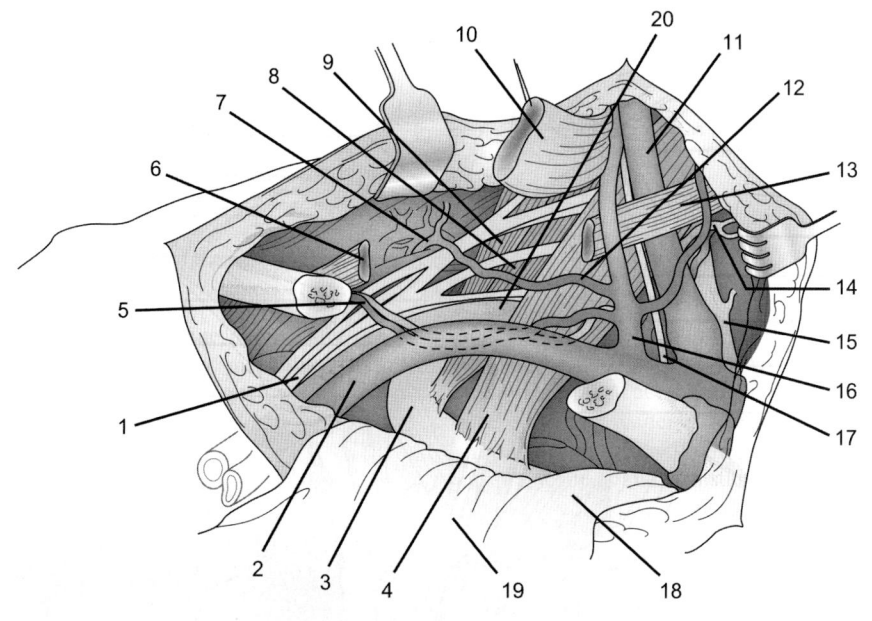

Fig. 4. Anatomic structures of zone I.

Important structures in this relatively inaccessible region include the distal cervical, petrous, and cavernous portions of the internal carotid artery, the vertebral artery, the external carotid artery and its major branches, the jugular veins, the prevertebral venous plexus, and the trunk of the facial nerve. Injuries involving zones I or III present difficult challenges with regard to diagnosis and surgical approach because of the overlap between the chest cavity and the intracranial cavity. Although the management of zone II injuries has been controversial, trauma to this relatively accessible region is usually readily managed once the diagnosis has been rendered.

Pathophysiology of gunshot wounds and ballistics

The wounding power of a projectile depends on several variables, including its size, shape, composition, stability, and most importantly, velocity. The energy imparted to the tissue by the projectile depends on the mass and velocity of the projectile according to the following equation:

$$KE = \frac{1}{2} MV^2$$

Thus high-velocity injuries result in greater damage because of the exponentially larger amounts of energy being transmitted to the tissue (velocity is squared). In addition, the power of the projectile is proportional to the conversion of kinetic energy into mechanical disruption, which in turn, causes indirect tissue damage. Low-velocity projectiles travel less than 2000 feet per second, characteristically create a small entrance and exit wound, and cause damage by lacerating and crushing the tissue. There is little transmission of energy, and therefore little damage is sustained beyond those structures that come in direct contact with the projectile. High-velocity projectiles are those that travel at speeds greater than 2000 feet per second, have an unpredictable course and exit wound, and create widespread objects that are applied with sufficient force to break through skin and into the subcutaneous tissues of the neck (Fig. 8). The trajectory of these stab wounds may be apparent from the history of the incident, and can be predictive of underlying neurovascular injury [50,51]. For example, cervical stab wounds have a higher incidence of subclavian vessel injury because the majority of these wounds occur in a downward direction and extend over the clavicle into the subclavian vessels [52].

A review of the senior author's institutional experience of 120 consecutive patients who had penetrating neck injuries, including a demographic analysis, was recently performed [2]. Typical of most trauma victims, the patients were predominantly male (M = 89, F = 31), had a mean age of 33.8 years (range = 4–92 years) and manifested varying injury severity (mean Injury Severity Scale (ISS) = 13.0; range = 1–50). The majority of the injuries resulted from an assault with a deadly weapon (n = 56); however, 36 injuries resulted from accidents and 28 injuries were self-inflicted. There were 31 patients who had gunshot wounds (GSW), 63 patients who had stab wounds (SW), 13 who had flying glass injuries, and 13 who were impaled with sharp objects (Fig. 9). Of the 120 patients, 55 presented with superficial injuries that did not penetrate the platysma. These patients were generally managed in the emergency department with wound debridement and closure. The primary study group consisted of 65 patients who sustained more significant injuries that violated the platysma, including deep, complex, or avulsive wounds, vascular injuries, or injuries to

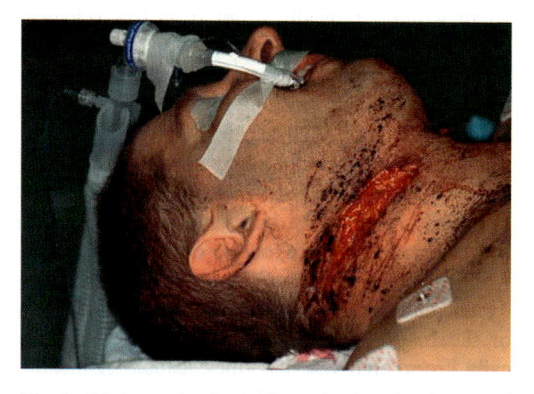

Fig. 8. Photograph of a patient who has a stab wound to the neck. The trajectory of wounds may be apparent from the history of the incident, and can be predictive of underlying neurovascular injury.

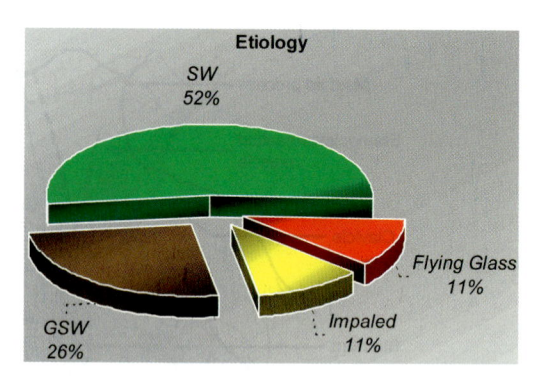

Fig. 9. Etiology of penetrating neck injuries, LEHHC, 2000–2005.

the aerodigestive tract, musculoskeletal system, cranial nerves, or thyroid gland. Of these, there were 13 zone I injuries (16%), 50 zone II injuries (64%) and 16 zone III injuries (20%). Deep neck wounds and vascular trauma were the most common; however, virtually every vital structure in the neck was represented.

Diagnosis

Physical examination

The initial evaluation of a trauma patient begins with the "ABCs" of trauma management as outlined by the *Advanced Trauma Life Support Manual* (ATLS) advocated by the American College of Surgeons: (1) establish a secure airway, (2) assure breathing/respiration, and (3) initiate volume resuscitation [53]. Particular importance should be placed on the airway because bleeding within the tight compartmentalized spaces of the neck may appear quiescent externally, but can cause progressive airway compromise and eventual complete obstruction (Fig. 10). Orotracheal intubation is recommended, and usually feasible; however, once the neck swelling is advanced, endotracheal intubation may be impossible. Emergency cricothyrotomy or trachestomy may be necessary to establish a patent airway.

In conjunction with the primary and secondary surveys, a thorough head and neck examination should be performed. The clinical evaluation should focus on signs and symptoms suggestive of injuries to major vessels, the aerodigestive tract, spinal cord, or cranial nerves or nerve roots. The surgeon should look for signs of entrance and exit wounds and classify them according to the level of injury. Based on the anatomic location of the entrance/exit wound, the suspected trajectory of the penetrating object, and the physical signs and symptoms, the surgeon should be able to direct attention to certain organ systems or structures.

Physical examination alone has been shown to be a reliable indicator of clinically significant vascular injury [39–42,53]. Hematoma is the most common sign of vascular injury, followed by shock and external bleeding. Other "hard" signs of vascular injury include absent carotid pulse, carotid bruit or thrill, shock not responsive to fluid resuscitation, and diminished radial pulse. Signs and symptoms of aerodigestive injuries include dysphagia, hoarseness, subcutaneous emphysema or crepitance, dyspnea, and air bubbling from a wound. Focal neurologic defects such as altered sensation within the anatomic distribution of known sensory nerves such as the greater auricular nerve, local motor defects such as tongue deviation indicative of hypoglossal nerve injury, or peripheral sensorimotor defects indicating brachial plexus injury are common.

Absence of these signs or symptoms, however, does not mean absence of injury. In Fogelman and Stewart's [15] classic paper on penetrating neck injuries, 43% of their patients who had significant vascular injury had no evidence of peripheral vascular collapse, and 70% had no evidence of bleeding at the time of admission. In addition, of the 13 patients who had obvious injury and penetration of the trachea and larynx, 4 failed to develop clinical signs or symptoms before surgical exploration and repair. A more recent study, however, by Azuaje and colleagues [54], reported on a series of 216 patients who had penetrating neck injuries, and demonstrated that physical examination alone boasted a 93% sensitivity and 97% negative predictive value for predicting vascular injuries. Based on the clinical evaluation, recommendations can be made regarding further diagnostic evaluation, observation, or immediate surgical intervention. It is clear that emergent surgical exploration is necessary for patients who have hard signs of vascular injury such as hemodynamic instability, exsanguinating hemorrhage, or expanding hematoma. Those patients who are hemodynamically stable and have no respiratory compromise should undergo further diagnostic evaluation. The indications for the various diagnostic modalities remain controversial, however, and the remainder of this article deals with a rationale for management.

Diagnostic evaluation

Angiography became the most reliable method of evaluation vascular injuries in a hemodynamically stable patient (Fig. 11). The patients would undergo direct contrast angiography. This technique has limitations, however, including its invasive nature and potential complications. The reported incidence of complications related to catheter angiography ranges between 0.2% to 2% [41,55–57]. Hematoma at the puncture site is the most common complication; however, vascular spasm, allergic reactions, embolization of atherosclerotic plaques, thrombosis, and arterial dissection can also be seen. The severity of the cardiovascular and central nervous system complications related to this method allows for questioning, especially in the hemodynamically stable patient, given the reported high frequency (over 70%) of negative test results [58–61].

The complications related to catheter angiography have led to the search for other noninvasive diagnostic methods for detection of vascular injuries. Color Doppler ultrasonography has emerged as a fast, safe, noninvasive method for evaluation of vascular flow and wall integrity. Several authors have compared this technique with catheter angiography, outlining the advantages and disadvantages of this method [60–62]. In most centers its use has been limited for the evaluation of penetrating neck injuries. The method is highly operator-dependent, which may result in a long examination time in the hands of the inexperienced operator. Physical examination findings related to the trauma such as hematoma, lacerations, or subcutaneous emphysema limit the reliability of the results. In addition, zones I and III and the vertebral arteries are often difficult to assess.

Despite the availability of advanced imaging modalities for the evaluation of penetrating neck trauma, physical examination techniques continue to be of significant value. In 1993 Demetriades and colleagues [39] looked at physical examination and selective conservative management in patients who had penetrating neck injuries. They prospectively evaluated 335 patients and examined the decision whether to operate or observe according to a protocol based mainly on physical examination. In their cohort of patients, 20% were subjected to emergency surgery, and angiography was used in only 3 patients. They concluded that physical examination is a reliable method for detecting significant

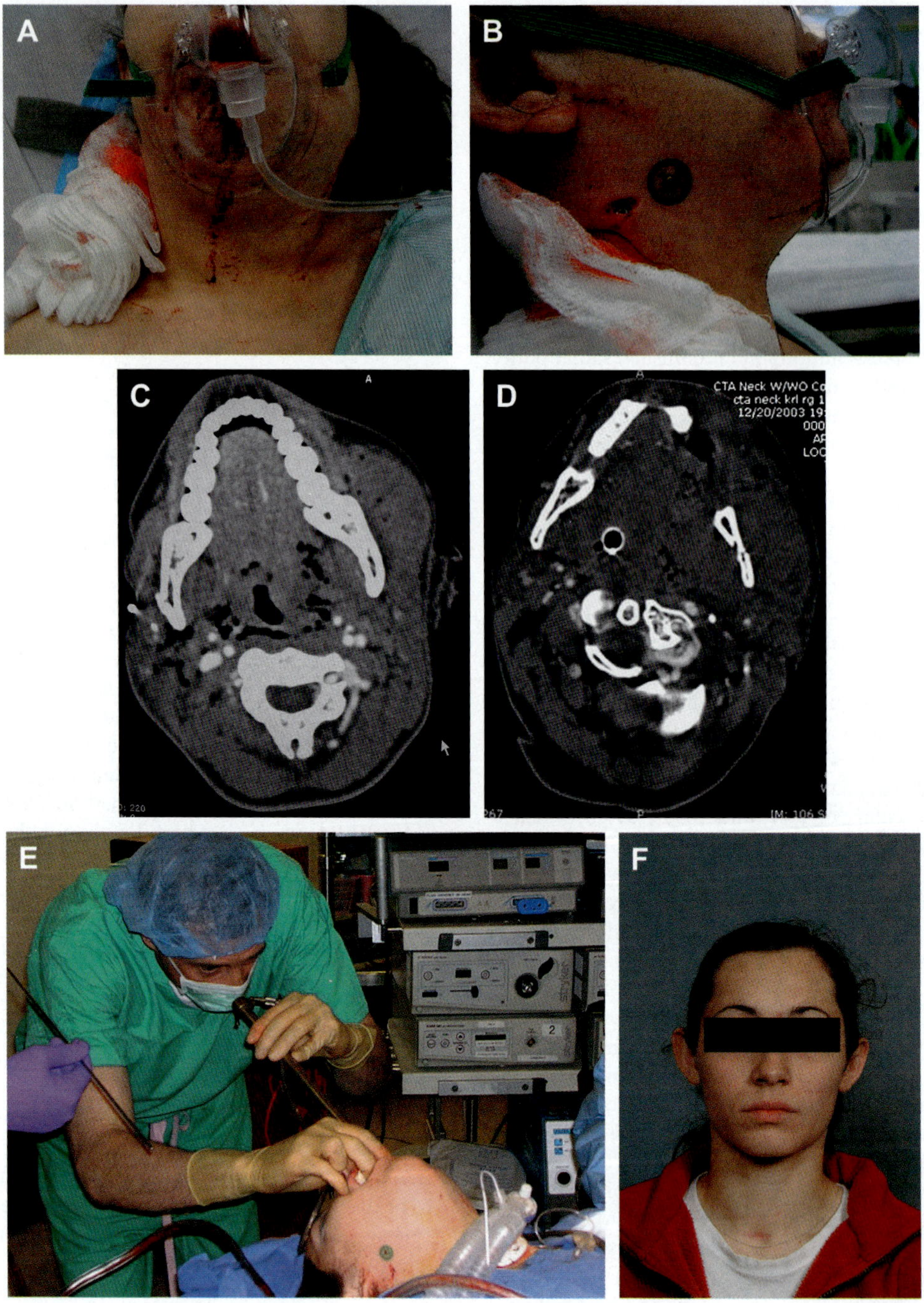
A
B
C
D
E
F

injuries following penetrating neck trauma, and suggest that angiography is rarely needed.

Magnetic resonance angiography (MRA) has developed in the last 2 decades as a useful imaging modality for evaluation of vascular injuries, both in the management of vascular trauma and also in the diagnosis and management of stroke victims. For the management of stroke, the combined method of MRI/MRA has become the gold standard because of the superior imaging resolution of the brain parenchyma that is critical for stroke evaluation, and the relatively accurate diagnosis of vascular injuries and anatomy; however, MR technology has not evolved as the gold standard in the evaluation of penetrating neck injuries because of several factors: (1) time-consuming scans limit it use in the acutely unstable patient, (2) the non-MR compatibility of much trauma equipment limits its use, (3) relative higher cost, (4) decreased ability to detect cervical spine fractures, and (5) decreased imaging resolution compared with recently introduced helical and multislice computed tomography angiography (CTA).

Helical and multislice CTA has emerged as a fast, minimally invasive, accurate study to evaluate penetrating neck injuries, with virtual elimination of the need for mandatory neck exploration [2,63–66]. Helical and multislice CTA is used to assess patients suffering from both penetrating and blunt trauma to the neck, extremities, mediastinum, and abdomen [63–72]. A significant advantage of helical and multislice CTA in trauma patients is the ability to obtain high-quality images in less than 1 minute. It has emerged as a important imaging modality in most hospital emergency rooms for diagnosis and management of trauma patients. Several factors have contribute to the emergence of this modality in modern trauma care: (1) the use of helical and multislice CTA technology to obtain reproducible and reliable images is easy and not operator-dependent, (2) it requires minimal support of additional nonphysician staff (in contrast to angiography), (3) it is readily available, (4) It is highly accurate for detection of vascular injuries, and (5) multiplanar and three-dimensionally–generated images are easily obtained, facilitating the traditionally more challenging interpretation of images in the axial plane. Munera and colleagues evaluated the use of helical and multislice CTA as an initial method for evaluating patients who had possible arterial injuries to the neck, reporting a sensitivity of 100% and a specificity of 98.6% [73,74].

In 2005, Woo and colleagues [64] examined how the management of penetrating neck trauma has changed with the advent of computed tomography angiography CTA. They retrospectively reviewed their experience over 10 years for 130 cases of penetrating neck trauma, with 34 undergoing CTA and 96 with no CTA. The CTA group had only one neck exploration (3%), versus 32 (33%) in the non-CTA group. Negative neck explorations were significantly higher in the group that did not receive a CTA.

In an effort to appreciate the affect that CTA has had on the management of penetrating neck injuries at the authors' trauma center, a study of 120 consecutive patients who had penetrating neck injuries presenting to Legacy Emanuel Hospital and Health Center (LEHHC) from 2000 to 2005 was performed, with the purpose of further elucidating the role of CTA in clinical decision-making and to assess patient outcome [2]. Of the

Fig. 10. Nineteen-year-old female who has a low-velocity, transpharyngeal gunshot wound. Low-velocity projectiles travel less than 2000 feet per second, characteristically create small entrance and exit wounds, and cause damage by lacerating and crushing the tissue. There is little transmission of energy and therefore little damage is sustained beyond those structures that come in direct contact with the projectile. (*A*) Frontal view demonstrating neck swelling, dyspnea, and impending airway obstruction. Orotracheal intubation is recommended and usually feasible; however, once the neck swelling is advanced, endotracheal intubation may be impossible. Emergency cricothyrotomy or trachestomy may be necessary to establish a patent airway. (*B*) Lateral view of the same patient demonstrating entrance wound. (*C*) CTA (axial image) of the same patient demonstrating the path of the bullet with transpharyngeal subcutaneous emphysema, right mandibular fractures, and no evidence of vascular injury. A marker is placed at the exit wound on the left side. (*D*) CTA (axial image) of the same patient, again demonstrating the transpharyngeal trajectory of the bullet, massive subcutaneous emphysema, and bilateral mandibular fractures. Despite lack of evidence of vascular injury, the bullet trajectory and findings of subcutaneous emphysema are highly suggestive of upper aerodigestive tract injury and mandate further interrogation. (*E*) Rigid esophagoscopy is performed to evaluation the hypopharynx and cervical esophagus to the level of the gastric introitus. Bilateral hypopharyngeal perforations were noted just above the pyriform recess. (*F*) Postoperative appearance of the patient 6 months following operative repair of her mandibular fractures and nonsurgical management of her transpharyngeal gunshot wounds.

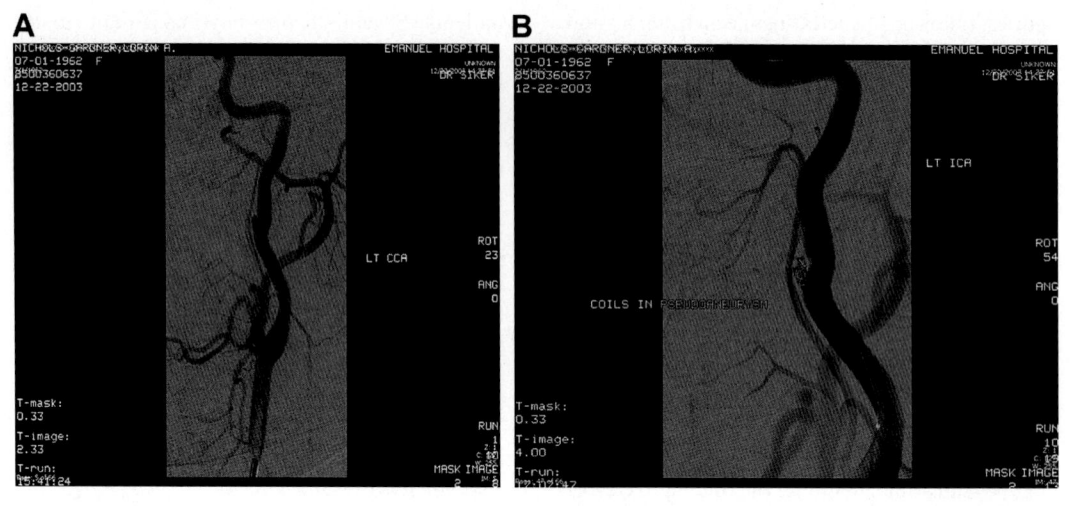

Fig. 11. Imaging of a patient who sustained a low-velocity gunshot wound to the neck involving zone III. The patient was neurologically intact and had no hard signs of vascular injury. (*A*) Carotid angiogram that demonstrates a 5 mm aneurysm or pseudoaneurysm involving the internal carotid artery at about the level of the 2nd cervical vertebra. (*B*) Post-endovascular repair arteriogram demonstrating coiling on the aneurysm.

120 patients, 55 were excluded from the study because either the patients' injuries were superficial, the patients died before operative intervention, or the patients underwent emergent neck exploration to control hemorrhage. CTA was used extensively at LEHHC beginning in 2003; therefore the 65 patients who had injuries penetrating the platysma and who met the inclusion criteria for the study were divided into groups and compared based upon having received CTA as part of the diagnostic evaluation. The results showed that the use of CTA in the study group resulted in significantly fewer formal neck explorations when compared with patients who did not receive CTA (CTA = 6 explorations versus no CTA = 27 explorations). In addition, the rate of negative neck exploration was significantly decreased from 48% in patients not receiving a CTA to 0% in those who did receive a CTA. At the authors' institutions, however, we continue the judicious use of various adjunctive studies to evaluate the upper aerodigestive tract (Fig. 12).

Management

For practical purposes, neck injuries are classified according to the scheme proposed by Monson and colleagues [1] in 1969. Traditionally, zone I and zone III injuries were managed selectively because of the difficulties associated with surgical access, and zone II injuries were routinely explored. This resulted in overtreatment of a significant number of zone II injuries (negative neck explorations) and undertreatment of zone I and III injuries (missed injuries). Today, the shift toward selective intervention for injuries involving all three zones when "hard signs" of vascular injury are absent has somewhat diminished the importance of the three zones of the neck.

There is no universal agreement with regards to selective versus mandatory exploration, the role of and type of preoperative diagnostic examinations, the rationale for ligation, observation, and revascularization of the injured carotid artery, or the role of endovascular repair of arterial injuries. Management should be based upon the surgeon's experience and, most importantly, the resources available at each particular center. As discussed previously, the approach at LEHHC over the last 5 years has generally been one of selective surgical management based upon physical examination and findings on CTA. All patients who have active bleeding, expanding hematoma, shock, massive subcutaneous emphysema, or significant airway compromise are surgically explored, regardless of the zone of injury. Indications for immediate surgical intervention include

Exsanguinating hemorrhage
Expanding hematoma
Shock
Airway compromise
Massive subcutaneous emphysema

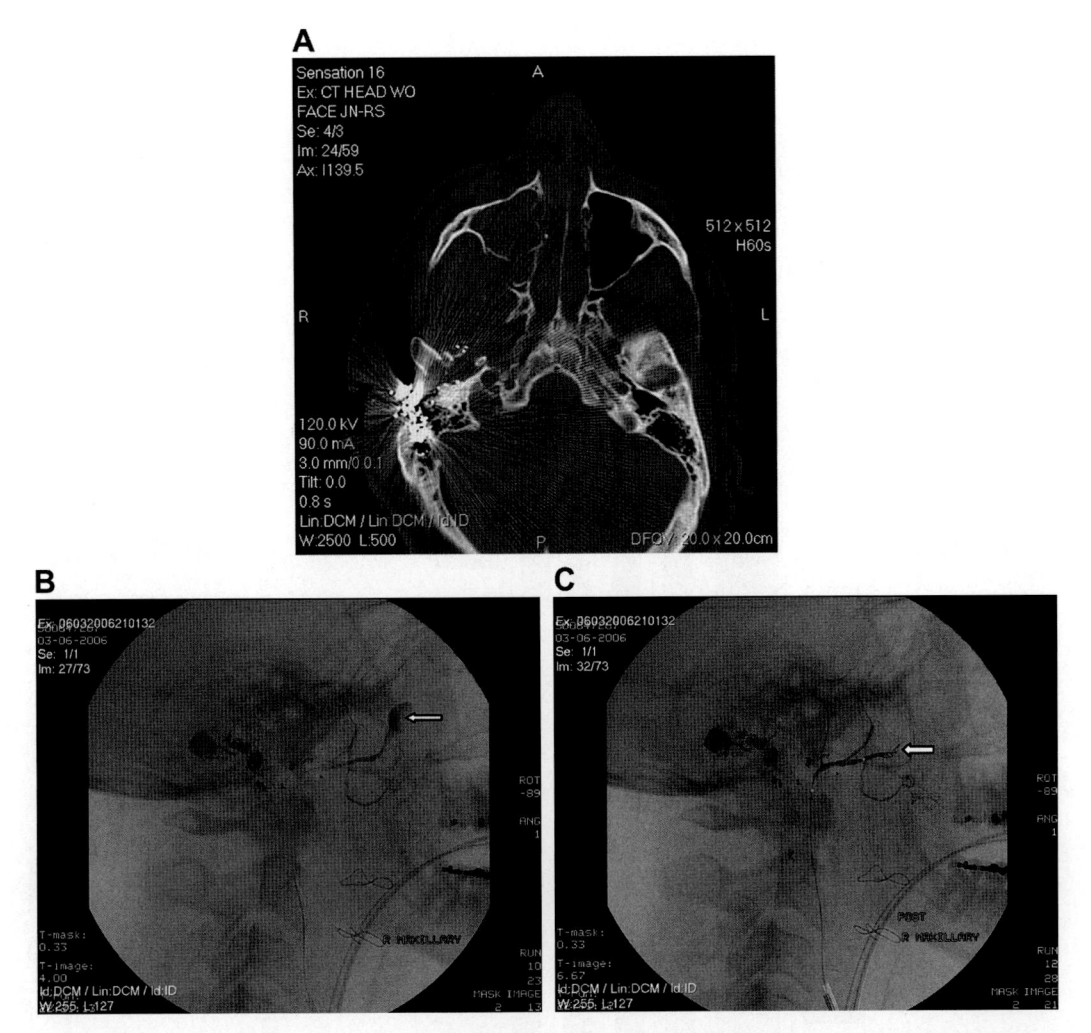

Fig. 12. Forty-three-year-old male who has a self-inflicted gunshot wound to the neck and face presenting with massive epistaxis. (*A*) CT scan demonstrating bullet trajectory through the maxillary sinus and multiple bullet fragments throughout the temporal bone, internal and external auditory canal. (*B*) Angiogram was obtained because of the trajectory and epistaxis to rule out vascular injury. Arrow points to a "blush" associated with the right internal maxillary artery, consistent with a pseudoaneurysm. (*C*) Angiogram following endovascular coiling of the right internal maxillary artery. Arrow points to the coil.

Patients who have injuries that penetrate the platysma and are hemodynamically stable are evaluated by CTA. Further diagnostic studies, such as angiography, esophagography, direct laryngoscopy, or rigid esophagoscopy, are used based on the CT findings. The use of CTA at the authors' institution has resulted in fewer formal neck explorations and virtual elimination of negative exploratory surgery. Thus far, however, it has not had a significant effect on the number of adjunctive diagnostic modalities performed in the preoperative setting. The management of specific anatomic injuries varies somewhat from surgeon to surgeon, but is generally based on the location and extent of the injury in addition to the neurologic status of the patient. Fig. 13 illustrates the management algorithm used at LEHHC for penetrating neck injuries, and provides an outline for the remainder of the article. Fig. 14 demonstrates the general trend in the use of CTA, neck exploration, and negative neck exploration in the patients treated at LEHHC between 2000 and 2005 [2].

If surgical exploration is deemed necessary, the neck may be approached by one of several

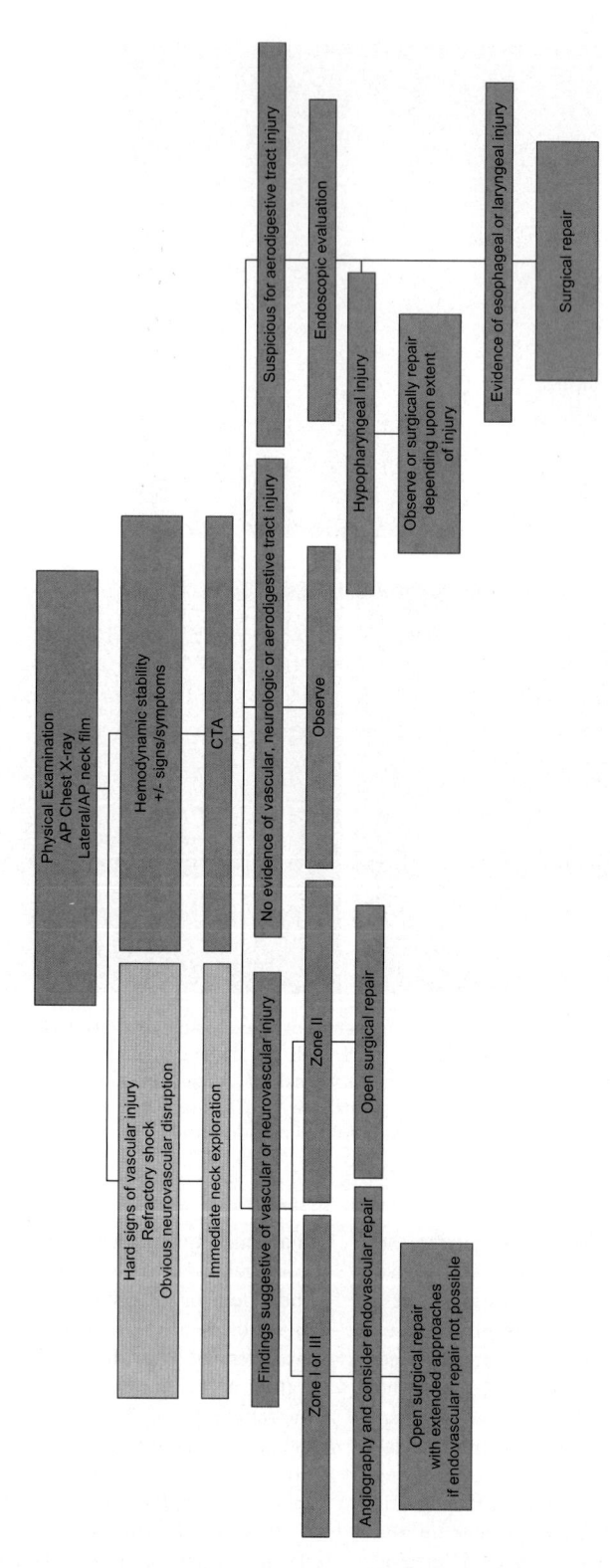

Fig. 13. LEHHC management guidelines for penetrating neck injuries.

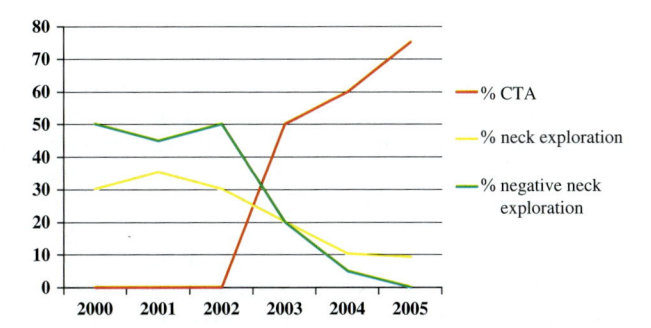

Fig. 14. Trends in the use of CTA, neck exploration, and the rate of negative neck exploration. The surgical management of these injuries is extremely complicated because of their location in the posterior neck encased within the cervical vertebral column.

incisions, based on the suspected injury and the zone of entry (see Fig. 6). The standard approach is a vertical incision along the anterior border of the sternocleidomastoid muscle extending from the angle of the mandible to the sternoclavicular junction. This incision may be modified with horizontal limbs extending to the mastoid for further exposure of zone III injuries or along the superior aspect of the clavicle for zone I injuries. Alternatively, horizontal incisions may be used, encompassing skin flaps developed in a subplatysmal plane superiorly and inferiorly, to provide maximum access to multiple zones, anteriorly and posteriorly. Once the skin flaps are developed, the marginal mandibular branch of the facial nerve is identified and protected, and the great vessels are approached by identifying and skeletonizing the anterior-medial aspect of the sternocleidomastoid muscle. Proximal and distal control of the carotid artery can then be attained from the base of the skull to the clavicle. This approach also provides wide access for repairing cranial nerves, the esophagus, and other vital structures. The horizontal incision can be carried to the opposite side as an "apron flap" to provide maximum exposure to both sides of the neck. For these reasons, a horizontal incision is the authors' preferred approach for most significant neck injuries when multiple structures or multiple zones are involved (ie: carotid artery and esophagus). Special consideration is given to the operative management of high carotid injuries at or above the skull base (zone III) that may require a vertical ramus osteotomy to provide access to the distal extracranial vessels [75]. Access may be improved by dividing the digastric and stylohyoid muscles or by disinserting the sternocleidomastoid muscle. Lower zone I injuries that involve the subclavian or innominate vessels may require a median sternotomy, disarticulation of the sternoclavicular joint, or anterolateral thoracotomy. Appropriate neurosurgical, vascular, and cardiothoracic surgical assistance is advised when managing these challenging injuries.

Extracranial vascular trauma

Vascular injuries are the most common injuries associated with penetrating neck trauma, occurring in 40% of patients; 10% of these injuries involve the carotid artery. The mortality rate associated with penetrating injury is 10% to 30%. Physical findings may be characterized by neruologic defects, including an ipsilateral Horner's syndrome or cranial nerve dysfunction. Penetrating injuries to the neck from gunshot wounds, stab wounds, or other lacerations can result in the formation of pseudoaneurysms, arteriovenous fistulae, vessel transections, intimal flaps, dissections, and occlusions to the carotid or vertebral arteries or jugular veins. Management paradigms are directed at rapidly identifying the injury and preventing cerebral ischemia. As stated previously, CTA has been shown to be highly efficacious for identifying vascular injuries of the head and neck, and has the additional advantage of simultaneously providing information on cerebral ischemia or infarct as well as other associated injuries. Once a vascular injury is identified, the decision must made to repair, bypass, ligate, or observe the lesion. Unilateral carotid artery occlusion can be well-tolerated in patients who have adequate collateral circulation to the brain; however, in patients who have an incomplete circle of Willis, contralateral occlusions or stenoses, or athrosclerotic disease, strong consideration should be given to revascularization. In recent years, endovascular therapy has altered the management of many of these patients, and the approach—whether medical, surgical or endovascular—is based upon hemodynamic stability, the extent of hemorrhage, the type and location of the injury, and the neurologic status of the patient.

There is general agreement that carotid injuries in neurologically intact patients should be repaired. When possible, primary repair of carotid artery injuries is preferred. Otherwise the use of saphenous vein or polytetrafluoroethylene (PTFE) can be considered. There are no conclusive studies to suggest the superiority of one method over the other for repair of vascular trauma from penetrating injuries of the neck. There appear to be no significantly increased rates of infection or thrombosis with the use of PTFE compared with saphenous vein grafts [76,77]. Controversy exists, however, with regards to the revascularization of carotid occlusion in patients who have a depressed state of consciousness or coma, and the management of an occlusive injury in an asymptomatic patient who would require a complex repair. The former controversy is based on experience with carotid artery arthroscerotic disease and the findings that some patients who have cerebral ischemia who are revascularized will develop hemorrhagic infarcts [78]. In 1974, Thal and coworkers [79] published their experience in the management of 60 patients who had penetrating carotid injuries based upon pretreatment neurologic status. Their findings suggested that patients who have no preoperative neurologic symptoms and those who have mild neurologic deficits should routinely undergo primary repair. Those patients who have severe neurologic deficits or coma should undergo repair only if distal carotid patency is demonstrated on angiography. Liekweg and Greenfield [80] similarly recommended that ligation of the carotid artery be reserved for the comatose patient who has no prograde flow and for cases in which primary repair is technically impossible. More recent studies have confirmed the efficacy of routine repair of carotid injuries in all but comatose patients [81–83]. In the asymptomatic patient who has an occlusive injury there is a small risk of thrombus propagation into the middle cerebral artery. Most trauma centers anticoagulate these patients if there is no contraindication to anticoagulation. Relatively minor injuries such as pseydoaneurysms less than 5 mm and small intimal defects may be observed and followed with repeat imaging in 1 to 2 weeks.

Exsanguinating hemorrhage at any level generally mandates rapid surgical exploration and repair, if possible. All injuries, regardless of location, are preferentially repaired surgically. Injuries of the common and internal carotid arteries are repaired by lateral arteriorrhaphy or resection of the injured vessel, with either primary re-anastomosis or replacement with an interpositional graft (Fig. 15). During repair, an interluminal shunt may be used to maintain prograde cerebral blood flow. Distal internal carotid injuries that are actively bleeding and cannot readily be exposed may be controlled with a balloon catheter (Fogarty) that is placed into the distal lumen of the artery. Once the balloon is inflated and the bleeding controlled, the vessel can be repaired directly or ligated. As stated earlier, however, ligation is indicated only in comatose patients.

Advances in endovascular therapy have altered the management of traumatic vascular injuries, and its role in the treatment of vascular lesions of the head and neck is evolving. There is some evidence to suggest that traumatic occlusions of the carotid artery may be repaired by endovascular revascularization, particularly in those patients in whom surgical repair is technically difficult or impossible [84–88]. No large series of long-term data are available regarding the safety and efficacy of this technique, despite its rapidly expanded use. Caution must be exercised until more data are available. A recent study by Cothren and coworkers [89] reported unfavorable

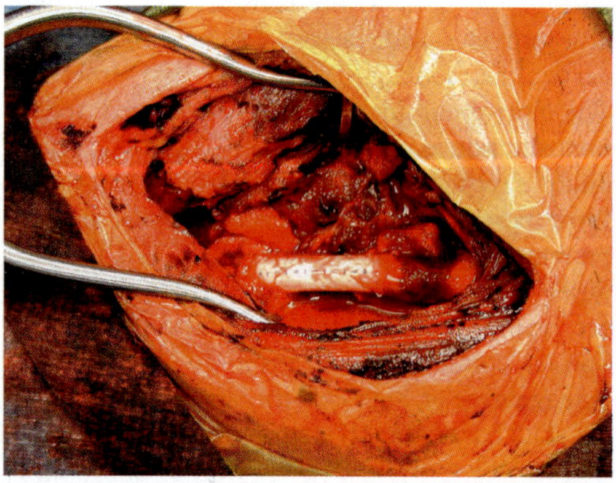

Fig. 15. Repair of an injured common carotid artery with an interpositional graft using polytetrafluoroethylene (PTFE) in a patient who sustained a zone II gunshot wound.

results for blunt trauma patients who had persistent carotid pseudoaneurysms that were treated with endovascular stenting. In this prospective analysis, 46 patients sustained blunt carotid pseuodoaneurysms; 23 of them underwent carotid stent placement with anticoagulation, and 23 were treated with anticoagulation alone. There were four complications in stented patients, including three strokes and one subclavian dissection. Carotid occlusion rates were significantly higher in the stented group (45% versus 5% in those who received antithrombotic agents alone). Until further data that support the routine use of endovascular therapy are available, the authors reserve its use for patients who have stable, intimal, high zone III carotid injuries and most vertebral artery injuries.

Vertebral artery injuries are much less common than carotid injuries. The surgical management of these injuries is extremely complicated because of their location in the posterior neck, encased within the cervical vertebral column (Fig. 16). Unilateral vertebral artery occlusion rarely results in a neurologic deficit if the contralateral vertebral artery is normal and the posterior inferior cerebellar artery is preserved. McConnell and Trunkey [90] recommend operative repair of the injured vertebral artery instead of ligation if the contralateral vertebral is hypoplastic or stenosed. Endovascular management of these injuries has gained popularity for vertebral injuries and its use seems promising.

Esophageal injury

Injury to the cervical esophagus is uncommon, but should be suspected in cases in which there is a penetrating injury in the proximity. It has been estimated that most busy trauma centers encounter only about five patients per year with these injuries [91]. Delay in diagnosis has been cited as the most important contributor for significant mortality of about 19% [92,93]. The American Association for the Surgery of Trauma supported the most significant multicenter study on penetrating esophageal injuries [94], and concluded that increased esophageal-related morbidity occurs with the diagnostic workup and its inherent delay in the operative repair of these injuries. The optimal safety period has not been established, but for centers practicing selective management of penetrating neck injuries, the highest priority should be given to identification and repair. The use of esophagoscopy and esophagography in combination with physical examination is highly sensitive in diagnosis of any injuries. There has been some debate over the use of flexible versus rigid esophagoscopy [95]; however, a recent retrospective study by Horwitz and colleagues [96] suggests that the flexible scope is highly sensitive, safe, and

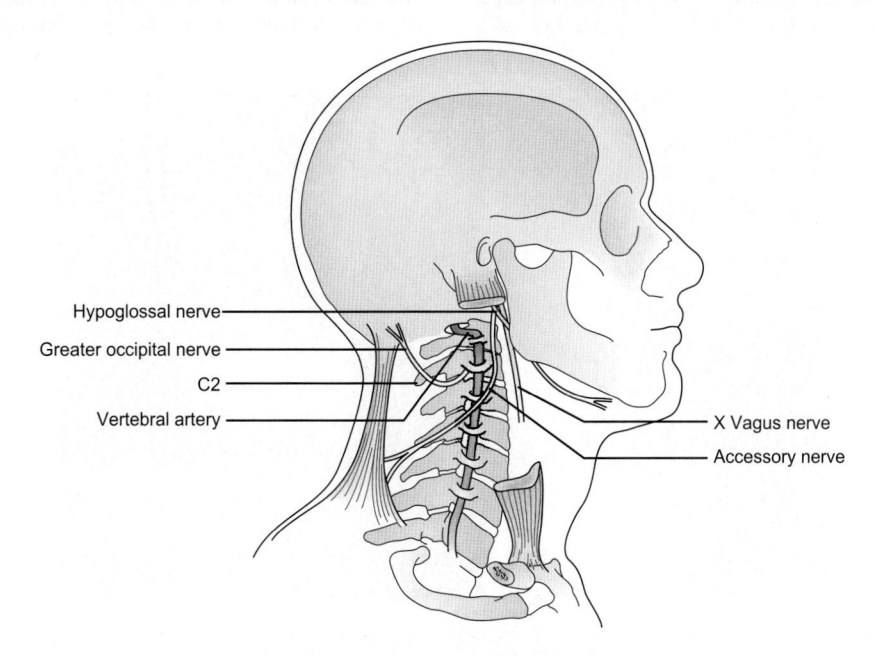

Fig. 16. Anatomy of the vertebral arteries.

accurate when used by an experienced operator. The cervical esophagus should be repaired directly whenever possible in a one- or two-layered fashion, depending on the extent of the injury. Adjunctive muscle flaps, such as a strap muscle or sternocleidomastoid muscle, can be used to buttress the repair, which should be liberally drained. Avulsive injuries that result from high-velocity weaponry occasionally require the use of microvascular free tissue transfer or other regional rotational flaps to effect adequate repair. The majority of patients who die secondary to esophageal injury do so because of mediastinitis and sepsis; therefore all treatments are to prevent abscess formation.

Laryngotracheal injury

Injury to the laryngotracheal structures in most commonly seen in the cervical trachea. The evidence of extensive subcutaneous emphysema on clinical examination (crepitus) or CTA imaging is highly suspicious of injury to the airway, although subcutaneous emphysema may also be caused by dissection of air into the subcutaneous tissue by the initial traumatic insult. The management of tracheal injuries is mainly dependent on the size of the injury. Small injuries may be primarily repaired. Larger defects may require a combination of tracheotomy, along with the use of synthetic materials, or local and regional flaps. Laryngeal injuries may be repaired with a combination of suturing of fractured segments, rigid internal fixation using miniplates, or placement of stents [97]. Please see the article by Bell, Verschueren, and Dierks in this issue for a thorough review of laryngeal injuries.

Endocrine injury

Clinically significant injuries to the thyroid and parathyroid glands are not common. Penetrating injuries that lacerate the gland do not significantly alter gland function. Vascular injuries are easily managed by cauterization or direct suturing of the offending vessels. Ligation of the inferior thyroid artery will control significant hemorrhage associated with the thyroid gland. Compromised thyroid hormone and calcium metabolism are rare; however, surveillance of calcium and thyroid hormone function can be considered.

Cervical spine injury

Penetrating injuries to the cervical spine can cause severe irreversible injuries, and despite prompt medical or surgical treatments, the outcome is primarily related to the severity of the initial traumatic insult (Fig. 17). Early intervention can prevent further injury. The diagnosis of patients presenting with cervical spine injury is generally easy to confirm by physical examination findings, and can range from minor to severe neurologic deficits that compromise, cardiovascular (most commonly manifesting as hypotension), or

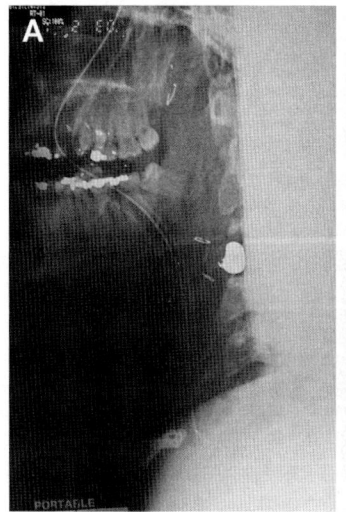

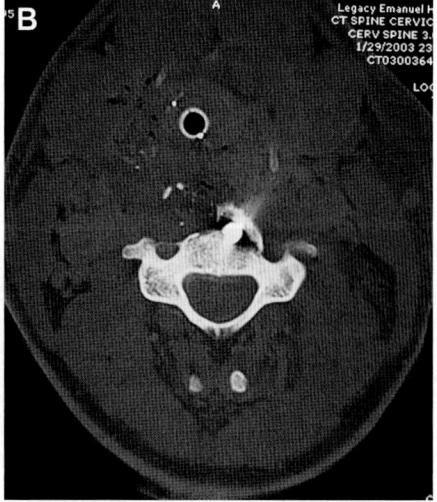

Fig. 17. Twenty-six-year-old male with a low-velocity gunshot wound to the neck. (*A*) Lateral cervical spine radiograph demonstrating bullet fragments within the neck. These films are good screening films but lack multidimensional perspective. (*B*) CT scan of the same patient demonstrating bullet fragments lodged within the body of the 4th cervical vertebra.

motor and sensory deficits. Hypotension in the presence of cervical spine injury may be caused by the compromised systemic arterial and venous vascular innervation, causing vasodilatation and subsequent hypotension; however, blood loss causing hypovolemic shock needs to be ruled out before consideration of other etiologies of shock.

The use of steroids in spinal injury remains to be fully elucidated. Currently, no studies have evaluated the use of steroids in penetrating neck injuries that result in cervical spine injury. In 1991 Bracken and colleagues [98] published the Results of the Second National Acute Spinal Cord Injury Study using a randomized, multicenter, placebo controlled trial of methylprednisolone in the treatment of acute spinal-cord injury. They administered methylprednisolone to 162 patients as a bolus of 30 mg per kilogram, followed by an infusion at 5.4 mg per kilogram for 23 hours. Placebos were given to 171 patients by bolus and infusion. After 6 months the patients who were treated with methylprednisolone within 8 hours of their injury had significant improvement in motor function and sensation to pinprick and touch as compared with those given placebo. The study authors concluded that in patients who have acute spinal-cord injury, treatment with methylprednisolone improves neurologic recovery when the medication is given in the first 8 hours. Subsequent studies have failed to show any significant improvement with the use of steroids [99,100]. There are no clear guidelines for the use of steroids in penetrating injuries of the cervical spine. Please see the article by Chen in this issue for a thorough review of management.

Summary

This article provides a timely review of current management trends for patients who have penetrating neck injuries. Management of these patients has evolved from that of frequent, obligatory surgical exploration to selective intervention based on physical examination and findings on CTA. The use of CTA as a guide to clinical decision-making has lead to a significant decrease in the number of neck explorations performed at the authors' institution and a virtual elimination of negative neck explorations. The authors believe that timely and aggressive surgical intervention is critical to successful outcomes. Despite trends toward less invasive surgery and fewer interventions, patients who have accessible vascular injuries, significant esophageal perforations, laryngeal fractures, and neurologic injuries are still best treated with direct open surgical repair. Endovascular techniques are helpful for small, stable, inaccessible (zone III) pseudoaneurysms or intimal injuries, but currently have little role for more significant injuries. At the end of the day, the treatment of each patient should be individualized and based on the patients' signs and symptoms, the experience of the surgeon, and the resources available at each institution.

References

[1] Monson DO, Saletta JD, Freeark RJ. Carotid vertebral trauma. J Trauma 1969;9:987–99.

[2] Bell RB, Osborn T, Dierks EJ, et al. Management of penetrating neck injuries: a new paradigm for civilian trauma. J Oral Maxillofac Surg 2007;65:691–705.

[3] Breasted JH. The Edwin Smith surgical papyrus. Chicago: University of Chicago Press; 1930.

[4] Key G, editor. The apologie and treatise of Ambroise Pare containing the ayages made into divers places with many writings upon surgery. London: Falcon Education Books; 1957.

[5] Fleming D. Case of rupture of the carotid artery and wounds of several of its branches, successfully treated by tying the common trunk of the carotid itself. Med Chir J Rev 1817;3:2.

[6] Watson WL, Silverstone SM. Ligature of the common carotid artery in cancer of the head and neck. Ann Surg 1939;109:1.

[7] Otis GA. Medical and surgical history of the War of Rebellion, part 3, vol. 2: surgical history. Washington, DC: US Government Printing Office; 1883.

[8] Medical Department of the United States Army in the World War, vol. 2. Washington, DC: US Government Printing office; 1927. p. 68.

[9] Bailey H. Surgery of modern warfare, vol. 2. 3rd edition. Baltimore (MD): Williams and Wilkins; 1944. p. 674.

[10] Halstead AE. IV. Report of a case of recovery after ligation of the first portion of the right subclavian artery for aneurism of the third portion. Ann Surg 1900;31(5):591–4.

[11] Blair VP. A note on the treatment of secondary hemorrhage from branches of the common carotid artery. Ann Surg 1921;74:313.

[12] Mooro A. A case of arteriovenous aneurysm of the neck. Lancet 1923;2:1186.

[13] Bigger IA, Lippert KM. Arteriovenous fistula involving common carotid artery and internal jugular vein. Surgery 1937;2:555.

[14] Porritt A. Treatment of war wounds, history of the Second World War: surgery. London: Her Maj Stat Off; 1953. p. 9–10.

[15] Fogelman MJ, Stewart RD. Penetrating wounds of the neck. Am J Surg 1956;91:581–93.

[16] Knightly JJ, Swaminathan AP, Rush BF. Management of penetrating injuries of the neck. Am J Surg 1973;126:575–80.
[17] Markey JC, Hines JL, Nance FC. Penetrating neck wounds: a review of 218 cases. Am J Surg 1975;130: 416–20.
[18] McInnis WD, Cruz AB, Aust JB. Penetrating injuries to the neck. Am J Surg 1975;130:416–20.
[19] Roon AJ, Christensen N. Evaluation and treatment of penetrating cervical injuries. J Trauma 1979;19:391–7.
[20] Hardaway RM. Surgical research in Vietnam. Mil Med 1967;132:873–87.
[21] Chipps JE, Canham RG, Makel HP. Intermediate treatment of maxillofacial injuries. U S Armed Forces Med J 1953;4:951.
[22] Thal ER. Injury to the neck. In: Mattox KL, Moore EE, Feliciano DV, editors. Trauma. Norwalk (CT): Appelton and Lange; 1988. p. 301.
[23] Asensio JA, Valenziano CP, Falcone RE, et al. Management of penetrating neck injuries. The controversy surrounding zone II injuries. Surg Clin North Am 1991;71(2):267–96.
[24] Almskog BA, Angeras U, Hall-Angeras M, et al. Penetrating wounds of the neck: experience from a Swedish hospital. Acta Chir Scand 1985;151:419.
[25] Ayuyao AM, Kaledzi YL, Parsa MH, et al. Penetrating neck wounds: mandatory versus selective exploration. Ann Surg 1985;202:563.
[26] Belinkie SA, Russell JC, Da Silva J, et al. Management of penetrating neck injuries. J Trauma 1983; 23:235.
[27] Bishara RA, Pasch AR, Douglas DD, et al. The necessity of mandatory exploration of penetrating zone II neck injuries. Surgery 1986;100:655.
[28] Cabasares HV. Selective surgical management of penetrating neck trauma: 15 year experience in a community hospital. Am Surg 1982;48:355.
[29] Campbell FC, Robbs JV. Penetrating injuries of the neck: a prospective study of 108 patients. Br J Surg 1980;67:582.
[30] Carducci B, Lowe RA, Dalsey W. Penetrating neck trauma: consensus and controversies. Ann Emerg Med 1986;15:208.
[31] Cohen ES, Breaux CW, Johnson PN, et al. Penetrating neck trauma: experience with selective exploration. South Med J 1987;80:26.
[32] De la Cruz A, Chandler JR. Management of penetrating wounds of the neck. Surg Gynecol Obstet 1973;137:458.
[33] Dunbar LL, Adkins RB, Waterhouse G. Penetrating injuries to the neck: selective management. Am Surg 1984;50:198.
[34] Ordog GJ. Penetrating neck trauma. J Trauma 1987;27:543.
[35] Ordog GJ, Albin D, Wasserberger J, et al. 110 bullet wounds to the neck. J Trauma 1985;25:238.
[36] Wood J, Fabian TC, Mangianate EC. Penetrating neck injuries: recommendations for selective management. J Trauma 1989;29:602.
[37] Mansour MA, Moore EE, Moore FA, et al. Validating the selective management of penetrating neck wounds. Am J Surg 1991;162:517–20.
[38] Roden DM, Pomerantz RA. Penetrating injuries to the neck: a safe, selective approach to management. Am Surg 1993;59:750–3.
[39] Demetriades D, Charalambides D, Lakhoo M. Physical examination and selective conservative management in patients with penetrating injuries of the neck. Br J Surg 1993;80:1534–6.
[40] Atteberry LR, Dennis JW, Menawat SS, et al. Physical examination alone is safe and accurate for evaluation of vascular injuries in penetrating zone II neck trauma. J Am Coll Surg 1994;179: 657–62.
[41] Jarvik JG, Philips GR, Schwab CW, et al. Penetrating neck trauma: sensitivity of clinical examination and cost-effectiveness of angiography. AJNR Am J Neuroradiol 1995;16:647–54.
[42] Sriussadaporn S, Rattaplee P, Tharavej C, et al. Selective management of penetrating neck injuries based on clinical presentation is safe and practical. Int Surg 2002;86:90–3.
[43] Gracias VH, Reilly PM, Philpott J, et al. Computed tomography in the evaluation of penetrating neck trauma. Arch Surg 2001;136:1232–6.
[44] Prgomet D, Danic D, Milicic D, et al. Management of war-related neck injuries during the war in Croatia, 1991–1992. Eur Arch Otorhinolaryngol 1996;253:294–6.
[45] Appenzeller GN. Injury patterns in peacekeeping missions: the Kosovo experience. Mil Med 2004; 169:187–91.
[46] Xydakis MS, Fravell MD, Nasser KE, et al. Analysis of battlefield head and neck injuries in Iraq and Afghanistan. Otolaryngol Head Neck Surg 2005; 133:497–504.
[47] Wade AL, Dye JL, Mohrle CR, et al. Face and neck injuries during operation Iraqi Freedom II: results from the US Navy-Marine Corps Combat Trauma Registry. J Trauma 2007;63:836–40.
[48] Rustemeyer J, Kranz V, Bremerich A. Injuries in combat from 1982–2005 with particular reference to those to the head and neck: a review. Br J Oral Maxillofac Surg 2007;45:556–60.
[49] Osborne TE, Bays RA. Pathophysiology and management of gunshot wounds to the face. In: Fonseca RJ, Walker RV, editors. Oral and maxillofacial trauma. 2nd edition. Philadelphia: WB Saunders Co.; 1997. p. 948–74.
[50] Holt R, Kostohryz G. Wound ballistics of gunshot injuries to the head and neck. Arch Otolaryngol 1983;109:313.
[51] Steinberg C. Gunshot wounds to the head and neck. Arch Otolaryngol 1992;118:592.

[52] Saletta J, Folk F, Freeark R. Trauma to the neck region. Surg Clin North Am 1973;53:73.
[53] Committee on Trauma, American College of Surgeons. Advanced trauma life support instructors manual. Chicago: American college of Surgeons; 2005.
[54] Azuaje RE, Jacogson LE, Glover J, et al. Reliability of physical examination as a predictor of vascular injury after penetrating neck trauma. Am Surg 2003;69:804–7.
[55] Willinsky RA, Taylor SM, ter Brugge K, et al. Neurologic complications of cerebral angiography: prospective analysis of 2899 procedures and review of literature. Radiology 2003;227:L522–8.
[56] Demetriades D, Theodorou D, Cornwell E, et al. Evaluation of penetrating injuries of the neck: prospective study of 223 patients. World J Surg 1997;21:41–7.
[57] Rivers SP, Patel Y, Delanby HM, et al. Limited role of arteriography in penetrating neck trauma. J Vasc Surg 1998;8:112–6.
[58] Eddy VA. Is routine angiography mandatory for penetrating injury to zone I of the neck? Zone I Penetrating Neck Injury Study Group. J Trauma 2000;48:213–4.
[59] Munera F, Soto JA, Palacio D, et al. Diagnosis of arterial injuries caused by penetrating trauma to the neck: comparison of helical CT angiography and conventional angiography. Radiology 2000; 216:356–62.
[60] Ginzburg E, Montalvo BM, Leblang S, et al. The use of duplex ultrasonography in penetrating neck trauma. Arch Surg 1996;131:691–3.
[61] Demetriades D, Theodorou D, Cornwell E, et al. Penetrating injuries to the neck in patients in stable condition: physical examination, angiography, or color flow Doppler imaging. Arch Surg 1995;130: 971–5.
[62] Corr P, Abdool Carrim AT, Robbs J. Colour-flow ultrasound in the detection of penetrating vascular injuries of the neck. S Afr Med J 1999;89:644–6.
[63] Munera F, Morales C, Soto JA, et al. Gunshot wounds of abdomen: evaluation of stable patients with triple contrast helical CT. Radiology 2004; 231:399–405.
[64] Woo K, Magner DP, Wilson MT, et al. CT angiography in penetrating neck trauma reduces the need for operative neck exploration. Am Surg 2005;71: 754–8.
[65] Stallmeyer MJ, Morales RE, Flanders AE. Imaging of traumatic neurovascular injury. Radiol Clin North Am 2006;44:13–39.
[66] Munera F, Soto JA, Nunez D. Penetrating injuries of the neck and the increasing role of CTA. Emerg Radiol 2004;10:303–9.
[67] Mazolewski PJ, Curry JD, Browder T, et al. Computed tomographic scan can be used for surgical decision making in zone II penetrating neck injuries. J Trauma 2001;51:315–9.

[68] Chiu WC, Shanmuganathan K, Mirvis SE, et al. Determining the need for laparotomy in penetrating torso trauma: a prospective study using triple-contrast enhanced abdominopelvic computed tomography. J Trauma 2001;51:860–9.
[69] Shanmuganathan K, Mirvis SE, Chiu WC, et al. Triple-contrast helical CT in penetrating torso trauma: a prospective study to determine peritoneal violation and the need for laparotomy. AJR Am J Roentgenol 2001;177:1247–50.
[70] Soto JA, Morales C, Munera F, et al. Penetrating stab wounds to the abdomen: use of serial US and contrast-enhanced CT in stable patients. Radiology 2001;220:1015–21.
[71] Soto JA, Munera F, Cardoso N, et al. Diagnostic performance of helical CT angiography in trauma of large arteries of the extremities. J Comput Assist Tomogr 1999;23:188–96.
[72] Hanpeter DE, Demetriades D, Asensio JA, et al. Helical computed tomographic scan in the evaluation of mediastinal gunshot wounds. J Trauma 2000;49:689–94 [discussion: 694–5].
[73] Munera F, Soto JA, Palacio DM, et al. Penetrating neck injuries: helical CT angiography for initial evaluation. Radiology 2002;224:366.
[74] Saletta JD, Lowe RJ, Lim LT, et al. Penetrating trauma of the neck. J Trauma 1976;16:579–87.
[75] Kumins NH, Tober JC, Larsen PE, et al. Vertical ramus osteotomy allows exposure of the distal internal carotid to the base of the skull. Am Surg 2001;15:225–31.
[76] Panayiotopoulous YP, Taylor PR. A paper for debate: vein versus PTFE for critical limb ischemia —an unfair comparision? Eur J Vasc Endovasc Surg 1997;14:191 1983.
[77] Shah PM, Ito K, Cluss RH, et al. Expanded microporus polytetrafluoroethylene (PTFE) grafts in contaminated woulds: experimental and clinical study. J Trauma 2003;23:1030.
[78] Wylie EJ, Hein MF, Adams JE. Intercranial hemorrhage following surgical revascularization for treatment of acute strokes. J Neurosurg 1964; 21:212.
[79] Thal ER, Snyder WH, Hays RA, et al. Management of carotid artery injuries. Surgery 1974; 76:955.
[80] Liekweg WG, Greenfield LJ. Management of penetrating carotid arterial injury. Ann Surg 1978;188: 582–92.
[81] Richardson JD, Simpson C, Miller FB. Management of carotid artery trauma. Surgery 1988;104: 673.
[82] Fabian RC, George SM, Croce MA, et al. Carotid artery trauma: management based on mechanism of injury. J Trauma 1990;30:953–61.
[83] Nanda A, Vannermreddy PS, Willis BK, et al. Management of carotid artery injuries: Louisiana State University Shreveport experience. Surg Neurol 2003;59:184–90.

[84] Joo JY, Ahn JY, Chung YS, et al. Therapeutic endovascular treatments for traumatic carotid artery injuries. J Trauma 2005;58:1159–66.

[85] Fanelli F, Salvatori FM, Ferrari R, et al. Stent repair of bilateral post-traumatic dissection of the internal carotid artery. J Endovasc Ther 2004;11:517–21.

[86] Biggs KL, Chiou AC, Hagino RT, et al. Endovascular repair of a spontaneous carotid artery dissection with carotid stent and coils. J Vasc Surg 2004;40:170–3.

[87] McNeil JD, Chiou AC, Gunlock MG, et al. Successful endovascular therapy of a penetrating zone III internal carotid injury. J Vasc Surg 2002;36:187–90.

[88] du Toit DF, Strauss DC, Blaszczyk M, et al. Endovascular treatment of penetrating thoracic outlet arterial injuries. Eur J Vasc Endovasc Surg 2000;19:489–95.

[89] Cothren CC, Moore EE, Ray CE Jr, et al. Carotid artery stents for blunt cerbrovascular injury: risks exceed benefits. Arch Surg 2005;140:480–5.

[90] McConnell DD, Trunkey DD. Management of penetrating trauma to the neck. Adv Surg 1994;27:97–127.

[91] Rohman M, Ivatury RR. Esophagus. In: Ivatury RR, Cayten CG, editors. Textbook of penetrating trauma. Baltimore (MD): Williams & Wilkins; 1996. p. 555–63.

[92] Cheadle W, Richardson JD. Options in management of trauma to the esophagus. Surg Gynecol Obstet 1982;155:380–4.

[93] Asensio JA, Berne JD, Demetriades D, et al. Penetrating esophageal injuries: time interval of safety for preoperative evaluation—how long is safe? J Trauma 1997;43:319–24.

[94] Asensio JA, Chahwan S, Forno W, et al. Penetrating esophageal injuries: multicenter study of the American Association for the Surgery of Trauma. J Trauma 2001;50(2):289–96.

[95] Weigelt JA, Thal ER, Snyder WH, et al. Diagnosis of penetrating cervical esophageal injuries. Am J Surg 1987;154:619–21.

[96] Horwitz B, Krevsky B, Buchman RF, et al. Endoscopic evalaution of penetrating esophageal injuries. Am J Gastroenterol 1993;88:1249.

[97] Verschueren D, Bell RB, Bagheri SC, et al. Management of laryngo-tracheal injuries associated with craniomaxillofacial trauma. J Oral Maxillofac Surg 2006;64:203–14.

[98] Bracken MB, Shepardd MJ, Collins WF, et al. A randomized, controlled trial of methylprednisolone or naloxone in the treatment of acute spinal-cord injury. Results of the Second National Acute Spinal Cord Injury Study. N Engl J Med 1991;322(20):1459–61.

[99] Prendergast MR, Saxe JM, Ledgerwood AM, et al. Massive steroids do not reduce the zone of injury after penetrating spinal cord injury. J Trauma 1994;37:576.

[100] Thompson EC, Porter JM, Fernandez LG. Penetrating neck trauma: an overview of management. J Oral Maxillofac Surg 2002;60:918–23.

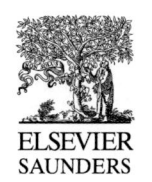

Management of Laryngeal Trauma

R. Bryan Bell, DDS, MD, FACS[a,b,*],
David S. Verschueren, DMD, MD[a,b],
Eric J. Dierks, DMD, MD, FACS[a,b]

[a]*Oral and Maxillofacial Surgery Service, Legacy Emanuel Hospital and Health Center, Portland, OR, USA*
[b]*Department of Oral and Maxillofacial Surgery, Oregon Health & Science University, Portland, OR, USA*

Laryngeal trauma is uncommon, occurring in approximately 1 patient per 14,000 to 30,000 emergency room visits [1–4] and 1 patient per 131,000 hospital admissions [5]. The incidence can be as high as 1 in 445 in seriously injured patients presenting to major urban trauma centers [6]. Laryngeal injuries often present in association with maxillofacial injuries and are potentially complicated by life threatening airway obstruction, impaired vocal function, dysphagia, chronic aspiration and death (Fig. 1). Surgeons managing patients who have maxillofacial injuries should be familiar with the diagnosis, airway management, complications, and treatment of patients who have laryngeal trauma. Functionally and anatomically complex, the larynx is partially protected by the mandible, sternum, and cervical spine. Once violated, it can rapidly become a tight space for airway compromise and collapse, requiring emergency airway stabilization and extensive reconstruction.

The most common cause of laryngeal injury is blunt trauma caused by motor vehicle collisions or sporting accidents, followed by penetrating neck injuries, such as gunshot wounds (Fig. 2) [3,5,6]. Sporting injuries, such as those associated with all-terrain vehicles (ATVs) and jet skis, are increasing in frequency and may be associated with increased risk for laryngeal injury [3]. In blunt trauma, the larynx is compressed between an intrusive object (eg, steering wheel or handlebars) and the cervical spine. Depending on the amount of compressive force and the degree of ossification of the larynx, this may result in a variety of injury patterns, ranging from simple isolated cartilaginous fractures of the thyroid cartilage requiring little or no treatment to a complex composite tissue injury with massive cartilaginous displacement, endolaryngeal disruption, or laryngotracheal separation.

The average age of patients who have laryngeal trauma has been reported to be approximately 37 years, although the distribution is wide and older patients (older than 70 years of age) tend to have poorer outcomes (Fig. 3) [5]. If the injury is severe enough to warrant surgical treatment, laryngeal trauma is associated with a longer than 13-day hospital stay and carries with it a mortality rate of approximately 1% [5].

Classification of laryngeal injuries

Injuries to the larynx can include the soft or hard tissues and may be described by the mode, site, structure, and degree [7]. The mode is either blunt or penetrating. The site of injury has been classified as supraglottic, glottic, subglottic, or a combination of all three. Additional description is provided by identifying the structures injured, such as the hyoid bone, thyroid cartilage, cricoid cartilage, and arytenoids. The degree of injury can also be appreciated by classifying the patient into a known scheme based on various clinical

* Corresponding author. Oral and Maxillofacial Surgery Service, Legacy Emanuel Hospital and Health Center, 1849 NW Kearney, Suite 300, Portland, OR 97209
E-mail address: bellb@hnsa1.com (R.B. Bell)

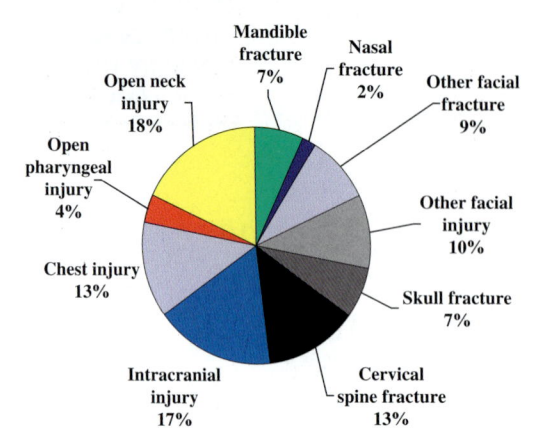

Fig. 1. Primary diagnoses, excluding external laryngeal trauma. (*Data from* Jewett BS, Shockley WW, Rutledge R. External laryngeal trauma analysis of 392 patients. Arch Otolaryngol Head Neck Surg 1999;125: 877.)

and radiographic factors. Schaefer and his colleagues [2] described the most well-known classification based on the severity of the injury and the level of management necessary, but they did so largely in the pre-CT scan era. The authors have subsequently modified this classification scheme slightly to incorporate technologic advances in imaging that serve to make a more contemporary management tool and a useful therapeutic guide (Fig. 4) [6].

Blunt trauma resulting from motor vehicle accidents accounts for most laryngeal injuries that are seen in civilian trauma centers [6]. Although penetrating injuries are seen less frequently outside of a war zone, it has been the authors' experience that they are typically more severe and result in greater endolaryngeal disruption and potentially poorer outcomes.

It is important to identify accurately the site of injury during assessment of the patient. Trauma to the supraglottic larynx may result in a variety of injuries, including epiglottic hematoma or avulsion, hyoid bone fracture, thyroid cartilage fracture, arytenoid dislocation or degloving, endolaryngeal edema, and airway obstruction. Epiglottic hematoma may progress to inspiratory stridor and voice changes (Fig. 5). Epiglottic avulsion may occur in association with fractures of the hyoid and thyroid cartilage and results in epiglottic displacement superiorly. The result is profound dysphagia and aspiration. Fiberoptic nasopharyngoscopy is generally diagnostic; however, concomitant bleeding and edema may make awake endoscopy challenging. Therefore, direct laryngoscopy under anesthesia may be necessary to appreciate fully the extent of endolaryngeal injury. Arytenoid subluxation is a common finding in patients who has significant laryngeal injuries and may result in vocal cord dysfunction. Fractures of the hyoid bone are relatively common in sporting injuries, such as baseball, jet skiing, and karate (Fig. 6). Severe painful dysphagia is the most common symptom. Isolated fractures of the hyoid may provide little in the way of physical findings, although the injury is readily identified on CT scan.

Patients who have glottic injuries often present with hoarseness that is generally associated with fractures of the thyroid cartilage (Fig. 7). Such injuries may result in vocal cord edema, endolaryngeal lacerations, or avulsion of the vocal cords from the anterior commissure. Shortening of the vocal cords is associated with seemingly minimal displacement of the thyroid cartilage and has the potential for significant vocal changes unless accurately reduced.

Subglottic injuries typically involve the cricoid cartilage and cervical trachea and often result in profound airway compromise immediately after the injury. Complete cricotracheal disruption with acute airway obstruction is associated with rapid death unless prompt corrective measures are used (Fig. 8). Immediate airway stabilization in the form of a tracheostomy is usually necessary and is often performed in the field. Among survivors, associated findings may include recurrent laryngeal

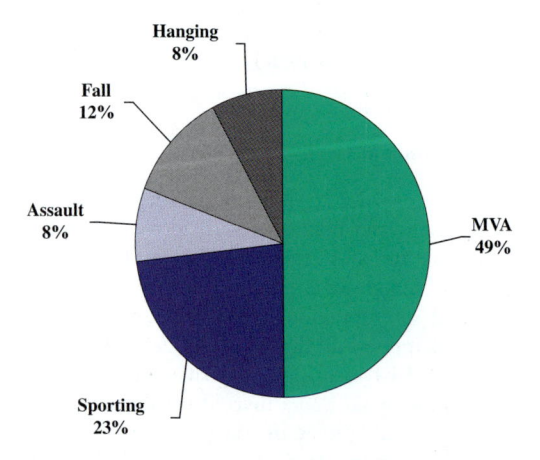

Fig. 2. Cause of laryngeal fractures: Legacy Emanuel Hospital and Health Center, 1992 to 2004. MVA, motor vehicle accident.

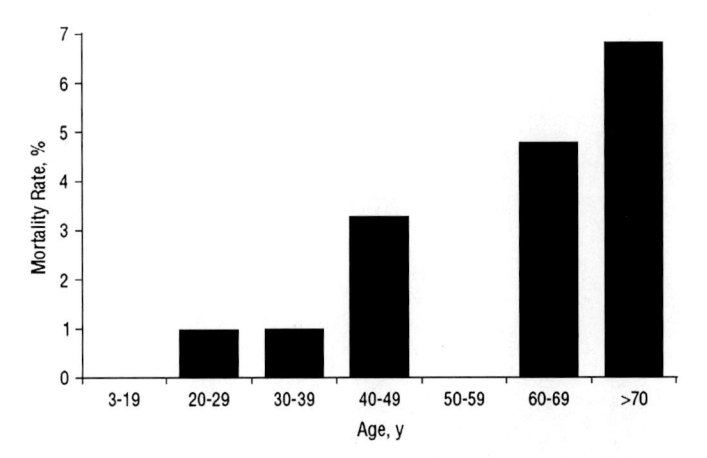

Fig. 3. External laryngeal trauma: age versus mortality. (*From* Jewett BS, Shockley WW, Rutledge R. External laryngeal trauma analysis of 392 patients. Arch Otolaryngol Head Neck Surg 1999;125:877; with permission.)

nerve injury, cricothyroid separation, and laryngotracheal separation.

Evaluation

The clinician should have a high suspicion for laryngeal injury in any patient who has blunt or penetrating neck trauma, particularly those patients presenting with cervical subcutaneous emphysema manifested as crepitus, or cervical ecchymosis (Fig. 9) [8]. Diagnosis of laryngeal injury in a timely manner is important for treatment and prognosis. Evaluation of laryngeal trauma begins with ensuring a patent airway. The force of the injury can cause significant soft tissue and cartilaginous disruption with minimal external signs of laryngeal trauma. As noted previously, common signs of laryngeal injury include stridor,

	Clinical Presentation	Diagnostic Findings	Management
Stage 1	Minor airway symptoms +/- voice changes	Minor hematomas Small Lacerations No detectable fractures	Observation Humidified air Head of bed elevation
Stage 2	Airway compromise Voice changes +/- subcutaneous emphysema	Edema/hematoma nondisplaced fracture Minor mucosal disruption No cartilage exposure	Direct laryngoscopy +/- ORIF
Stage 3	Airway compromise Palpable laryngeal fx Subcutaneous emphysema Voice changes	Massive edema Mucosal tears Class 2 Exposed cartilage Vocal cord immobility	Direct laryngoscopy Exploration/ORIF
Stage 4	Airway compromise Palpable laryngeal fx Subcutaneous emphysema Voice changes	Massive edema Mucosal tears Multiple displaced fractures Skeletal instability Exposed cartilage Vocal cord immobility	Direct laryngoscopy Exploration/ORIF Consider stent

Stage 2-4 receive immediate, "awake" tracheostomy if airway not already secured in the field

Fig. 4. Legacy Emanuel Hospital and Health Center laryngeal injury classification. fx, fracture.

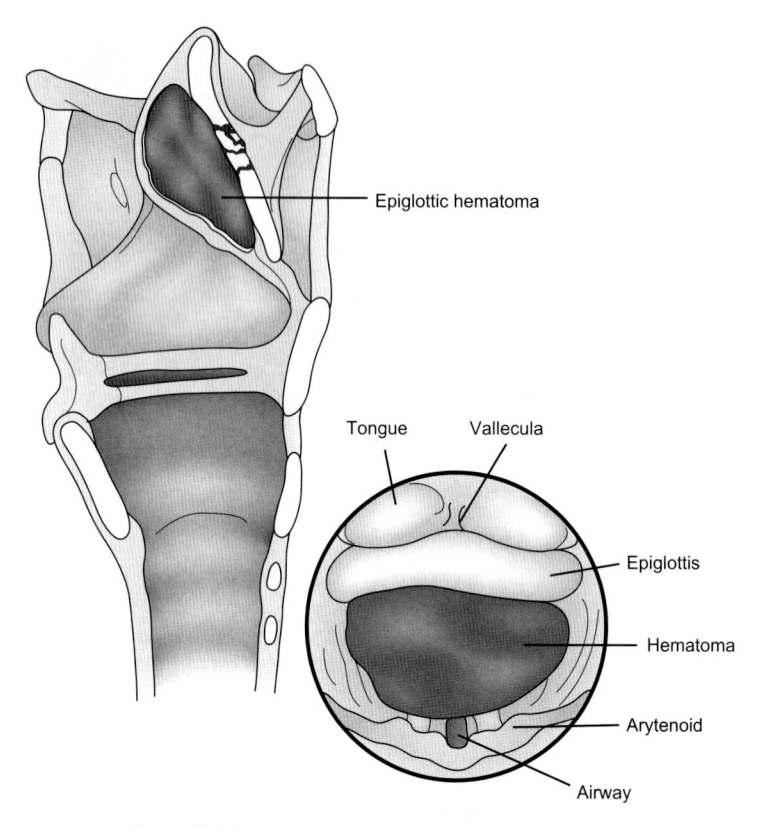

Fig. 5. Epiglottic hematoma causing airway obstruction.

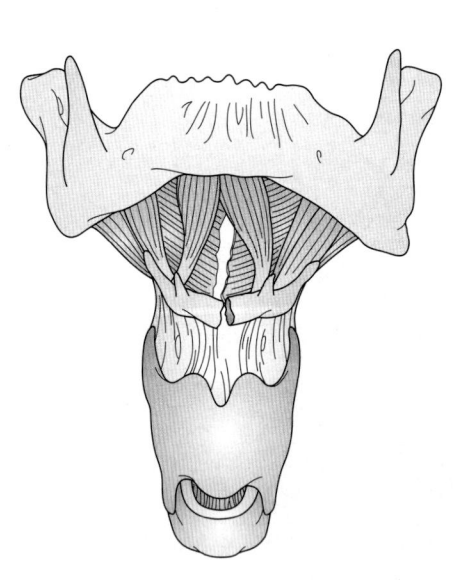

Fig. 6. Fracture of the hyoid bone. Asymptomatic patients require no specific treatment. Pain and odynophagia are treated by open reduction and internal fixation or partial hyoid resection.

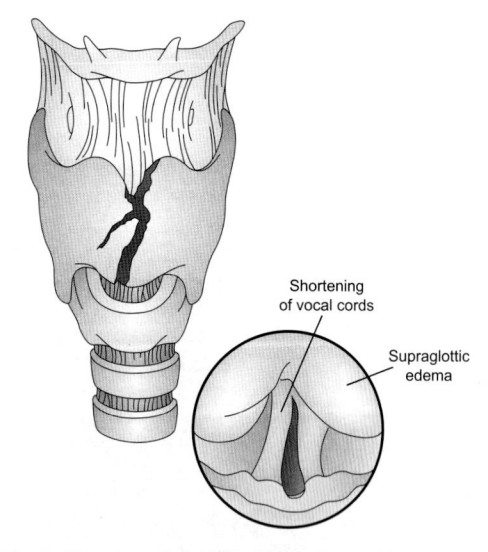

Fig. 7. Fracture of the thyroid cartilage with associated glottic injuries resulting in vocal cord edema, endolaryngeal lacerations, or avulsion from the anterior commissure. Shortening of the vocal cords is associated with seemingly minimal displacement of the thyroid cartilage and has the potential for significant vocal changes unless accurately reduced.

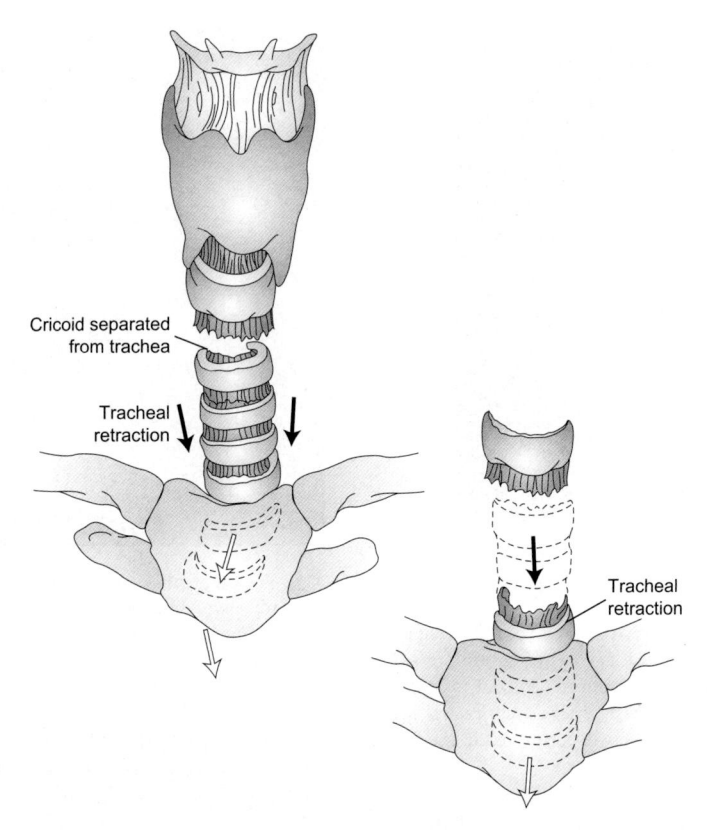

Fig. 8. Laryngotracheal separation causes upward retraction of the larynx and downward retraction of the trachea and commonly results in fatal airway obstruction.

vocal changes, subcutaneous emphysema, hemoptysis, hematoma, ecchymosis, laryngeal tenderness, vocal cord immobility, loss of anatomic landmarks, crepitus, and difficulty in swallowing. The preferred artificial airway in patients who have a laryngeal fracture is a tracheostomy, which should be performed with the patient awake under local anesthesia if possible [9]. Although oral endotracheal intubation is not contraindicated, care must be taken to avoid further disruption of the endolaryngeal structures, creation of a "false passage" into a submucosal pocket, or facilitation of potentially catastrophic laryngotracheal separation. Once the airway has been secured, associated cervical spine, esophageal, and vascular injuries can then be evaluated.

The workup of laryngeal trauma includes physical examination, radiologic examination, and panendoscopy. A thorough physical examination, particularly focused on neck tenderness, crepitus secondary to subcutaneous emphysema, soft tissue edema, and loss of anatomic landmarks, is part of the standard secondary survey according to the American College of Surgeons Advanced Trauma Life Support (ATLS) guidelines. In stable patients, this may include flexible fiberoptic laryngoscopy to examine the extent of endolaryngeal injury and to provide valuable information about vocal cord function and mobility (Fig. 10). Fiberoptic examination can also help to determine if the patient's airway is adequate before placing the patient in the CT scanner.

CT is the single most important diagnostic tool currently available [10]. Fine-cut CT imaging allows rapid and precise anatomic evaluation of the cartilaginous framework, even in minimally displaced cartilaginous fractures, and provides evidence of upper aerodigestive tract injury with subcutaneous emphysema (Fig. 11). Angiography can also be added when needed for penetrating injuries to help evaluate vascular injuries.

Formal endoscopic evaluation using direct laryngoscopy, esophagoscopy, and bronchoscopy allows the treating surgeon to visualize the upper aerodigestive tract and extent of mucosal injury

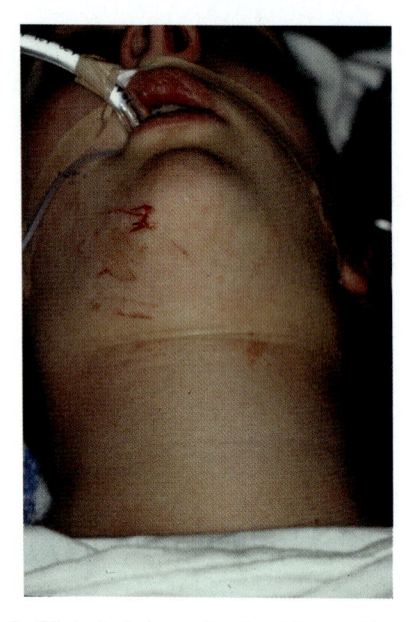

Fig. 9. Clinical photograph of a 19-year-old woman with a significantly displaced laryngeal fracture presenting with cervical edema and crepitus, loss of anatomic landmarks in the neck, and progressive dyspnea and stridor. Endotracheal intubation was performed in the field before the diagnosis.

fully. CT, direct laryngoscopy, and rigid esophagoscopy are the most effective tools to define or clarify the nature of the upper aerodigestive tract. The authors recently published their experience

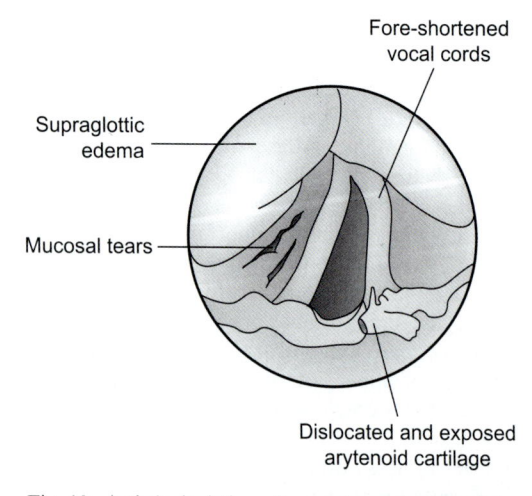

Fig. 10. Artist's depiction of an endoscopic view of the glottic larynx demonstrates distortion of normal anatomy, shortening of the vocal cords, mucosal disruption, and dislocation of the arytenoid cartilage.

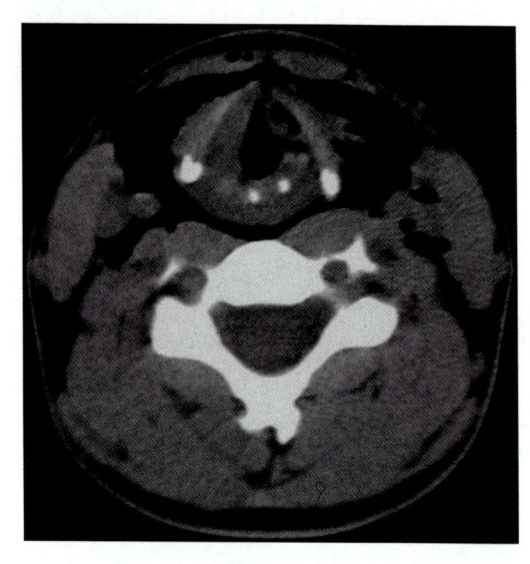

Fig. 11. CT scan of a patient who has a laryngeal fracture involving the thyroid and cricoid cartilage demonstrates subcutaneous emphysema.

with laryngotracheal injuries at Legacy Emanuel Hospital in Portland, Oregon, which incorporated these advancements into a classification scheme and a protocol for the management of patients who have laryngeal fractures based on airway status, high-definition CT, and physical examination (Fig. 12) [6]. The remainder of this article further defines this management protocol and provides the reader with a rational therapeutic approach.

Management

Historical perspectives

Management of laryngeal trauma may include nonsurgical or surgical treatment depending on the status of the airway, CT or CT angiography (CTA) findings, and the amount of cartilaginous displacement (Fig. 13). Advances in diagnostic imaging and refinements in surgical technique have altered the management of patients who have laryngotracheal injuries. The goal of treatment is to restore the three primary functions of the larynx—airway, voice, and swallowing—and to prevent complications, such as airway embarrassment, dysphonia, tracheal or laryngeal stenosis, and dysphagia.

Because of the infrequency of laryngeal trauma, few individuals have extensive experience with the management of complex laryngotracheal

MANAGEMENT OF LARYNGEAL TRAUMA 421

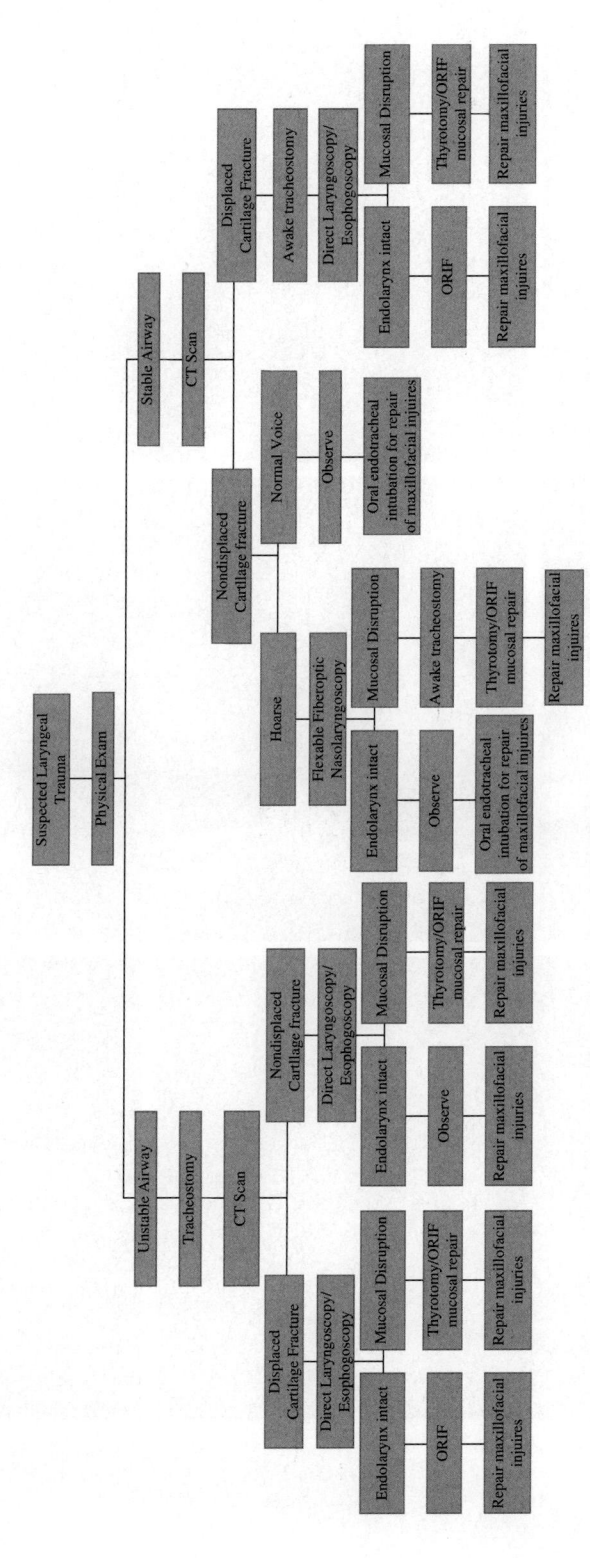

Fig. 12. Legacy Emanuel Hospital and Health Center protocol for the management of laryngotracheal injuries. ORIF, open reduction and internal fixation.

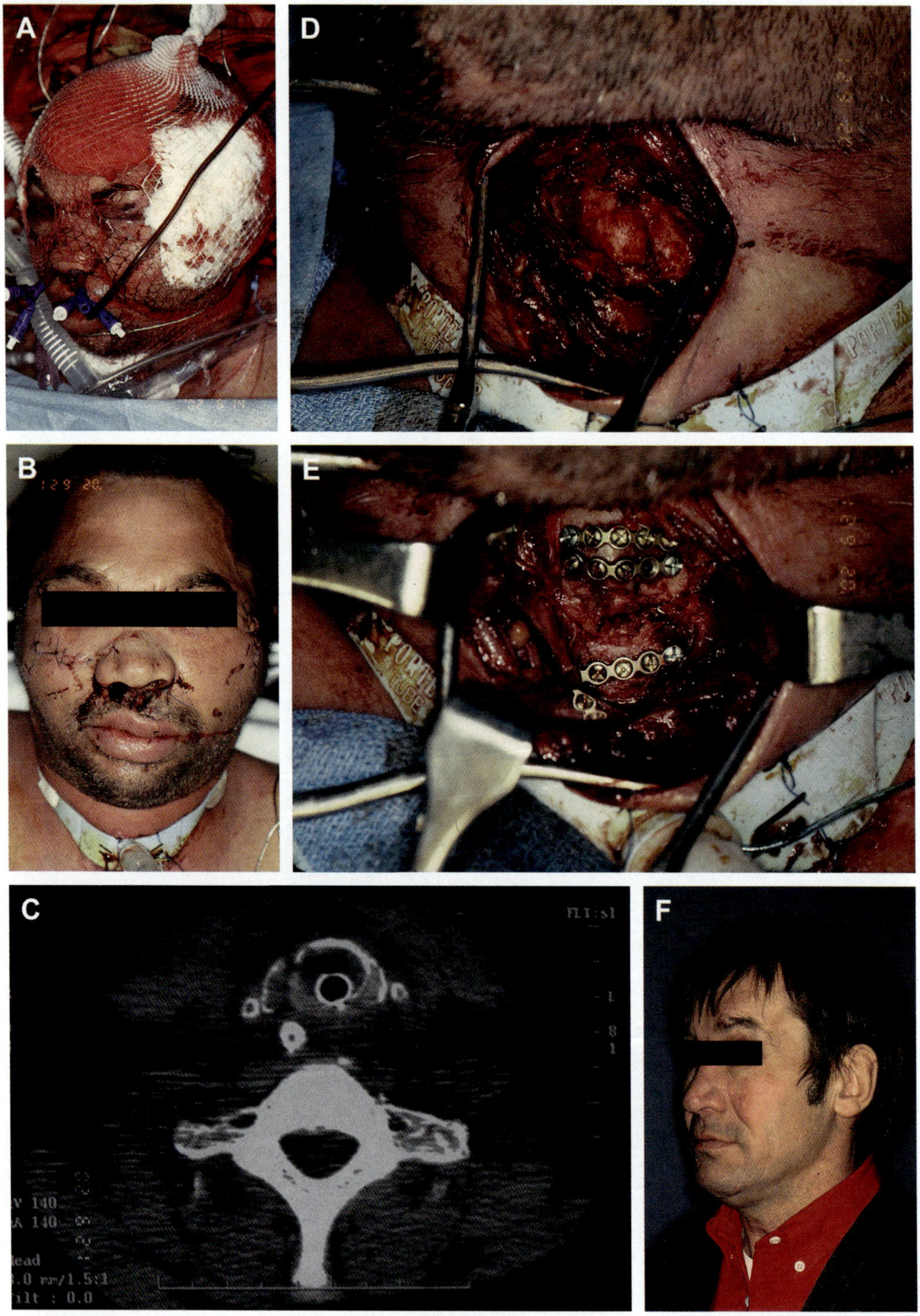
A
D
B
E
C
F

injuries; therefore, most treatment recommendations emanate from retrospective reviews of single-surgeon experience [1–6,11–25]. In 1983, Leopold [3] reviewed more than 200 cases in the literature and analyzed surgical versus medical treatment, type and duration of stenting techniques, and time interval between injury and surgery. He concluded that laryngeal trauma treated medically within 24 hours, without a stent, and without penetrating trauma resulted in better voice and airway function compared with patients managed surgically after 48 hours with a stent and with blunt trauma. Leopold [3] also concluded that the best results were obtained when stents were used for only 2 to 4 weeks.

In 1986, Gussack and colleagues [4] reviewed 12 case series with a combined total of 392 cases of laryngeal trauma and compared that with their own experience. These investigators concluded that laryngotracheal trauma is rare and that complications like laryngeal stenosis and voice changes occur in as many as 40% of the cases. Decannulation and airway patency were assured without stenosis or significant granulation tissue in most patients.

In 1993, Bent and colleagues [23] reviewed their treatment of 77 patients who have laryngeal trauma. These authors concluded that conservative treatment of Schaefer group 1 and 2 injuries is 100% effective and that surgical repair within 48 hours greatly reduced poor outcomes. The investigators determined that based on the Schaefer classification of degree of injury, one can roughly predict patient outcome for voice and airway function. In addition, they concluded that penetrating trauma is neither more common nor less serious than blunt trauma and that almost all patients are decannulated with functional speech and normal deglutination.

To date, Schaefer and his colleagues [1,2,12] have reported the most extensive experience in the English literature, describing outcomes in 139 patients treated at Parkland Memorial Hospital in Dallas, Texas from 1965 to 1991. He concluded that there was an increase in penetrating assault trauma and a decrease in motor vehicle collisions but found no difference in voice or airway outcome between blunt versus penetrating trauma specifically. He noted, however, that patients who had penetrating trauma tended to have worse overall injuries. He recommended conservation of all anatomy when possible and the use of flexible fiberoptic laryngoscopy as a diagnostic tool. Although most of his experience occurred before the high-resolution CT scan era, he questioned the use of CT when physical examination obviously demonstrated the need for surgical intervention. Rigid esophagoscopy was considered more sensitive than flexible endoscopy for evaluating injuries in the pharyngoesophageal region. Oral intubation was considered hazardous because of the possibility of serious iatrogenic complications; therefore, tracheotomy under local anesthesia for all patients suspected of having laryngeal trauma requiring airway support was recommended. Patients in Schaefer groups 1 and 2 generally experienced full recovery without surgical intervention. Surgical intervention in groups 3 and 4 within 24 hours was efficacious with open reduction and internal fixation (ORIF) of cartilaginous fractures. Stents were avoided when possible.

Most recently, the authors reviewed their single-institution experience at an urban, level 1 trauma center and specifically examined the incidence of concomitant maxillofacial injuries in association with laryngeal trauma [6]. They also modified Schaefer's classification scheme by incorporating a more contemporary view of CT imaging (see Fig. 4). Laryngeal injuries occurred in 1 per 445 severely injured patients presenting to a level 1 trauma center with head, face, or neck injuries (incidence = 0.002). Ninety-six percent (26 of 27) of the patients who had laryngotracheal trauma also had maxillofacial injuries. These findings suggest that laryngeal injuries may be under-recognized at dedicated trauma care centers and emphasize the importance of airway management

---

Fig. 13. A 42-year-old male assault victim with severe multisystem trauma, including panfacial fractures and highly disrupted fractures of the thyroid and cricoid cartilage. (*A*) Clinical appearance after initial stabilization that included emergent tracheostomy and nasal packing for severe epistaxis. (*B*) Clinical appearance 1 week before definitive management of his laryngeal injuries and facial injuries. Treatment was delayed because of concomitant systemic injuries, systemic inflammatory response, and disseminated intravascular coagulation. (*C*) CT scan of the same patient demonstrates fractures involving the thyroid cartilage. (*D*) Intraoperative exposure for repair of laryngeal injuries. (*E*) ORIF of thyroid cartilage and cricoid ring. There was no significant endolaryngeal injury. (*F*) Postoperative appearance of patient 6 months after injury.

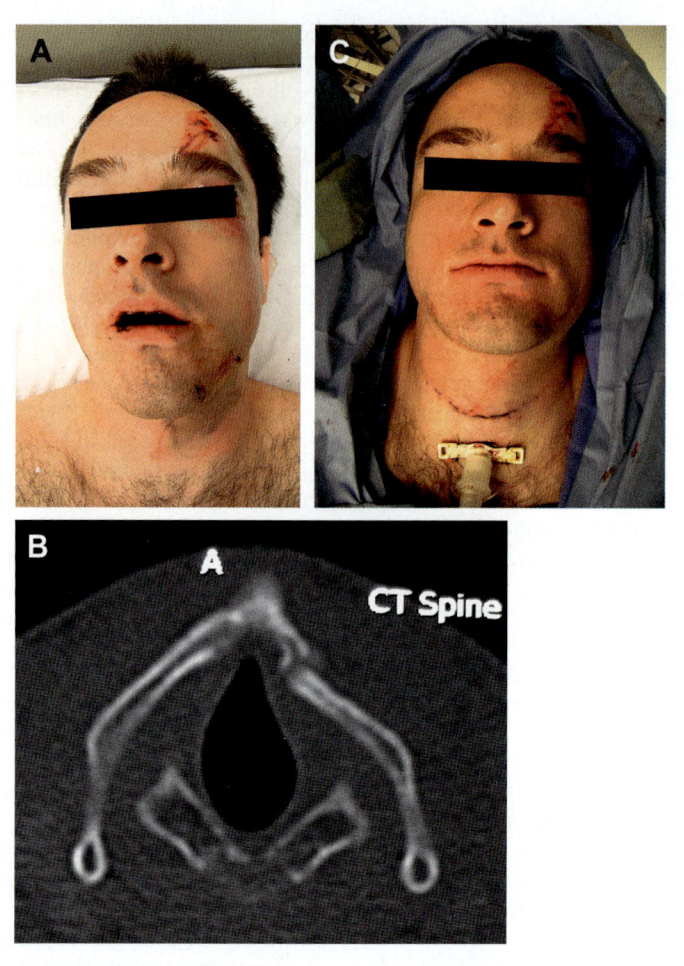

Fig. 14. A 36-year-old man involved in a bicycle accident sustained a displaced mandibular fracture in addition to laryngeal injuries. (*A*) Clinical appearance at presentation to the emergency room demonstrates cervical ecchymosis and edema, stridor, and malocclusion. (*B*) CT scan of the same patient demonstrates displaced fracture of the thyroid cartilage. (*C*) Postoperative appearance of the same patient immediately after awake tracheostomy, repair of the laryngeal injuries by ORIF of the thyroid cartilage, and ORIF of the mandibular fracture.

to all clinicians charged with caring for patients at a trauma center. Most patients in this study required an advanced airway, generally a tracheostomy, which is similar to other published reports [1–5]. Because of the fragile nature of the endolarynx, upper airway intervention takes precedence over repair of facial injuries. This study demonstrates that function and form can be restored to the larynx and the maxillofacial skeleton by adherence to a sound management protocol. All patients in this series who returned for follow-up had a functional voice and were successfully decannulated. Most patients (93%) thought that they had normal deglutition. Delayed treatment of all facial injuries did not result in unfavorable facial esthetics or occlusal function. Because of the limited number of patients who presented to follow-up, the authors were unable to draw statistically significant data from the study population. Nevertheless, there was a general trend among the current patient population suggesting a positive correlation between complications, such as hoarseness, and the severity of injury as assessed by the Emanuel laryngeal injury classification.

Nonsurgical treatment

Nonsurgical management should be limited to patients who have minor mucosal injuries and no airway compromise. This generally involves head of bed elevation to 30° to 45°, bed rest, voice rest, humidified air, clear liquid diet, corticosteroids, antibiotics, and antireflux medications (eg, H_2 antagonists, proton pump inhibitors) that help to reduce granulation tissue formation.

Surgical technique

The rationale for surgery in patients who have laryngotracheal trauma has been discussed previously. Various treatment approaches have been advocated, depending on the extent of the endolaryngeal injury and the amount of cartilaginous displacement, which include nonoperative management, open reduction with wire fixation, open reduction with rigid plate fixation, and the placement of endolaryngeal stents [1–31].

If surgery of any significance is indicated, the authors recommend a tracheostomy before repair of the laryngeal structures. Repair should be undertaken urgently, ideally within 24 hours of the injury. Significant delays, some of which cannot be avoided in patients who have severe multisystem injuries and coagulopathy, are likely to increase the chances of laryngeal stenosis, scarring, and granulation formation.

Step 1: Tracheostomy

If the patient has not already had an emergency airway placed, and the airway is relatively stable, he or she is taken directly to the operating room for an awake tracheostomy performed under local anesthesia and in the presence of an anesthesiologist (Fig. 14). Using cervical spine precautions if indicated, or a shoulder roll if tolerated, a standard horizontal tracheostomy incision is made approximately half of the way between the sternal notch and the cricothyroid membrane. Injury permitting, the tracheotomy is made between the second and third tracheal rings. A single-lumen cuffed tracheostomy tube of appropriate diameter (generally size 6, 7, or 8 in adults) or a reinforced flexible endotracheal tube is placed and sutured to the skin.

Step 2: Endoscopic evaluation

Once the airway is stabilized, a direct laryngoscopy is performed using an anterior commissure scope to evaluate the oropharynx, hypopharynx, supraglottic larynx, and larynx. After this, an esophagoscopy is performed to evaluate the cervical esophagus, which may be concomitantly injured. The authors' preference has been to use a rigid esophagoscope; however, other investigators prefer a flexible scope, and the decision is one of surgeon comfort and experience. Although flexible endoscopy allows the option of photographic documentation of injuries, there is no convincing evidence that one option is better than the other [32]. A rigid or flexible bronchoscopy may also be helpful to ascertain the full extent of the injury, particularly in more complex laryngotracheal trauma. On completion of the endoscopic evaluation, a surgical plan may be finalized before formal neck exploration.

Step 3: Neck exploration

A horizontal, middle, or low cervical incision is made extending between the anterior borders of the sternocleidomastoid muscles at a level midway between the sternal notch and the thyroid cartilage (see Fig. 14C). Superior and inferior skin flaps are developed in a subplatysmal plane, extending from the sternal notch to the hyoid bone, and sutured to the adjacent skin. The strap muscles are separated in the midline and retracted laterally. If esophageal injury is noted or suspected by clinical or radiographic examination, it is wise to skeletonize the anterior-medial aspect of the sternocleidomastoid and identify, preserve, and protect the carotid artery, jugular vein, and vagus nerve. The thyroid cartilage is identified, and the extent of cartilaginous injury is determined (Fig. 15). Depending on the amount of disruption, a midline thyrotomy may be necessary for endolaryngeal repair. A midline thyrotomy is performed with an oscillating saw and carried to the anterior commissure, which is divided with a number 12 scalpel, thus facilitating lateral

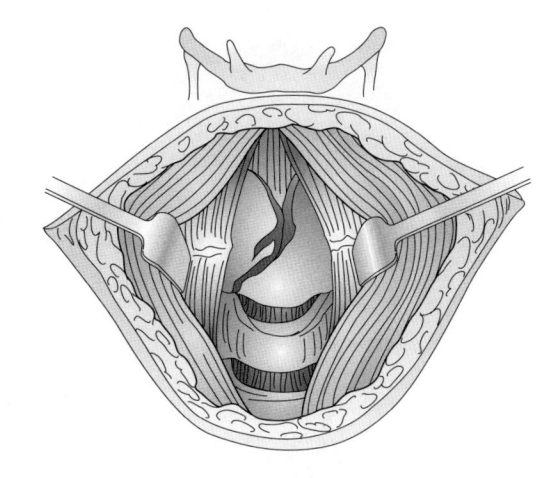

Fig. 15. Thyroid and cricoid cartilage is identified by careful dissection and retraction of the strap muscles, and the extent of cartilaginous injury is determined.

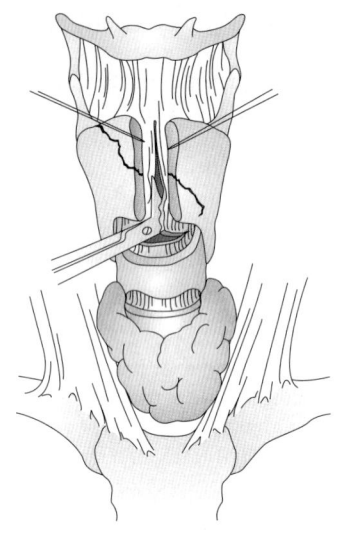

Fig. 16. Midline thyrotomy is performed with an oscillating saw and carried to the anterior commissure, which is divided with a number 12 scalpel or scissors, thus facilitating lateral retraction of the thyroid or cricoid cartilage and allowing visualization of the endolaryngeal structures.

retraction of the thyroid or cricoid cartilage and allowing visualization of the endolaryngeal structures (Fig. 16). If exploration of the neck or endoscopic evaluation demonstrates an esophageal injury, the esophagus is repaired primarily, before addressing the laryngeal injury. A nasogastric tube or appropriately sized Bougie tube is inserted into the esophagus to facilitate repair.

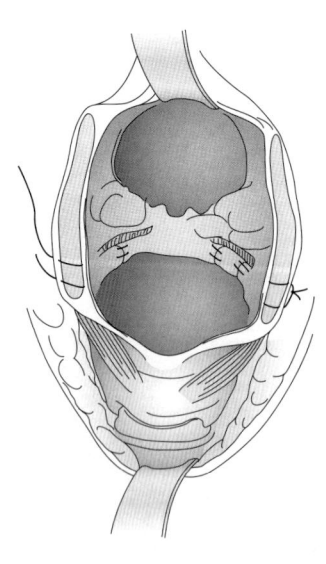

Fig. 17. View of the endolarynx demonstrates mucosal lacerations that are closed with 3-0 or 4-0 chromic sutures.

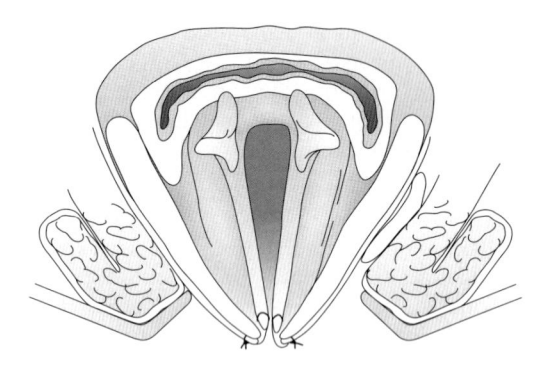

Fig. 18. Anterior attachment of the vocal cord to the thyroid cartilage (Broyle's ligament) is resuspended to the external perichondrium with 4-0 PDS suture.

Step 4: Laryngotracheal repair

As stated previously, a laryngofissure is occasionally necessary to visualize the endolarynx directly so as to repair mucosal lacerations or to resuspend disrupted arytenoids. The authors have found that a formal laryngofissure is not necessary in most significantly displaced laryngeal fractures, because the exposure is already facilitated by the injury. Once identified, endolaryngeal mucosal lacerations are closed with 4-0 chromic sutures (Fig. 17). If the arytenoid has been dislocated, an attempt should be made to manipulate it into its normal anatomic position. If the anterior attachment of the vocal cord to the thyroid cartilage (Broyle's ligament) is disrupted, it should be

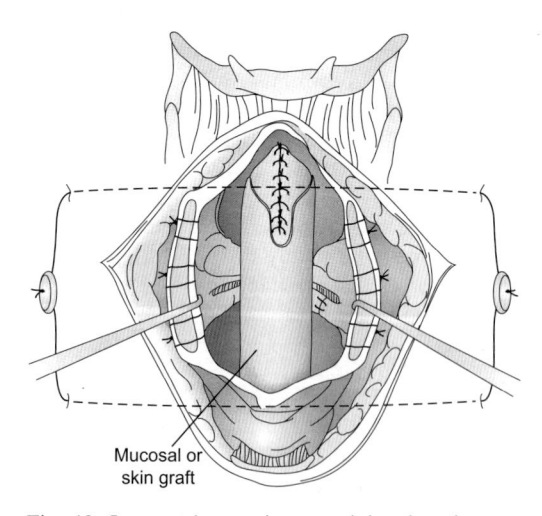

Fig. 19. Laryngeal stent is secured in place by two sutures placed through the skin, thyroid lamina, and subglottic space and out through the opposite thyroid lamina and skin. The sutures are tied loosely over silicone buttons.

resuspended to the external perichondrium with 4-0 PDS suture (Fig. 18). If primary repair of the mucosal or vocal cord injury is not possible, consideration must be given to placing a stent, with or without a skin graft (Fig. 19). The laryngeal stent is secured in place by two sutures placed through the skin, thyroid lamina, and subglottic space and out through the opposite thyroid lamina and skin. The sutures are tied loosely over silicone buttons. There is no universally accepted length of time that a laryngeal stent should be left in place [1,3–5]. The authors generally recommend 2 weeks, which allows for adequate mucosalization and cartilaginous healing (Fig. 20).

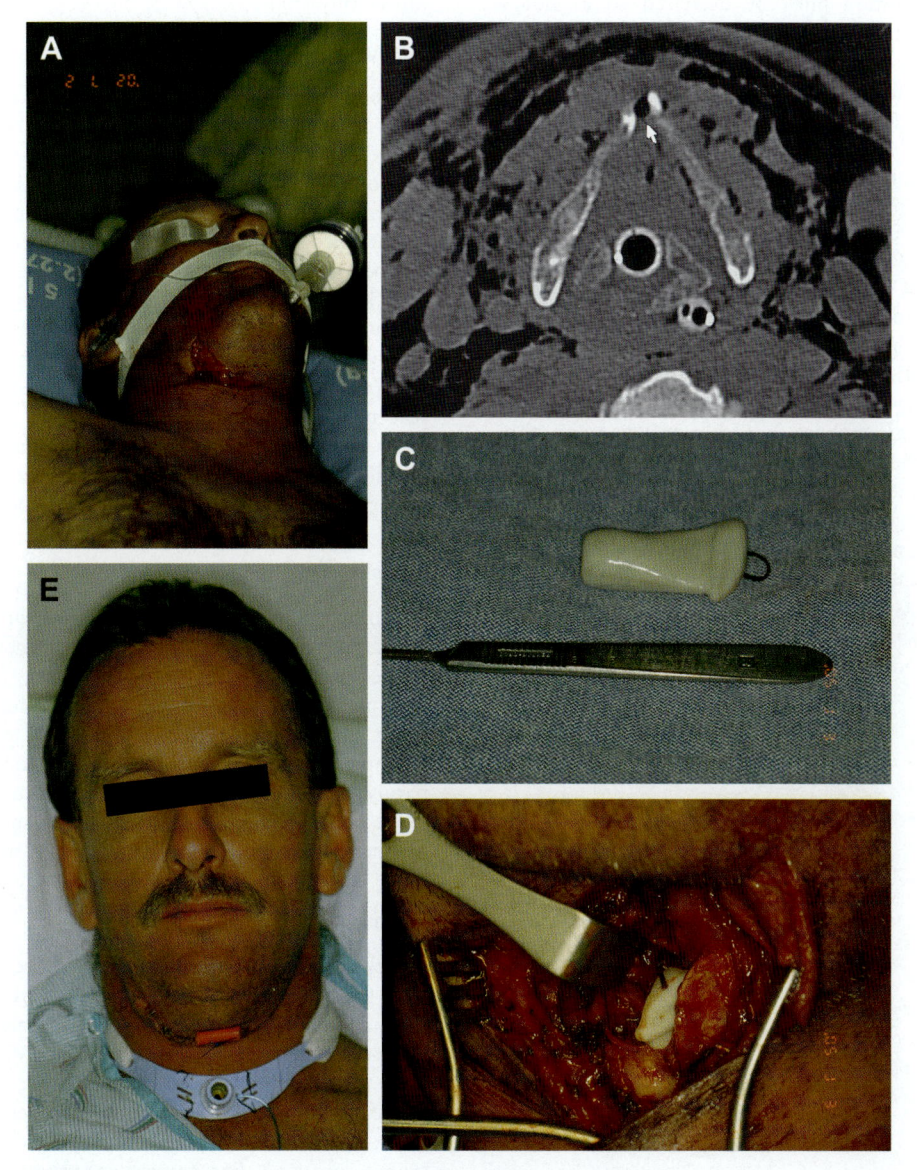

Fig. 20. A 43-year-old longshoreman involved in a "clothesline-like" boating accident. (*A*) Preoperative appearance of the patient on arrival to the emergency room. The patient was intubated in the field because of upper airway obstruction. (*B*) CT scan of the same patient demonstrates massive subcutaneous emphysema suggestive of upper aerodigestive tract injury. (*C*) Montgomery stent. (*D*) Laryngeal stent is secured in place by two sutures placed through the skin, thyroid lamina, and subglottic space and out through the opposite thyroid lamina and skin. The sutures are tied loosely over silicone buttons. (*E*) Postoperative appearance of the same patient 1 week after treatment.

Although rarely encountered, the most severe injury is complete laryngotracheal separation. Patients often die of airway obstruction before reaching a hospital. The tracheal stump may be mobilized cephalad into the neck using Babcock forceps. Anterior and posterior dissection of the trachea can be facilitated by flexing the neck forward. An infrahyoid myotomy is rarely necessary. Caution must be exercised so as not to dissect the tracheoesophageal groove extensively laterally, which contains the blood supply to the trachea and the recurrent laryngeal nerves. Once mobilized, a tension-free anastomosis of the tracheal stump to the cricoid ring is performed using 2-0 Prolene or wire suture. Suspensory sutures to the prevertebral fascia are also helpful.

Step 5: Cartilage stabilization

After repair of the internal larynx, attention is turned to repair of the cartilaginous elements. The thyroid and cricoid cartilages are anatomically reduced and stabilized with titanium or biodegradable miniplate and screw fixation (Fig. 21). Particular emphasis is paid to reducing and stabilizing the cricoid cartilage anatomically, because this is the only circumferential ring in the airway. If the hyoid bone is fractured, this is repaired as well. Some investigators have advocated removal of a central portion of the bone to prevent the segments from rubbing together [7]. Although treatment is not always required, the authors prefer to reduce displaced fractures anatomically and provide rigid internal fixation with titanium plates and screws. Once the external larynx is closed, the wound is closed in layers by first reapproximating the strap muscles in the midline. The superior and inferior skin flaps are then closed by reapproximating the platysma layer and skin closure achieved with nylon or staples. A Penrose drain is placed to drain fluids and to avoid subcutaneous emphysema.

Postoperative care

The authors' preference is to avoid oral intake with nasogastric tube feeding for approximately 2 weeks after significant laryngoesophageal disruption. In isolated laryngeal injuries, however, a clear liquid diet is initiated whenever practical. The tracheostomy tube is left in place for at least 5 to 7 days. Decannulation is accomplished whenever feasible, depending on the severity of the injury, and often occurs after hospital discharge. Antibiotics are continued for 7 days after surgery. Removal of the stent occurs 2 to 3 weeks after placement. Endoscopic laser excision of granulation tissue is commonly needed after severe injuries. Referral to a laryngologist is optimal for postoperative re-evaluation and subsequent care.

Complications

Complications for complex injuries are common and can be divided into acute and chronic. Acute complications include upper airway obstruction and asphyxiation, recurrent laryngeal nerve injury, postoperative hematoma, and infection. Chronic complications include vocal cord paralysis and hoarseness; recurrent granulation tissue formation; supraglottic, glottic, subglottic or tracheal stenosis; and chronic aspiration.

Summary

Several common conclusions can be drawn from the existing literature, all of which are limited by small sample size and retrospective nature. First, early intervention within the first 24 to 48 hours leads to the best results for the airway and voice. These findings support early repair of mucosal and cartilaginous anatomy that theoretically decreases granulation and fibrous tissue formation. The authors support this contention and recommend early repair of all laryngeal injuries, preferably in the first 24 hours of presentation.

Second, for patients who have Emanuel laryngeal injury stage 2 or greater, the preferred airway

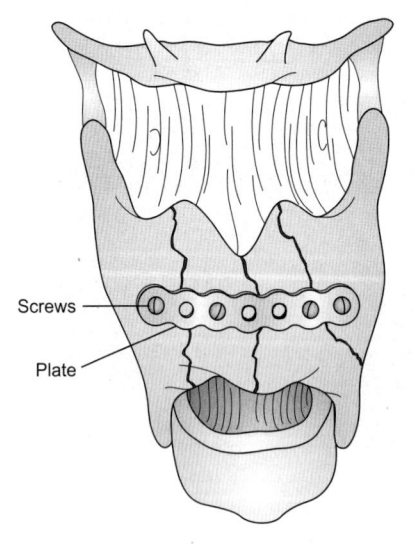

Fig. 21. Cartilaginous fragments are anatomically reduced and stabilized with titanium or biodegradable plates and screws.

is a tracheostomy. Of course, with acute airway obstruction and impending death, any airway is a good airway and ventilation should be secured by any means possible. Commonly, patients present to the emergency department with progressive respiratory failure or with significant laryngeal trauma and a currently stable airway. It is in these patients that an awake tracheostomy, performed under local anesthesia, can circumvent the potential iatrogenic sequelae of oral endotracheal intubation.

Third, patients managed conservatively have more favorable results. This conclusion has often been repeated in prior studies and should probably be considered inaccurate. It is important to recognize that patients who received nonoperative treatment usually had less severe injuries, and, subsequently, the rate of suboptimal outcomes increased with the severity of laryngeal injuries. It is more accurate to state that "less severe injuries have more favorable outcome, and surgical repair is rarely required for less severe injuries." It is the authors' opinion that laryngeal fractures, or those with Emanuel laryngeal injury stage 2, 3, or 4 injuries (or Schaefer group 2–4 injuries), should be managed with aggressive surgery to prevent the complications of hoarseness, laryngeal stenosis, and dysphagia. Although the authors prefer to avoid the use of endolaryngeal stents, if the injury involves complex endolaryngeal mucosal and arytenoid disruption, a stent may be required.

Fourth, successful decannulation, airway patency, a functional voice, and normal deglutition can be expected in most patients who have laryngeal injuries and are managed with prompt airway stabilization and proper surgical repair when indicated [1,3–5].

Fractures of the larynx are uncommon injuries that may be associated with maxillofacial trauma. Clinicians treating maxillofacial injuries should be familiar with the signs and symptoms of laryngeal fractures and with proper airway management. A timely evaluation of the larynx, rapid airway intervention, and proper surgical repair are essential for a successful outcome.

References

[1] Schaefer SD. The acute management of external laryngeal trauma. A 27-year experience. Arch Otolaryngol Head Neck Surg 1992;118(6):598–604.
[2] Trone TH, Schaefer SD, Carder HM. Blunt and penetrating laryngeal trauma: a 13-year review. Otolaryngol Head Neck Surg 1980;88(3):257–61.
[3] Leopold DA. Laryngeal trauma. A historical comparison of treatment methods. Arch Otolaryngol 1983;109(2):106–12.
[4] Gussack GS, Jurkovich GJ, Luterman A. Laryngotracheal trauma: a protocol approach to a rare injury. Laryngoscope 1986;96:660–5.
[5] Jewett BS, Shockley WW, Rutledge R. External laryngeal trauma analysis of 392 patients. Arch Otolaryngol Head Neck Surg 1999;125:877–80.
[6] Verschueren DS, Bell RB, Bagheri SB, et al. Management of laryngo-tracheal injuries associated with craniomaxillofacial trauma. J Oral Maxillofac Surg 2006;64:203–14.
[7] Shockley WW. Repair of laryngeal fractures. In: Shockley WW, Pillsbury HC, editors. The neck: diagnosis and surgery. St. Louis (MO): Mosby; 1994. p. 603–11.
[8] Goudy SL, Miller FB, Bumpous JM. Neck crepitans: evaluation and management of suspected upper aerodigestive tract injury. Laryngoscope 2002;112(5):791–5.
[9] Granholm T, Farmer DL. The surgical airway. Respir Care Clin N Am 2001;7(1):13–23.
[10] Lupetin AR, Hollander M, Rao VM. CT evaluation of laryngotracheal trauma. Semin Musculoskelet Radiol 1998;2(1):105–16.
[11] Bent JP III, Porubsky ES. The management of blunt fractures of the thyroid cartilage. Otolaryngol Head Neck Surg 1994;110(2):195–202.
[12] Schaefer SD. The treatment of acute external laryngeal injuries. 'State of the art.' Arch Otolaryngol Head Neck Surg 1991;117(1):35–9.
[13] Fuhrman GM, Stieg FH, Buerk CA. Blunt laryngeal trauma: classification and management protocol. J Trauma 1990;30:87–92.
[14] Hwang SY, Yeak SC. Management dilemmas in laryngeal trauma. J Laryngol Otol 2004;118(5): 325–8.
[15] de Mello-Filho FV, Carrau RL. The management of laryngeal fractures using internal fixation. Laryngoscope 2000;110(12):2143–6.
[16] Klotz PL, Fisher J. Evaluation of laryngeal trauma in the living. Ann Med Leg Criminol Police Sci Toxicol 1952;32(1):62–75.
[17] Kuttenberger JJ, Hardt N, Schlegel C. Diagnosis and initial management of laryngotracheal injuries associated with facial fractures. J Craniomaxillofac Surg 2004;32(2):80–4.
[18] Merritt RM, Bent JP, Porubsky ES. Acute laryngeal trauma in the pediatric patient. Ann Otol Rhinol Laryngol 1998;107(2):104–6.
[19] Schild JA, Denneny EC. Evaluation and treatment of acute laryngeal fractures. Head Neck 1989; 11(6):491–6.
[20] Ganzel TM, Mumford LA. Diagnosis and management of acute laryngeal trauma. Am Surg 1989; 55(5):303–6.
[21] Myers EM, Iko BO. The management of acute laryngeal trauma. J Trauma 1987;4:448–52.

[22] Minard G, Kudsk KA, Croce MA, et al. Laryngotracheal trauma. Am Surg 1992;59:181–7.
[23] Bent JP, Silver JR, Porubsky ES. Acute laryngeal trauma: a review of 77 patients. Otolaryngol Head Neck Surg 1993;109:441–9.
[24] Yen PT, Lee HY, Tsai MH, et al. Clinical analysis of external laryngeal trauma. J Laryngol Otol 1994;108:221–5.
[25] Cherlan TA, Raman R. External laryngeal trauma: analysis of thirty cases. J Laryngol Otol 1993;107:920–3.
[26] Bhanot S, Alex JC, Lowlicht RA, et al. The efficacy of resorbable plates in head and neck reconstruction. Laryngoscope 2002;112(5):890–8.
[27] Pou AM, Shoemaker DL, Carrau RL, et al. Repair of laryngeal fractures using adaptation plates. Head Neck 1998;20(8):707–13.
[28] Lykins CL, Pinczower EF. The comparative strength of laryngeal fracture fixation. Am J Otolaryngol 1998;19(3):158–62.
[29] LeJeune FE Jr, Weir DF. A laryngeal stent for repair of laryngeal fractures. Laryngoscope 1983;93(10):1359.
[30] Woo P. Laryngeal framework reconstruction with miniplates. Ann Otol Rhinol Laryngol 1990;99(10 Pt 1):772–7.
[31] Sasaki CT, Marotta JC, Lowlicht RA, et al. Efficacy of resorbable plates for reduction and stabilization of laryngeal fractures. Ann Otol Rhinol Laryngol 2003;112(9 Pt 1):745–50.
[32] Weigelt JA, Thal ER, Snyder WH, et al. Diagnosis of penetrating cervical esophageal injuries. Am J Surg 1987;154:619–22.

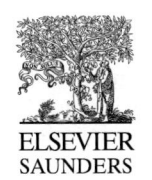

Thyroid Disorders: Evaluation and Management of Thyroid Nodules

James I. Cohen, MD, PhD[a],*, Kelli D. Salter, MD, PhD[b]

[a]Department of Otolaryngology/Head and Neck Surgery, Oregon Health & Science University, 3181 SW Sam Jackson Park Road, PV-01, Portland, OR 97239-3098, USA
[b]Department of General Surgery, Oregon Health & Science University, 3181 SW Sam Jackson Park Road, L223, Portland, OR 97239-3098, USA

Although it is well documented that thyroid nodules are a common clinical disorder, significant controversy persists as to ideal management strategies. Population studies suggest that approximately 3% to 7% of adults have asymptomatic palpable thyroid nodules, and that the number of nodules, including asymptomatic and symptomatic, increases with age [1–6]. However, the advent and implementation of high-resolution radiographic imaging has significantly impacted the discrepancy between clinically evident disease and incidentally discovered disease. High-resolution ultrasound (US) can detect thyroid nodules in 20% to 67% of randomly selected individuals, with a higher frequency in women and the elderly [3–8]. Moreover, 20% to 48% of patients who have a single palpable nodule have additional nodules identified on US. This discrepancy is further supported by data from autopsies conducted for medical reasons unrelated to thyroid disorders. Such data suggest that the prevalence of thyroid nodules in clinically normal glands is approximately 50% to 70% [3–6,9]. Therefore, the true prevalence of nodular thyroid disease in the general population remains unknown.

As the incidence of thyroid nodules has exhibited a steady rise over the past decade, so too has the incidence of thyroid cancer. The National Cancer Institute estimates the number of new cases and deaths from thyroid cancer in the United States in 2007 to be 33,550 and 1,530, respectively [10]. These numbers have steadily increased from the reported 13,000 number of new cases and 1000 thyroid cancer–associated deaths in 1994 [10–12]. However, despite the notable increase in the number of new cases, mortality rates have remained constant [10–12]. Most experts in the field of cancer agree that the increasing incidence of thyroid cancer likely reflects the implementation of technology with increased sensitivity and specificity for detecting thyroid nodules. Such technology increases the need for physicians to improve their ability to differentiate benign from malignant thyroid lesions, because the clinical importance of thyroid nodules rests on the need to exclude thyroid cancer.

Incidentally discovered nodules present the same risk for malignancy (~10%) as palpable nodules if they are equivalent in size [3–6,13]. Therefore, the physician who finds an incidental thyroid nodule is faced with the challenge of determining the clinical significance of the lesion. Differentiating a benign nodule, which may require observation only and no specific treatment, from a malignant nodule, which requires more aggressive treatment, presents a diagnostic dilemma. Because of the high prevalence of incidental disease, it is neither economically feasible nor necessary to surgically excise all, or even most, thyroid nodules. It is essential that the physician develop and follow a reliable, cost-effective strategy for diagnosis and treatment of incidentally found thyroid nodules. This article provides practical guidelines, algorithms, and current recommendations for the effective diagnosis and management of thyroid nodules incidentally discovered by physicians

* Corresponding author.
E-mail address: cohenj@ohsu.edu (J.I. Cohen)

managing patients for other medical reasons. Important elements of the history and physical examination, laboratory evaluation, and imaging modalities are reviewed, and a suggested management strategy is presented. This outline is not intended to be all inclusive, nor does it preclude additional evaluation, according to the specific clinical situation. Furthermore, the specific management of hypothyroidism, hyperthyroidism, or thyroid malignancies is beyond the scope of this article. These lesions should be specifically managed by a multidisciplinary team, including, at a minimum, an endocrinologist and surgeon who specialize in the treatment of such disorders.

Diagnosis

No reliable noninvasive way exists to distinguish a benign thyroid nodule from a thyroid carcinoma. Multiple diagnostic methods must be used to increase the accuracy of the diagnosis. Fig. 1 provides a basic algorithm of diagnostic modalities typically used in the initial evaluation of a thyroid nodule. Generally, the inability to accurately differentiate benign from malignant nodules warrants operative removal of the lesion.

History and physical examination

The history and physical examination, including that of adjacent cervical lymph nodes, remain the diagnostic cornerstone in evaluating a patient who has a thyroid nodule. Unfortunately, neither the history nor the physical examination is highly sensitive or specific for detecting malignancy. However, several well-documented factors are associated with an increased risk for malignancy and, therefore, warrant further discussion [3–6]. Factors that present a high risk for thyroid cancer include: history of head and neck or total body radiation; family history; rapid growth; hard, fixed nodule; and/or regional, cervical lymphadenopathy. Factors that present a moderate risk include: male gender; age younger than 30 or older than 60 years; and/or persistent local symptoms (hoarseness, dysphagia, dysphonia, dyspnea).

A history of head and neck or total body irradiation is a well-known risk factor for subsequent development of thyroid cancer. The incidence of thyroid malignancy in a patient who has a nodule and a previous history of radiation has been reported to range from 20% to 50% [2–6,14–18]. Therefore, the incidental finding of a thyroid nodule in a patient who has had prior radiation exposure requires careful and complete evaluation, although by itself it does not justify removal if the workup should prove negative.

Despite high levels of intraobserver and interobserver variations, careful inspection and palpation of the thyroid, the anterior neck compartments, and the lateral neck compartments should always be performed. Texture and size of the nodule should be documented. A firm or hard, solitary or dominant nodule with an increased

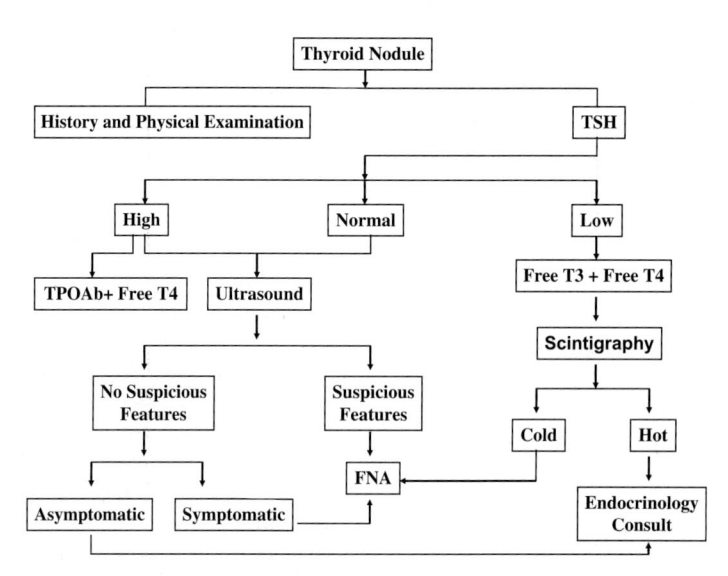

Fig. 1. Diagnosis and management of thyroid nodules. FNA, fine-needle aspiration; T_3, triiodothyronine; T_4, thyroxine; TPOAb, thyroid peroxidase antibody; TSH, thyroid-stimulating hormone (thyrotropin).

rate of growth that clearly differs from the rest of the gland suggests an increased risk for malignancy [2,4,6]. The presence of multiple nodules (symptomatic or asymptomatic) does not decrease the likelihood that any one of them is a carcinoma, as was once thought, although the overall incidence of malignancy in a multinodular gland is the same as that for any given nodule (~10%) [3–6,19,20]. Each nodule should be evaluated on its own merit regardless of the number of nodules present. Finally, ipsilateral or contralateral cervical lymphadenopathy is worrisome in the setting of a thyroid nodule and significantly increases the risk for malignancy.

Thyroid cancer may present as a familial trait or syndrome [21–24]. Although medullary thyroid carcinoma (MTC) accounts for only approximately 10% of all thyroid carcinomas, 25% of MTCs occur secondary to an inherited cancer risk, namely familial MTC (<2%) and multiple endocrine neoplasia (MEN 2A, ~25% or MEN 2B, <2%) [23–25]. Mutations in the *RET* proto-oncogene are responsible for all three conditions [23–25]. Patients diagnosed with MTC should undergo genetic testing to determine if mutations in the *RET* proto-oncogene are present.

Papillary and follicular carcinomas, the two most common forms of thyroid cancer, may also present as a family trait or syndrome [21,22,25]. Patients who have familial adenomatous polyposis (FAP) syndrome or Gardner syndrome (a variant of FAP), Cowden syndrome, and Werner (adult progeroid) syndrome are at increased risk for development of thyroid cancer [21,22,25]. Families with adenomatous polyposis (FAP or Gardner syndrome) show an increased incidence (2%) of papillary thyroid cancers, which tend to be multicentric (65%), exhibit a higher female-to-male ratio (6:1), and develop at a younger age (third decade) [21,22,25]. Patients who have Cowden syndrome have up to a 10% lifetime risk for follicular or papillary thyroid cancer, with follicular being the most common [21,22,25]. Approximately 70% to 85% of people with Cowden syndrome will have benign thyroid changes, including multinodular goiter, adenomatous nodules, and follicular nodules [21,22,25]. Thyroid cancer associated with Werner syndrome, an autosomal connective tissue disorder, occurs a decade earlier than in the general population, with a mean age of 34 years. Variability in the type of non-MTC occurring in patients who have Werner syndrome has been observed among ethnic groups. Although papillary (84%), follicular (14%), and anaplastic (2%) forms have been observed in Japanese patients, only papillary appears to occur in Caucasian patients [25]. Finally, papillary thyroid carcinoma can occur in families independent of syndromes such as FAP, Cowden, or Werner [21,22,25]. This form of thyroid cancer is believed to be inherited as an autosomal dominant condition. However, a specific genetic mutation has not been identified. Therefore, genetic testing is not currently available for these families.

Extremes of age (<30 or >60) and male gender are associated with an increased risk for thyroid cancer if a nodule is present [2–6]. Thyroid nodules during childhood and adolescence should induce caution, because the rate of malignancy is twofold higher in children than in adult patients [2–6]. Furthermore, although thyroid nodules are four times more common in women and increase with age, men are at greater risk for malignancy than women [2–6].

Most patients who have thyroid nodules have few or no symptoms. When present, symptoms are generally nonspecific. No defined relationship exists between nodule histology or size and the reported symptoms. However, persistent local symptoms of hoarseness, dysphagia, dysphonia, dyspnea, or cough should raise the suspicion of malignancy and warrant further investigation, including an evaluation for thyroid cancer [2–6].

Finally, iodine deficiency and socioeconomic status have been proposed as independent risk factors for thyroid carcinoma [6,26–29]. Population-based studies conducted from the 1960s to the 1990s on residents living in areas of endemic goiter indicated that iodine deficiency was an associated risk factor for thyroid cancer, primarily of the follicular and papillary subtypes [26–29]. Lower socioeconomic status additionally was identified as an independent risk factor for more advanced disease secondary to limited access to appropriate health care [26–29].

Laboratory evaluation

Because clinical evaluation is not sensitive for thyroid gland disease, laboratory examination is necessary. Measurement of the serum thyrotropin or thyroid-stimulating hormone (TSH) concentration is the single most useful test, and may be the only one warranted, in the initial evaluation of thyroid nodules [2–6]. The TSH assay has a high sensitivity in detecting even subtle thyroid dysfunction [30]. If the serum TSH level is within the normal range, the measurement of free thyroid hormones adds no further relevant information. Abnormal serum TSH levels, however, generally warrant further laboratory testing (see Fig. 1). If the serum TSH level is high, a free thyroxine (T_4) and thyroglobulin or thyroid peroxidase antibody (TPOAb) should be obtained to evaluate for hypothyroidism or thyroiditis [2–6]. In both these situations, the thyroid gland can be enlarged or nodular. By contrast, if the serum TSH level is low, a free T_4 and free triiodothyronine (T_3) level should be obtained to evaluate for hyperthyroidism, such as an autonomic functioning gland or thyrotoxicosis [2–6].

Serum thyroglobulin, a protein normally produced by the thyroid gland, correlates with the iodine status and the size of the thyroid gland rather than the nature (malignant versus benign) of a thyroid nodule. Many factors, including the degree of thyrotropin receptor stimulation, the volume of the gland, inflammation, radiation, multinodular goiter, biopsy, or surgery, may falsely elevate or decrease levels of thyroglobulin [4–6,31]. Furthermore, the presence of TPOAb, which attack the thyroglobulin protein, may decrease the reliability of the thyroglobulin assay [4–6,31,32]. Such antibodies may be present in 10% of normal subjects, 15% to 30% of patients who have differentiated thyroid cancer, 89% to 98% of patients who have Grave's disease, and 100% of patients who have Hashimoto's thyroiditis [4–6,31,32]. Additionally, autoimmune thyroid diseases are associated with several other organ-specific and systemic autoimmune disorders [32]. Therefore, a preoperative assay cannot be used to diagnose or exclude cancerous lesions. Although commonly implemented as a means of monitoring for recurrence of thyroid cancer in patients following thyroidectomy, measurement of serum thyroglobulin should not be used in the routine assessment of thyroid nodules.

Routine measurement of calcitonin, a useful serum marker of MTC, in all patients is not cost-effective [4–6]. However, the incidence of sporadic MTC in patients who have nodular thyroid glands can be as high as 1.5% [23,25]. Furthermore, unlike familial MTC which often is diagnosed early secondary to family history and genetic testing, sporadic MTC usually presents at a later stage with regional metastasis because of increased difficulty in diagnosis due to various morphologies [23,25]. Therefore, although not recommended in routine assessment of thyroid nodules, a calcitonin level should be considered in patients who have factors suspicious for sporadic MTC and is imperative in those patients who have a suspected familial MTC or a familial MEN syndrome.

Imaging modalities

High-resolution ultrasound

High resolution ultrasonography (US) is the cornerstone of imaging for assessment of thyroid nodules. To date, it is the most accurate test available to evaluate such lesions, measure their dimensions, identify their structure, and evaluate diffuse changes in the thyroid gland [4–6]. However, because of the high prevalence of clinically inapparent, small thyroid nodules, routine US is not recommended as a screening test in the general population unless well-known risk factors are present.

Many studies have been published debating the ability of US to distinguish between benign and cancerous lesions [13,32–38]. In 2005, the Society of Radiologists in Ultrasound convened a panel of specialists from a variety of medical disciplines to formulate a consensus regarding management of thyroid nodules identified by ultrasonography in adult patients [39]. The likelihood of cancer in a thyroid nodule was shown to be the same regardless of the size measured at US [13,32–39]. Furthermore, sonographic features suggestive of malignancy were found to vary between types of thyroid carcinomas [13,32–39]. Despite these discrepancies, several sonographic features were found to be suggestive of an increased risk for malignancy (Fig. 2, Table 1), including microcalcifications, hypoechogenicity, irregular margins, absence of nodule halo, predominant solid composition, and intranodular vascularity [13,32–39]. However, the sensitivities, specificities, positive predictive values and negative predictive values for these criteria were variable between studies [13,32–39]. No US feature was found to have both a high sensitivity and positive predictive value but the combination of factors was shown to improve the positive predictive value of US to some degree. Therefore, patients who have palpable thyroid nodules or incidentally discovered nodules with concerning patient demographics or risk factors should undergo US to evaluate for sonographic features suggestive of malignancy, baseline characteristics and volume of the nodule, coincidental thyroid nodules, and baseline characteristics and volume of the remaining thyroid gland. In addition the cervical lymph nodes

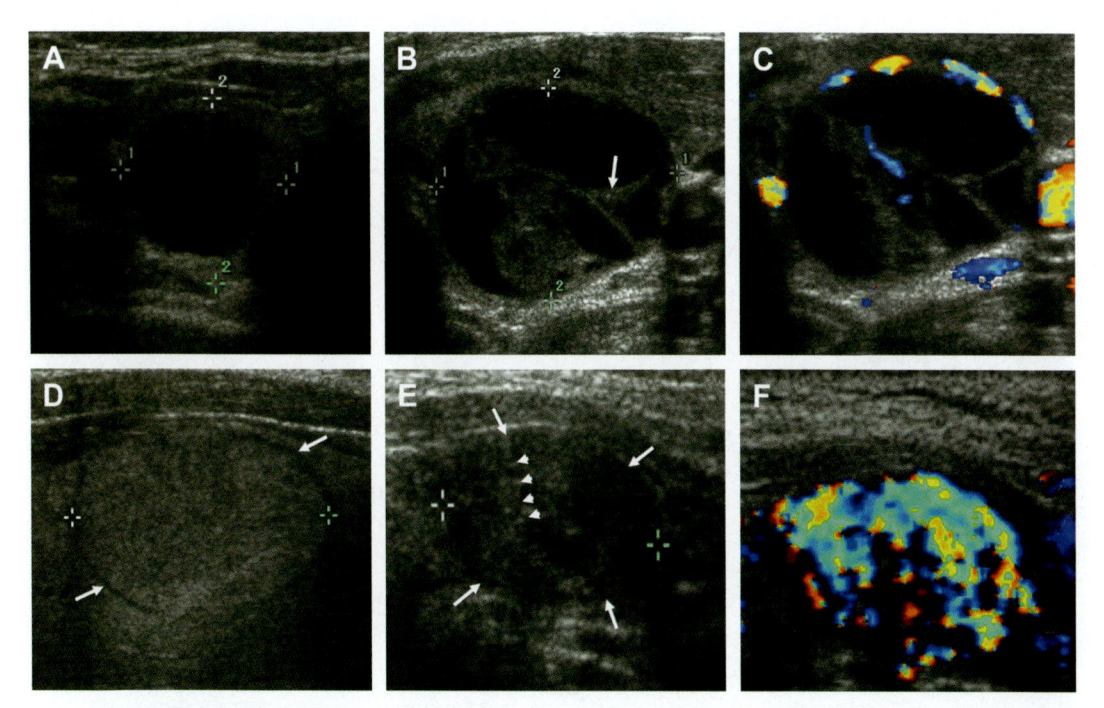

Fig. 2. Ultrasound images of thyroid nodules of varying parenchymal composition (cystic to solid) and vascularity. (*A*) Gray-scale image of predominately cystic nodule (*calipers*) that proved to be benign at cytologic examination (fine-needle aspiration [FNA]). (*B*) Gray-scale image of mixed solid and cystic nodule (*calipers*) with septate (*arrow*). (*C*) Addition of color Doppler mode did not demonstrate marked internal vascularity. The lesion was benign at cytologic examination (FNA). (*D*) Gray-scale image of predominately solid nodule (*calipers*) with surrounding halo (*arrows*) that proved to be benign at cytologic examination (FNA) and surgery. (*E*) Gray-scale image of predominately solid nodule (*calipers*) with irregular margins (*arrows*) and multiple fine echogenicities (*arrowheads*). (*F*) Addition of color Doppler mode demonstrated marked internal vascularity indicating increased likelihood that nodule is malignant. FNA and surgery confirmed papillary carcinoma.

beds should be evaluated by ultrasonography as warranted.

Despite recommendations from the Society of Radiologists in Ultrasound Consensus Conference Statement, ultrasonography cannot reliably distinguish between benign and cancerous lesions without adjunct testing. Therefore, patients who have risk factors and ultrasonographic characteristics concerning for malignancy should undergo cytohistologic analysis of a representative tissue sample obtained by way of either fine-needle aspiration (FNA) or coarse-needle biopsy (CNB) [39]. In general, FNA is preferred over CNB because it is extremely accurate and less invasive and allows for

Table 1
Sonographic features associated with thyroid cancer

US feature	Sensitivity (%)	Specificity (%)	PPV (%)	NPV (%)
Microcalcifications	26–59	86–95	24–71	42–94
Hypoechogenecity	27–87	43–94	11–68	74–94
Irregular margins or halo absence	17–78	39–85	9–60	39–98
Solid composition	69–75	53–56	16–27	88–92
Intranodular vascularity	54–74	79–81	24–42	86–97

Abbreviations: NPV, negative predictive value; PPV, positive predictive value.

Modified from Frates MC, Benson CB, Charboneau JW, et al. Management of thyroid nodules detected at US: Society of Radiologists in Ultrasound consensus conference statement. Radiology 2005;237:794–800.

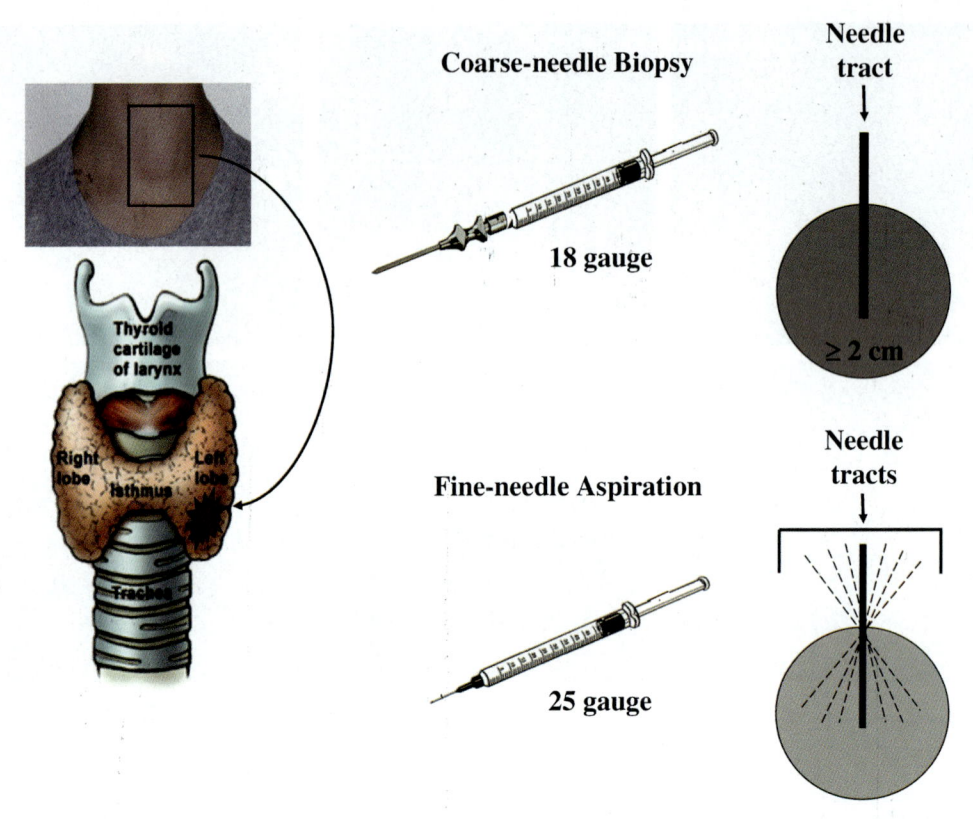

Fig. 3. Methods for obtaining thyroid tissue for cytohistologic analysis. A CNB uses a larger needle (16 or 18 gauge) and requires that the thyroid nodule be at least 2 cm in size. By contrast, an FNA uses a smaller needle (25 or 27 gauge) and allows for more complete sampling of the nodule because of the multiple passes taken through the nodule.

more complete sampling of the nodule because of the multiple passes taken through the nodule (Fig. 3) [4–6]. Additionally, US should be performed in all patients who have a history of familial thyroid cancer, MEN II, or childhood cervical irradiation, even if palpation yields normal findings [39]. Furthermore, the physical finding of adenopathy suspicious for malignant involvement in the anterior or lateral neck compartments warrants US examination of the lymph nodes and thyroid gland because of the risk for a lymph node metastatic lesion from an unrecognized thyroid carcinoma [39].

Radionuclide scintigraphy

Radionuclide scintigraphy (iodine 123 [^{123}I] or technetium-99m pertechnetate), once the cornerstone for thyroid imaging, has now been replaced by high-resolution ultrasonography as the imaging modality of choice for evaluating thyroid nodules [4–6]. Such scans, in the current status of thyroid imaging, are used primarily as adjuncts to ultrasonography for differentiating hyperfunctioning ("hot") from hypofunctioning ("cold") nodules (Fig. 4) [4–6,40,41]. Hyperfunctioning nodules represent approximately 5% of thyroid nodules and present a low risk for malignancy ($\leq 1\%$) [4–6]. Hypofunctioning nodules have a reported malignant risk of 5% to 25% and represent approximately 75% to 95% of thyroid nodules [4–6]. The remaining 10% to 15% of nodules are indeterminate, with a variable risk for malignancy [4–6]. Because most thyroid lesions are "cold" and few of these lesions are malignant, the predictive value of hypofunctioning nodules for the presence of malignant involvement is low. The diagnostic specificity is further reduced in small lesions (<1 cm), which may not be identified by scintigraphy. For these reasons, thyroid scintigraphy is not usually useful as a first-step diagnostic study in the evaluation of thyroid nodules. Indications that may warrant use of thyroid scintigraphy include identification of a solitary thyroid nodule in the setting of decreased serum thyrotropin, an indeterminate FNA or

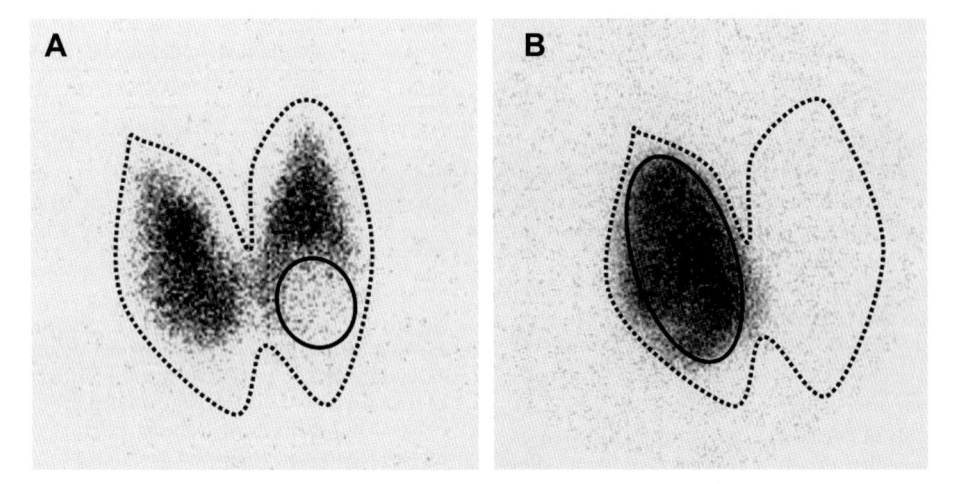

Fig. 4. Iodine 123 (^{123}I) thyroid scintigraphy patterns in thyroid glands (*dashed lines*) with "cold" and "hot" nodules. (*A*) Nonfunctioning "cold" nodule in the lower left thyroid lobe (*solid line*). (*B*) Hyperfunctioning "hot" right thyroid nodule (*solid line*), with suppressed serum TSH level and suppressed uptake of ^{123}I in the remainder of the thyroid gland.

CNB of a thyroid nodule, and for the detection of nonspecific neck masses or lymphadenopathy [4–6,40,41].

CT and MRI

CT and MRI, like other imaging modalities, cannot reliably differentiate between malignant and benign nodules [4–6,42]. Therefore, these tests are rarely indicated in the initial evaluation of a thyroid nodule. However, such imaging modalities may be used as secondary adjuncts if warranted. A CT scan can be used to evaluate nodules in a difficult-to-palpate, diffusely enlarged gland, to assist in detection of mediastinal thyroid tissue, and to assess for extrathyroidal invasion and cervical lymphadenopathy (Fig. 5). By contrast, MRI demonstrates exquisite soft tissue details and vascular anatomy, and thus, allows for identification of extraglandular invasion and involvement of the great vessels, respectively. Therefore, either of these imaging modalities may be implemented in preoperative staging. CT contrast medium contains iodine which reduces subsequent uptake of iodine molecules and thus may interfere with nuclear scintigraphy (^{123}I) or postoperative radioiodine ablation therapy (^{131}I) for malignant nodules. MRI uses contrast medium (gadolinium) that does not interfere with nuclear scintigraphy.

Incidental clinically silent thyroid nodules are commonly discovered in patients undergoing CT or MRI for medical reasons unrelated to thyroid disorders. The decision to pursue further workup of such nodules depends on several factors already discussed, including history and physical, laboratory analysis, and associated known risk factors. Although abnormalities of the thyroid gland can be detected on CT and MRI, sonography provides important additional information that may be useful in guiding further clinical management. Therefore, patients who have an incidentally discovered thyroid nodule on CT or MRI and

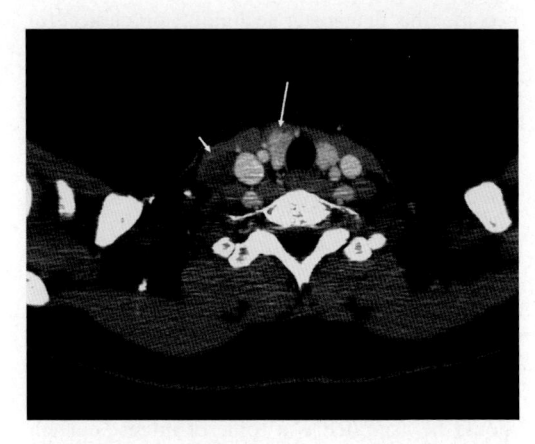

Fig. 5. CT scan of the neck demonstrating a metastatic right thyroid lobe carcinoma. The anterior aspect of the right thyroid lobe has a nodular exophytic mass (*long arrow*) near the junction with the isthmus. On the right side is a heterogeneous low-density enlarged lymph node (*short arrow*) that contains septations and nodules of high density. Fine-needle aspiration and surgery of the mass demonstrated papillary carcinoma with metastasis to the right paratracheal and lateral neck lymph nodes.

concerning clinical features should undergo ultrasonography to determine the need for biopsy and further analysis.

Cytohistochemistry analysis

A cytohistochemistry analysis should be performed on thyroid nodules with associated features concerning for malignancy. Tissue for such analysis is obtained by way of either FNA or CNB (see Fig. 3). Detailed reviews of aspiration biopsy of thyroid nodules have been published previously [4–6,43–45]. In general, FNA is the removal of a few clusters of individual thyroid cells by means of a small needle (usually a 25- or 27-gauge 1.5-in needle). By contrast, CNB uses a larger needle (usually a 16- or 18-gauge needle) and is more difficult to perform, and fewer physicians have experience in this procedure. In addition, the large size of the needle may cause a small amount of bleeding ($\leq 1\%$), injury to the trachea, or injury to the recurrent laryngeal nerves. Furthermore, unlike FNA, which can be performed on all types of nodules, the nodule must be at least 2 cm in size to perform a CNB successfully. Finally, although CNB provides a larger tissue sample that retains it cellular architecture, it rarely provides a more precise histologic diagnosis than FNA. Therefore, because of its minimal invasiveness, accuracy ($\sim 95\%$) and cost effectiveness, US-guided FNA has now become the diagnostic technique of choice for evaluating thyroid nodules [4–6]. For these reasons, only the role of FNA in the evaluation of thyroid nodules will be discussed in this article. The accuracy of FNA or CNB is only as good as the person performing the procedure and the person who analyzes and reports the cytologic findings. However, when performed by experienced personnel, the sensitivity and specificity (Table 2) of thyroid FNA are excellent [4–6].

Fine-needle aspiration

Not every patient who has a thyroid nodule should undergo FNA. Which thyroid nodule should be aspirated is a topic of intense current debate among multiple medical specialties. As stated in the 2005 Society of Radiologists in Ultrasound Consensus Conference Statement, the decision to perform or defer FNA in a given patient should be made according to the individual circumstances [39]. Several recommendations (Table 3) based on current literature and common practice strategies were made by the committee to assist physicians in their decision-making process

Table 2
Statistical features of thyroid fine-needle aspiration

Statistical feature	Mean (%)	Range (%)
Sensitivity	83	65–98
Specificity	92	72–100
PPV	75	50–96
False-negative rate	5	1–11
False-positive rate	5	0–7

Abbreviation: PPV, positive predictive value.

Modified from AACE/AME Task Force on Thyroid Nodules. American Association of Clinical Endocrinologists and Associazione Medici Endocrinologi medical guidelines for clinical practice for the diagnosis and management of thyroid nodules. Endocr Prac 2006;12(1):63–102; Gharib H, Papini E. Thyroid nodules: clinical importance, assessment, and treatment. Endocrinol Metab Clin N Am 2007;36:707–35; with permission.

[4–6,39]. As a general rule, a solitary thyroid nodule larger than 1 cm in diameter with microcalcifications should be biopsied [4–6,39]. A solitary thyroid nodule that is at least 1.5 cm in diameter and solid, or almost entirely solid, or with coarse calcifications should be biopsied [4–6,39]. Management of mixed solid and cystic (or almost entirely cystic) nodules is more controversial than that of solid nodules. FNA is likely unnecessary if the nodule is almost entirely cystic and without US features concerning for malignancy (see Table 1) [4–6,39]. However, it is generally recommended that FNA be performed on a mixed

Table 3
Recommendations for thyroid nodules greater than or equal to 1 cm in maximum diameter

Ultrasound features	Recommendation [4–6,39]
Solitary node	
Microcalcifications	≥ 1.0 cm: US-guided FNA
Solid (or mostly solid)	≥ 1.5 cm: US-guided FNA
Mixed	≥ 2.0 cm: US-guided FNA
None of the above but substantial growth	Consider US-guided FNA
Mostly cystic and none of the above	FNA probably not warranted
Multiple nodules	Consider US-guided FNA of one or more nodules based on above criteria; sampling should be focused on lesions with suspicious US features rather than size

or almost entirely cystic nodule with a solid mural component of at least 2 cm in size [4–6,39]. Finally, any nodule that exhibits substantial growth should be biopsied [4–6,39].

Controversy remains regarding the optimal management of patients who have multiple thyroid nodules. Some advocate routine FNA of all nodules larger than 10 mm, whereas others recommended FNA of only the largest nodule. The American Thyroid Association Guidelines Taskforce currently recommended that in the presence of two or more thyroid nodules larger than 1 to 1.5 cm, those with suspicious sonographic appearance should be aspirated preferentially [5]. If none of the nodules exhibits suspicious sonographic appearance and multiple sonographically similar coalescent nodules are present, only the largest nodule should be aspirated [5]. This lack of a consistent recommendation stems in part from the absence of studies investigating the prevalence and location of thyroid cancer in patients who have multiple thyroid nodules. Recently, a retrospective observational cohort study conducted from 1995 to 2003 investigated the prevalence and distribution of carcinoma in patients who have solitary and multiple thyroid nodules on sonography [20]. A total of 1985 patients underwent FNA of 3483 nodules. The prevalence of thyroid cancer was similar between patients who had a solitary nodule (14.8%) and patients who had multiple nodules (14.9%) [20]. Sonographic characteristics were unable to distinguish benign from malignant disease accurately. Consistent with previous evidence, solitary nodules were found to have a higher likelihood of malignancy than nonsolitary (cystic or mixed) nodules [20]. Cancer was multifocal in 46% of patients who had multiple nodules larger than 10 mm [20]. Seventy-two percent of cancers occurred in the largest nodule [20]. However, as the number of nodules increased, the frequency of cancer in the largest nodule decreased, and thus reduced the predictive value of FNA of the largest nodule. A strategy of biopsying the largest nodule detected only 86% of patients who had two nodules, one of which contained cancer, and only approximately 50% of patients who had three or more nodules, one of which contained cancer [20]. Thus, for confident exclusion of thyroid cancer in a gland with multiple nodules larger than 10 mm, it was recommended that FNA be performed in up to three or four nodules larger than 10 mm [20].

Management of thyroid nodules following biopsy depends on the cytohistologic diagnosis (Fig. 6). However, before making a cytohistologic diagnosis, the FNA specimen first must be evaluated for adequacy and classified as either adequate or inadequate (or unsatisfactory) [46–48]. If the specimen is considered inadequate or

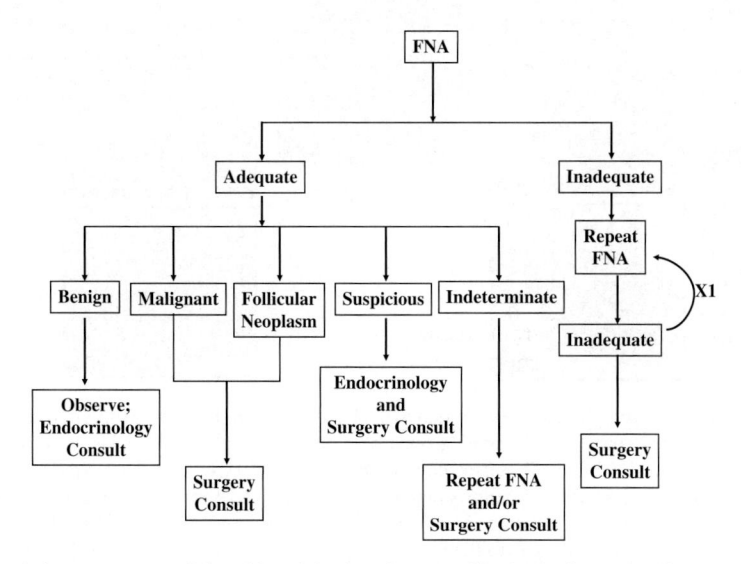

Fig. 6. Recommended management of thyroid nodules based on cytohistologic diagnosis. Tissue samples must first be evaluated for adequacy. If the specimen is considered inadequate or unsatisfactory, the FNA should be repeated with ultrasound guidance. A second indeterminate classification generally warrants surgical excision for accurate tissue analysis if the nodule has any features that are worrisome for malignancy.

unsatisfactory, the FNA should be repeated with US guidance, because the risk for malignancy in such samples reportedly ranges from 2% to 37%, depending on patient demographics and preoperative analysis [49–53]. A second inadequate classification generally warrants surgical excision for accurate tissue analysis if the nodule has any features that are worrisome for malignancy. Once the FNA specimen is considered adequate, it can be evaluated further by the pathologists and categorized into one of five cytohistologic diagnostic categories (Fig. 7) [4–6,46–48]: (1) benign or nonneoplastic, (2) malignant (usually papillary carcinoma), (3) suspicious for cancer, (4) follicular neoplasm, or (5) indeterminate. Approximately 70% of FNA specimens are classified as benign, 10% as suspicious, 5% as malignant, and 10% to 15% as indeterminate [4–6,46–48].

Benign nodules, usually of macrofollicular pattern, are characterized by abundant colloid, including watery colloid, which leads to red blood cell rouleau formation, and variably sized groups of cytologically bland follicular epithelial cells. They often have a cystic component, defined as cyst fluid (absence of rouleau formation) with conspicuous histiocytes. Cytopuncture of cyst fluid is a source of scant biopsies, leading to false-negative diagnosis. In general, benign

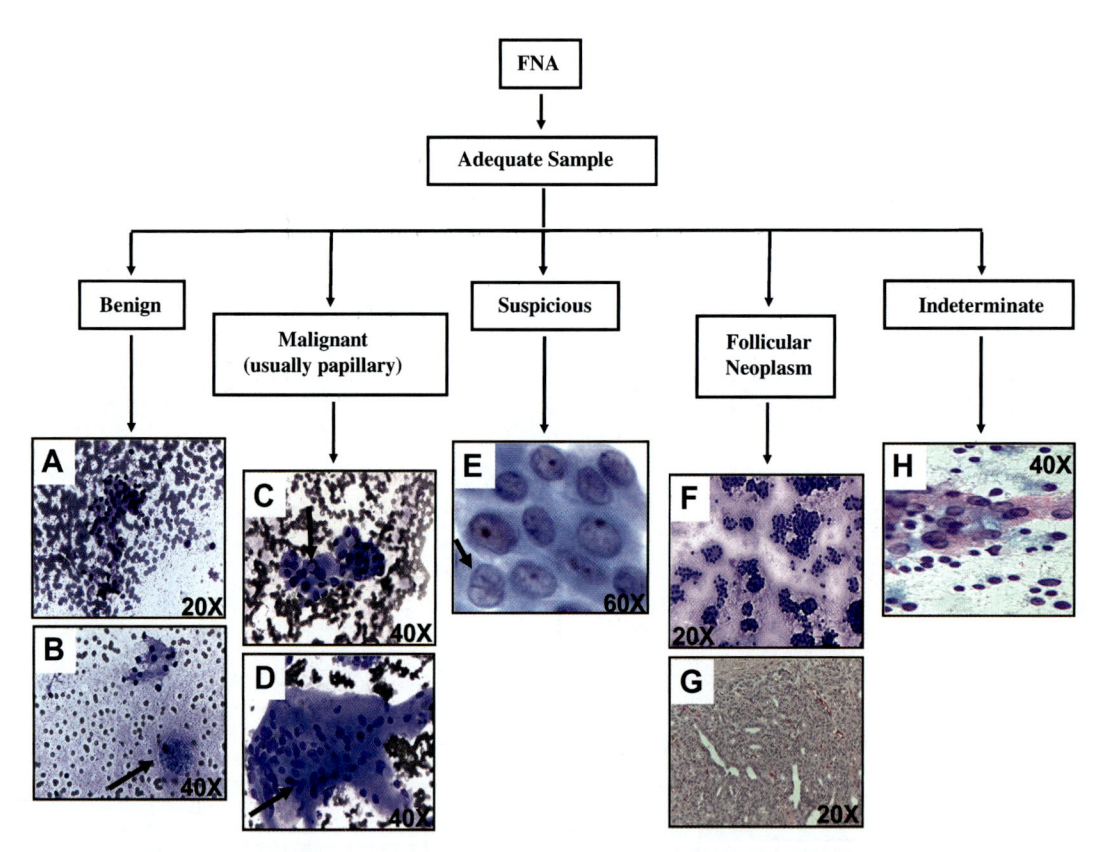

Fig. 7. Common thyroid cytology based on FNA analysis. (*A*) Benign thyroid nodule with abundant colloid, including watery colloid (shown here), and variably sized groups of cytologically bland follicular epithelial cells. (*B*) Cystic component of benign thyroid nodule with conspicuous histiocytes (*arrow*). (*C*) Papillary carcinoma with intranuclear cytoplasmic pseudoinclusions (*arrow*) and dense squamoid cytoplasm. (*D*) Bizarre multinucleated giant cells (*arrow*) of papillary carcinoma (compare with histiocyte in *A*). (*E*) Suspicious for papillary carcinoma lesion with many features of papillary carcinoma, including enlarged follicular cells with enlarged and prominent nuclei, powdery chromatin, nuclear grooves (*arrow*), and intranuclear cytoplasmic inclusions. (*F*) Follicular neoplasm with repetitive microfollicular groups and minimal amount of colloid, as would be expected given the cellular neoplasm with scant colloid seen in the accompanying histologic section of the follicular adenoma (*G*). (*H*) Indeterminate lesion exhibiting suboptimal cellularity but with features suggestive of papillary carcinoma.

thyroid nodules can be followed by an endocrinologist with clinical examination and ultrasonography [4–6].

Malignant lesions or those suspicious for cancer (usually papillary carcinomas or follicular neoplasms) warrant surgical excision [4–6]. Papillary thyroid carcinoma on cytohistologic examination may have moderate amounts of colloid and a cystic component similar to benign nodules but it is characterized by the combination of intranuclear cytoplasmic pseudoinclusions, dense squamoid cytoplasm, and papillary architecture. Other minor criteria that may support the diagnosis of papillary carcinoma include bizarre, multinucleated giant cells, psammoma bodies, thick "bubble-gum" colloid, nuclear membrane irregularities (so-called nuclear grooves), and nuclear enlargement. By contrast, follicular neoplasms, including follicular adenoma, follicular carcinoma, follicular variant of papillary carcinoma, and Hurthle cell neoplasm, are characterized by a cellular aspirate with repetitive microfollicular groups and minimal amount of colloid. Currently, no noninvasive methods reliably differentiate between follicular adenoma and follicular carcinoma.

Indeterminate lesions exhibit cellularity suboptimal for making a definitive diagnosis but generally show features suggestive of one of the above categories. Patients who have such lesions may undergo a second FNA or be directly triaged to surgery. The decision to repeat the FNA or surgically excise the lesion must be based on a combination of factors, including patient preference, physician recommendations, and clinical history of the lesion [4–6,46–48].

Summary

Thyroid nodules are a common clinical entity. Most nodules are discovered incidentally in patients undergoing surveillance for medical reasons unrelated to thyroid disorders. The physician who identifies an incidental thyroid nodule is faced with the challenge of determining the clinical significance of the lesion, with the primary objective being to evaluate the nodule for malignancy. Using a reliable, cost-effective strategy for diagnosis and treatment of incidentally discovered thyroid nodules improves the ability to differentiate benign from malignant nodules. This article provides practical guidelines and a suggested management strategy for the effective diagnosis and management of incidentally discovered thyroid nodules.

Appendix 1 contains a summary of key aspects for examination of thyroid nodules, as recommended by the American Thyroid Association [5], the American Association of Clinical Endocrinologists [6], the Associazione Medici Endocrinologi [6], and the Society of Radiologists in Ultrasound [39].

Appendix 1

Summary of key factors and recommendations regarding thyroid nodule examination

History and physical examination

About 90% to 95% of thyroid nodules are benign.
Risk for cancer is similar in solitary nodules and multinodular goiter.
Absence of symptoms does not exclude malignancy.
Pertinent patient demographics and physical examination factors should be assessed:
History of head and neck or total body irradiation
Family history of thyroid carcinoma in first-degree relative
Rapid growth and hoarseness
Ipsilateral cervical lymphadenopathy
Fixation of nodule to surrounding tissue
Vocal cord paralysis
TSH level should be obtained.

Diagnostic imaging

US of thyroid nodules should be performed in high-risk patients who have pertinent patient demographics or physical examination factors.
Nodules should be identified for FNA biopsy.

Cytohistochemistry analysis

Biopsy should be obtained from all solitary, firm, or hard nodules.
FNA should be performed:
Nodules of any size in patients who have concerning patient demographics or physical examination findings suggestive of malignancy
All hypoechoic nodules greater than or equal to 1 cm with microcalcifications, irregular margins, intranodular vascularity, absence of halo, or predominately solid consistency

Solid (or mostly solid) nodules (independent of size) with substantial or extracapsular growth or metastatic cervical lymph nodes

References

[1] Vander JB, Gaston EA, Dawber TR. The significance of nontoxic thyroid nodules: final report of a 15-year study of the incidence of thyroid malignancy. Ann Intern Med 1968;69:537–40.

[2] Hegedus L. Clinical practice: the thyroid nodule. N Engl J Med 2004;351(17):1764–71.

[3] Datta RV, Petrelli NJ, Ramzy J. Evaluation and management of incidentally discovered thyroid nodules. Surg Oncol 2006;15:33–42.

[4] Gharib H, Papini E. Thyroid nodules: clinical importance, assessment, and treatment. Endocrinol Metab Clin North Am 2007;36:707–35.

[5] Cooper DS, Doherty GM, Haugen BR, et al. The American Thyroid Association Guidelines Taskforce. Management guidelines for patients with thyroid nodules and differentiated thyroid cancer. Thyroid 2006;16(2):109–42.

[6] AACE/AME Task Force on Thyroid Nodules. American Association of Clinical Endocrinologists and Associazione Medici Endocrinologi medical guidelines for clinical practice for the diagnosis and management of thyroid nodules. Endocr Pract 2006;12(1):63–102.

[7] Tan GH, Gharib H. Thyroid incidentalomas: management approaches to nonpalpable nodules discovered incidentally on thyroid imaging. Ann Intern Med 1997;126:226–31.

[8] Ezzat S, Sarti DA, Cain DR, et al. Thyroid incidentalomas: prevalence by palpation and ultrasonography. Arch Intern Med 1994;154:1838–40.

[9] Mortensen JD, Woolner LB, Bennett WA. Gross and microscopic findings in clinically normal thyroid glands. J Clin Endocrinol Metab 1955;15:1270–80.

[10] Jemal A, Siegal R, Ward E, et al. Cancer statistics, 2007. CA Cancer J Clin 2007;57:43–66.

[11] Hundahl SA, Fleming ID, Fremgen AM, et al. A national cancer data base report on 53,856 cases of thyroid carcinoma treated in the U.S., 1985–1995. Cancer 1998;83:2638–48.

[12] Howe HL, Wingo PA, Thun MJ, et al. Annual report to the nation on the status of cancer (1973 through 1998) featuring cancers with recent increasing trends. J Natl Cancer Inst 2001;93:824–42.

[13] Papini E, Guglielmi R, Bianchini A, et al. Risk of malignancy in nonpalpable thyroid nodules: predictive value of ultrasound and color-Doppler features. J Clin Endocrinol Metab 2002;87(5):1941–6.

[14] Racini F, Vorontsova T, Demidchik E, et al. Post-Chernobyl thyroid carcinoma in Belarus children and adolescents: comparison with naturally occurring thyroid carcinoma in Italy and France. J Clin Endocrinol Metab 1997;81:3563–9.

[15] Acharya S, Sarafoglou K, LaQuaglia M, et al. Thyroid neoplasms after therapeutic radiation for malignancies during childhood or adolescence. Cancer 2003;97:2397–403.

[16] Tronko MD, Howe GR, Bogdanova TI, et al. A cohort study of thyroid cancer and other thyroid diseases after the Chornobyl accident: thyroid cancer in Ukraine detected during first screening. J Natl Cancer Inst 2006;98:897–903.

[17] Sigurdson AJ, Ronckers CM, Mertens AC, et al. Primary thyroid cancer after a first tumour in childhood (the childhood cancer survivor study): a nested case-control study. Lancet 2005;365:2014–23.

[18] Ronckers CM, Sigurdson AJ, Stovall M, et al. Thyroid cancer in childhood cancer survivors: a detailed evaluation of radiation dose response and its modifiers. Radiat Res 2006;166:618–28.

[19] Kim WB, Han SM, Kim Ty, et al. Ultrasonographic screening for detection of thyroid cancer in patients with Graves' disease. Clin Endocrinol 2004;60:719–25.

[20] Frates MC, Benson CB, Doubilet PM, et al. Prevalence and distribution of carcinoma in patients with solitary and multiple thyroid nodules on sonography. J Clin Endocrinol Metab 2006;91:3411–7.

[21] Houlston RS. Genetic predisposition to nonmedullary thyroid cancer. Nucl Med Commun 1998;19:911–3.

[22] Sippel RS, Caron NR, Clark OH. An evidence-based approach to familial nonmedullary thyroid cancer: screening, clinical management, and followup. World J Surg 2007;31:924–33.

[23] Moley JF, Fialkowski EA. Evidence-based approach to the management of sporadic medullary thyroid carcinoma. World J Surg 2007;31:946–56.

[24] Machens A, Dralle H. Genotype-phenotype based surgical concept of hereditary medullary thyroid carcinoma. World J Surg 2007;31:957–68.

[25] Alsanea O, Clark OH. Familial thyroid cancer. Curr Opin Oncol 2001;13:44–51.

[26] Pettersson B, Coleman MP, Ron E, et al. Iodine supplementation in Sweden and regional trends in thyroid cancer incidence by histopathologic type. Int J Cancer 1996;65:13–9.

[27] Szybinski Z, Huszno B, Zemla B, et al. Incidence of thyroid cancer in the selected areas of iodine deficiency in Poland. J Endocrinol Invest 2003;26(Suppl 2):63–70.

[28] Shakhtarin VV, Tsyb AF, Stepanenko VF, et al. Iodine deficiency, radiation dose, and the risk of thyroid cancer among children and adolescents in the Bryansk region of Russia following the Chernobyl power station accident. Int J Epidemiol 2003;32:584–91.

[29] Sehestedt T, Knudsen N, Perrild H, et al. Iodine intake and incidence of thyroid cancer in Denmark. Clin Endocrinol 2006;65:229–33.

[30] Christ-Crain M, Meier C, Roth CB, et al. Basal TSH levels compared with TRH-stimulated TSH levels to diagnose different degrees of TSH suppression: diagnostic and therapeutic impact of assay performance. Eur J Clin Invest 2002;32(12):931–7.

[31] Mazzaferri EL, Robbins RJ, Spencer CA, et al. A consensus report on the role of serum thyroglobulin as a monitoring method for low-risk patients with papillary thyroid carcinoma. J Clin Endocrinol Metab 2003;88:1433–41.

[32] Sinclair D. Clinical and laboratory aspects of thyroid autoantibodies. Ann Clin Biochem 2006;43:173–83.

[33] Khoo JL, Asa LS, Witterick IJ, et al. Thyroid calcification and its association with thyroid carcinoma. Head Neck 2002;24:651–5.

[34] Kim EK, Park CS, Chung Wy, et al. New sonographic criteria for recommending fine-needle aspiration biopsy of nonpalpable solid nodules of the thyroid. Am J Roentgenol 2002;178:687–91.

[35] Peccin S, de Castro JA, Furlanetto TW, et al. Ultrasonography: is it useful in the diagnosis of cancer in thyroid nodules? J Endocrinol Invest 2002;25:39–43.

[36] Frates MC, Benson CB, Doubilet PM, et al. Can color Doppler sonography aid in the prediction of malignancy of thyroid nodules? J Ultrasound Med 2003;22:127–31.

[37] Alexander EK, Marqusee E, Orcutt J, et al. Thyroid nodule shape and prediction of malignancy. Thyroid 2004;14:953–8.

[38] Iannuccilli JD, Cronan JJ, Monchik JM. Risk for malignancy of thyroid nodules as assessed by sonographic criteria. J Ultrasound Med 2004;23:1455–64.

[39] Frates MC, Benson CB, Charboneau JW, et al. Management of thyroid nodules detected at US: Society of Radiologist in Ultrasound consensus conference statement. Radiology 2005;237:794–800.

[40] McHenry CR, Slusarczyk SJ, Askari AT, et al. Refined use of scintigraphy in the evaluation of nodular thyroid disease. Surgery 1998;124:656–61.

[41] Meller J, Becker W. The continuing importance of thyroid scintigraphy in the era of high-resolution ultrasound. Eur J Nucl Med Mol Imaging 2002; 29(Suppl 2):S425–38.

[42] Shetty SK, Maher MM, Hahn PF, et al. Significance of incidental thyroid lesions detected on CT: correlation among CT, sonography and pathology. Am J Roentgenol 2006;187(5):1349–56.

[43] Gharib H. Fine-needle aspiration biopsy of thyroid nodules: advantages, limitations, and effect. Mayo Clin Proc 1994;69(1):44–9.

[44] Castro MR, Gharib H. Thyroid fine-needle aspiration biopsy: progress, practice, and pitfalls. Endocr Pract 2003;9:128–36.

[45] Baskin HJ. Ultrasound-guided fine-needle aspiration biopsy of thyroid nodules and multinodular goiter. Endocr Pract 2004;10(3):242–5.

[46] Baloch ZW, LiVolsi VA. Fine-needle aspiration of thyroid nodules: past, present and future. Endocr Pract 2004;10(3):234–41.

[47] Oertel YC. Cytopathology reports from fine needle aspirations of the thyroid gland: can they be improved? Thyroid 2007;17(1):33–5.

[48] Oertel YC. Fine-needle aspiration of the thyroid: technique and terminology. Endocrinol Metab Clin North Am 2007;36:737–51.

[49] McHenry CR, Walfish PG, Rosen IB. Nondiagnostic fine needle aspiration biopsy: a dilemma in management of nodular thyroid disease. Am Surg 1993;59:415–9.

[50] Burch HB, Burman KD, Reed HL, et al. Fine needle aspiration of thyroid nodules. Determinants of insufficiency rate and malignancy yield at thyroidectomy. Acta Cytol 1996;40:1176–83.

[51] MacDonald L, Yazdi HM. Nondiagnostic fine needle aspiration biopsy of the thyroid gland: a diagnostic dilemma. Acta Cytol 1996;40:423–8.

[52] Schmidt T, Riggs MW, Speights VO Jr. Significance of nondiagnostic fine-needle aspiration biopsy of thyroid nodules. South Med J 1997;90:1183–6.

[53] Chow LS, Gharib H, Goellner JR, et al. Nondiagnostic thyroid fine-needle aspiration cytology: management dilemmas. Thyroid 2001;11(12): 1147–51.

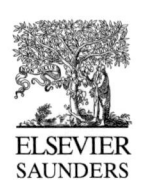

Clinical Implications of the Neck in Salivary Gland Disease

Andrew R. Salama, DDS, MD*, Robert A. Ord, DDS, MD, FRCS, FACS

Department of Oral and Maxillofacial Surgery, University of Maryland Medical Center, Baltimore College of Dental Surgery, 650 West Baltimore Street, Suite 1401, Baltimore, MD 21201, USA

Few regions of the human body are as anatomically and functionally complex as the neck. The proximity of the salivary glands to the neck compels clinicians to comprehensively understand the multitude of disease processes in the neck that relate to salivary tissue. Because the embryogenesis of the major salivary glands is intrinsically related to the development of the neck, it is not surprising that salivary tissue can occasionally be found within the neck distinct from the major salivary glands. The submandibular gland and parotid tail are confined to the anatomic boundaries of the neck and serve as the source of neoplastic and nonneoplastic processes. The neck also serves as a primary lymphatic drainage basin for the major and minor salivary glands. This article reviews the clinical spectrum of benign and malignant processes related to salivary gland tissues in the neck.

Heterotopic salivary gland tissue

The developmental complexity of the head and neck, particularly the propinquity to major salivary glands, makes them common sites for aberrant tissue growth. Among the major salivary glands, the parenchyma of the parotid gland, which is derived from oral epithelium, typically develops first. Encapsulation of glandular tissues, however, is a late embryologic event and occurs last in the parotid gland.

This temporal sequence gives rise to the unique phenomenon of intraglandular lymph nodes and extracapsular salivary tissue. Heterotopic salivary gland tissue (HSGT) is defined as salivary tissue not contained in either major or minor salivary glands. Although rare, this phenomenon has been reported in a multitude of head and neck sites and even distantly in the digestive tract [1]. Most heterotopic implantations occur along lines of embryologic fusion, commonly along the sternocleidomastoid muscle and the sternoclavicular joint and may even be bilateral [2].

Daniel and McGuirt [3], however, found HSGT to be more common in the periparotid region. A slight right-sided predilection seems to occur. The most commonly supported hypothesis is that HSGT develops from vestigial portions or ectodermal heteroplasia of the precervical sinus of His. Other proposed mechanisms are the developmental entrapment of salivary gland tissue in cervical lymph nodes, or embryologic migration of salivary tissue.

An underlying genetic basis is suggested by the association of HSGT with branchio-oto-renal syndrome [4]. Lesions typically appear in infancy and manifest as cervical cysts, masses, or productive sinuses that drain serous and mucoid secretions. Some disagreement exists regarding their association with branchial cleft cysts. Although salivary gland tissue may be found in branchial cleft cysts, HSGT lacks lining epithelium typically found in branchial cleft cysts.

Clinical features that distinguish HSGT from developmental cysts include absence of infection, drainage of clear fluid associated with eating, and absence of communication into the pharynx [5].

---

* Corresponding author.
E-mail address: arsalama@umaryland.edu (A.R. Salama).

Absolute distinction is only possible with histologic examination.

Histologically, HSGT largely resembles normal salivary gland tissue, but has a marked absence of excretory ducts. HSGT without its own duct system is called *aberrant glands*, and *accessory glands* when a duct system is present. This distinction has treatment implications, because surgery for HSGT is simple compared with the potential complexity of branchial clefts cysts. The differential diagnosis should include branchial cyst anomalies, accessory salivary glands, and neoplasia.

Neoplastic transformation in HSGT is uncommon, but the pathologic diversity is the same as that of orthotopic salivary glands [3,6]. Nearly 80% of neoplasms arising in HSGT are benign; the most common is Warthin's tumor, although various benign and malignant tumors have been reported [7]. HSGT can be simply excised; however, with neoplasia, the surgical treatment depends on the histologic nature of the underlying tissue.

The plunging ranula

A ranula is simply a mucocele in the floor of the mouth, notably in the lingual gutter. The term's origin is Latin, *ranula* (frog), because the clinical presentation resembles the bulging underbelly of a frog [8].

Ranula commonly arise from the sublingual gland and represent a mucus extravasation after trauma or obstruction of the sublingual duct. A limited number of patients actually report a history of surgery or trauma in the affected area.

The swelling or extravasation typically expands the surrounding tissue, which may be confined within the oral cavity, occur simultaneously in the oral cavity and neck, and occasionally be present in the neck without an intraoral component [9]. *Plunging* or *diving* ranula describes the extension of the swelling to involve the submandibular or parapharyngeal spaces [10].

Clinically, ranula manifest as painless, fluctuant lateral neck swellings that do not change shape or size with swallowing or eating (Fig. 1A, B). Average size is 4 to 10 cm, but they can extend to the skull base or the retropharyngeal space or toward the supraclavicular region [11]. Approximately 80% are associated with an intraoral component.

Extension into the neck occurs through two mechanisms. Extravasated secretions may dissect along the deep lobe of the submandibular gland between the mylohyoid and hyoglossus muscles. Alternatively, a dehiscence in the mylohyoid muscle allows for unimpeded flow from the sublingual to the submandibular space [12]. One study showed fenestrations in the mylohyoid in 36% to 45% of cadaver dissections [13].

The diagnosis is clinical and fairly straightforward when a cystic swelling in the lateral portion of the neck is accompanied by the prototypical swelling of the floor of the mouth. Diagnosis can be more difficult in the absence of an intraoral component. Fine needle aspiration cytology (FNAC) may be helpful. Analysis of the fluid shows high levels of amylase and may also show histiocytes, which are common in the wall of the pseudocyst [14].

The differential diagnosis should include epidermoid cyst, dermoid cyst, cystic branchial anomalies, cervical lymphangiomas, and malignancy. Cervical metastases, particularly from oropharyngeal cancer, may present as a cystic neck mass, which in patients older than 40 years should be considered malignant until proven otherwise.

CT is valuable diagnostic tool. Cystic swellings in the submandibular or parapharyngeal space that abut or extend into the sublingual space suggest a plunging ranula [10]. The "tail sign" is a radiographic description of a radiolucent duct-like extension between the cervical component and sublingual gland, and is usually located at the posterior margin or through the mylohyoid (Fig. 1C, D) [15].

The most commonly advocated surgical approach is excision of the sublingual gland. Removing the source of the extravasation has lower recurrence rates than other methods. Incision, drainage, and marsupialization generally do not have high rates of success. Recurrence rates reported by Crysdale and colleagues [16] were 61% with simple marsupialization, 100% with incision and drainage, and 0% with sublingual gland excision.

Treating the neck component of the plunging ranula does not require a cervical approach in most cases, and remains somewhat controversial. Drainage rather than excision of the neck component has yielded comparably low rates of recurrence when combined with excision of the sublingual gland [17]. Intraoral sublingual gland removal should be performed, followed by drainage of the neck pseudocyst, which may be approached intraorally using suction catheters,

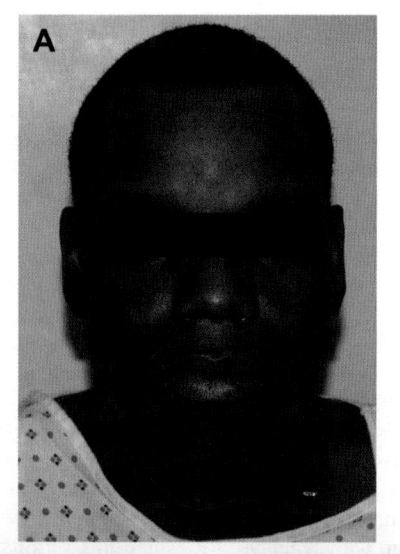

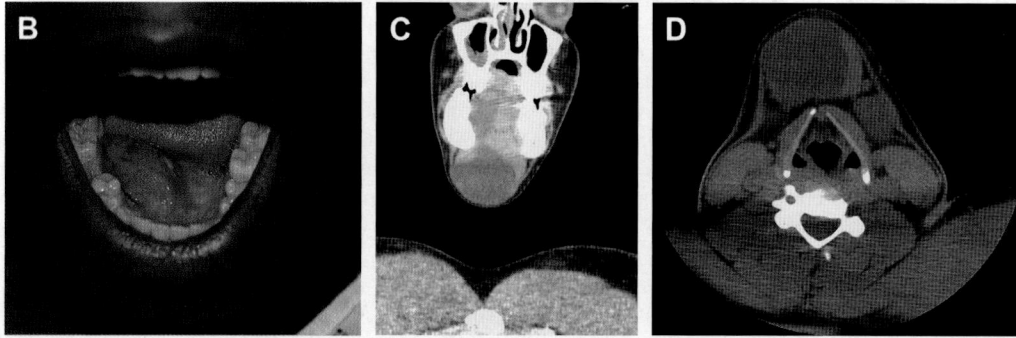

Fig. 1. (*A*, *B*) A 23-year-old African American man who has a recurrent ranula after experiencing a low-velocity gunshot wound 2 years prior. Progression of the ranula manifested as a fluctuant submental swelling. (*C*, *D*) Axial and coronal CT showing an in-continuity cystic lesion extending from the floor of the mouth into the neck with a dehiscence of the mylohyoid muscle. He underwent a right sublingual gland excision and transoral decompression of the neck component.

or transcervically with needle decompression. Compression dressings or surgical suction drains are helpful in preventing fluid reaccumulation in the neck. Closure of the mylohyoid dehiscence is not necessary, but may help eliminate neck recurrence [18].

Rho and colleagues [19] showed complete shrinkage and resolution of plunging ranulae in 33% of patients after one treatment with OK-432, a sclerosant used to treat cervical lymphangiomas. The described technique required multiple reinjections yielding a final recurrence rate of 14%. Fukase and colleagues [20] showed disappearance or marked reduction in 97% of patients treated with OK-432 injections. Another nonsurgical approach is to use Botulinum toxin, which has shown some efficacy in treating floor of mouth ranulae [21].

Extraparotid Warthin's tumor

Warthin's tumor (papillary cystadenoma lymphomatosum) is a slow-growing tumor arising almost exclusively in the parotid, typically in the tail [14]. It comprises 6% to 10% of all benign salivary glands tumors and is most common in white men in their 50s and 60s. The gender distribution has changed over time with a near-equal distribution among men and women [22].

A strong statistical relationship exists between Warthin's tumor and tobacco smoke. Klussmann and colleagues [23] report that 89% of 185 patients in their series were smokers and that smoking was a statistically significant factor in the development of bilateral lesions. It has a broad spectrum of clinical presentation, including bilateralism, multicentricity, and extraparenchymal tumor implantation [24]. Several etiopathogenic theories have been suggested.

One explanation is that salivary gland tissue becomes entrapped in the periparotid or intraparotid lymph nodes and develops into tumors. Theoretically, this phenomenon stems from the late developmental encapsulation of the parotid gland, which allows intermingling of lymphoid and salivary tissue. Another possible mechanism purports that Warthin's tumors arise as a reactive process to degenerated oncocytes.

Extraparotid Warthin's tumor (EPWT) is a rare event and is commonly seen in the periparotid lymph nodes. Among 14 cases of EPWT, Snyderman and colleagues [25] reported that nearly half were incidental pathologic findings in neck dissection specimens performed for malignancy, and one third presented as solitary neck masses. EPWTs not associated with synchronous lesions of the parotid appear as solitary cystic masses along the jugular lymph node chain (levels II and III) [24]. A parotid tail mass may be difficult to distinguish from one located in level II of the neck through clinical examination alone.

CT or MRI may be used to localize a mass and define tumor architecture (cystic versus solid) (Fig. 2). Technetium 99m pertechnetate scintigraphy is particular sensitive in detecting Warthin's tumor and even distinguishing between benign and malignant salivary gland neoplasms. The epithelial cells in Warthin's have the ability to concentrate large anions (pertechnetate). When large cystic spaces are present, the value of technetium 99m scintigraphy is diminished. Diffusion-weighted and dynamic contrast-enhanced MRI have been shown to be more predictive of Warthin's than technetium 99m scintigraphy [26].

EPWT should be included in the differential diagnosis of a cystic neck mass, particularly when found in conjunction with a synchronous parotid mass. A fine-needle aspiration biopsy (FNAB) may help evaluate an EPWT, because its sensitivity approaches 90% [27]. A review of 97 cases reported the accuracy to be 74% because of confounding variables in the specimen (squamous metaplasia/atypia, mucoid/mucinous background, spindle-shaped cells, and cystic/inflammatory debris) [28].

Warthin's tumors and EPWT are slow-growing and typically treated surgically. An extracapsular dissection is recommended for surgical management of EPWT. With multifocal intraparotid lesions, a superficial parotidectomy is advocated. Alternatively, an extracapsular dissection may be performed for a single tumor focus within the parotid gland. An evaluation of the role of extracapsular dissection for parotid tumors showed nearly equivalent 5- and 10-year survival rates, with decreased morbidity, compared to superficial parotidectomy [29].

Because most parotid lymph nodes are found in the tail, Warthin's tumors often occur in this region and may be mistaken for a neck mass [30]. The preferred treatment for these tumors is partial

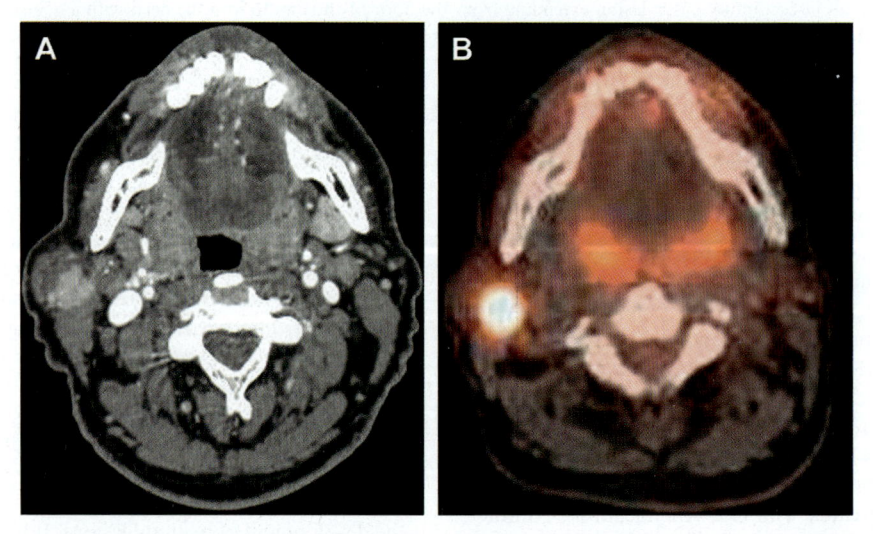

Fig. 2. (*A*, *B*) A CT and PET/CT showing a well-defined mass of the parotid tail. The standard uptake value of the mass was 22. Fine needle aspiration showed atypia without overt malignancy. The final pathology after superficial parotidectomy was Warthin's tumor. (*Courtesy of* Steven Engroff, DDS, MD, State College, PA).

parotidectomy with dissection of the cervical and mandibular branches of the facial nerve. Malignant transformation within Warthin's tumors is reported to be extremely rare; management should be based on the nature of the underlying malignancy.

Pleomorphic adenoma

Pleomorphic adenoma (PA), which is a benign mixed tumor, is the most common salivary gland tumor and accounts for approximately 80% of parotid tumors. These occur over a wide age range, although are most common in the 30s and 40s [14]. PA has been reported in various anatomic locations within the maxillofacial region, including the neck. In a review from the archives of the Armed Forces Institute of Pathology (AFIP) that included 6880 cases of PA, 89 (1.3%) were localized to the cervical lymph nodes.

PA may be found in the neck in several clinical scenarios. PAs of the parotid tail may encroach on level II of the neck. The origin of a mass in this location may be difficult to clinically distinguish as a parotid tail mass, submandibular gland mass, or cervical lymph node. Pedunculated masses arising from the inferior pole of the parotid have been referred to as "earring lesions." No anatomic divisions exist between the parotid tail and the main body of the parotid gland.

Hamilton and colleagues [31] consider the tail to be the inferior 2.0 cm of the gland. Nearly three quarters of parotid tail tumors are benign, with a near-equal distribution between PA and Warthin's tumors. Localizing lesions to the parotid gland in these instances is important to avoid a surgical approach that would injure the marginal mandibular branch of the facial nerve.

A superficial parotidectomy is nearly universally accepted in the surgical management of benign parotid tumors. When used in the management of small (<4 cm) mobile PAs confined to the superficial lobe, recurrence rates range from 1% to 4% [32]. A more conservative surgical approach is a subtotal resection of the superficial lobe, which does not dissect all branches of the facial nerve and removes less nontumorous tissue.

The primary difference between a partial superficial parotid resection and extracapsular dissection is the identification and dissection of the facial nerve and the removal of a margin of uninvolved glandular tissue (Fig. 3). Several authors have shown that partial parotidectomy and extracapsular dissection of a benign PA can be performed with comparable rates of local recurrence. A meta-analysis by Witt [32] did not show a difference in rates of recurrence between superficial parotidectomy and extracapsular dissection.

Although PA displays extracapsular tumor extension, the value of margins has been questioned in relation to local recurrence. Natvig and Soberg [33] did not find a difference in recurrence based on histologic margin status.

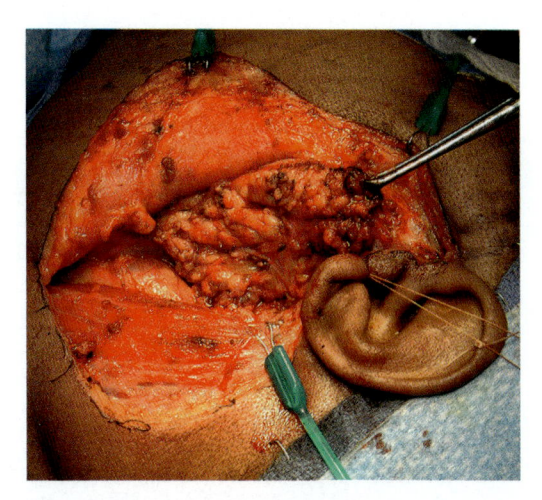

Fig. 3. 44-year-old African American woman who has a parotid tail mass. The cervical and marginal mandibular branches of the facial nerve have been dissected to perform a partial superficial parotidectomy.

Metastasizing pleomorphic adenoma

Although benign, PAs have been reported to metastasize regionally and distantly. Metastasizing pleomorphic adenoma (MPA) displays identical histologic features to their primary site counterparts. El-Naggar and colleagues [34] question the true benign nature of MPA and draw attention to the atypia found in reviewed cases. They believe that the histologic diversity of PA increases chances for sampling errors and misinterpretation and suggest that MPA may represent an unclassified malignant neoplasm.

An overwhelming association exists between incomplete excision of the primary tumor and repeated surgical procedures in the development of MPA [35]. Local recurrence is notably associated with enucleation and capsular rupture during surgery. Most reported cases occur after surgery for a primary tumor, typically in the parotid, minor salivary, or submandibular glands. Experts have suggested that surgical manipulation of tumors allows tumor cells to enter the bloodstream and spread hematogenously [36].

Up to 90% of patients who have MPA have concomitant local recurrence [37]. Metastases typically present several years after the primary is diagnosed. Nouraei and colleagues [38] reported the mean time of metastasis to be 16 years in patients who had a history of local recurrence. The median age of patients who have MPA is approximately 60 years, and no sex predilection is apparent.

Hematogenous metastasis to distant sites is more common than regional cervical metastasis. The most common sites of metastases are bone, head and neck, lungs, and abdomen. Metastatic sites within the head and neck are nearly equally distributed among the cervical lymph nodes and nonlymphatic sites. Metastases at multiple sites and those that occur within 10 years of the primary tumor are associated with a poor prognosis.

Despite the benignity of the tumor, patients who have MPA have 5-year disease-specific survival rates of 58%. Surgical treatment of metastases generally offers the most favorable degree of disease-free survival [35,39]. The value of a therapeutic neck dissection in the presence of cervical metastasis is unclear.

Malignant mixed tumors

Carcinoma ex pleomorphic adenoma (CExPA) is a rare, epithelial malignancy of salivary gland origin that accounts for 3.6% of all salivary neoplasms, 6.2% of all mixed tumors, and 11.6% of malignant salivary neoplasms [40]. Unlike carcinosarcomas of the salivary glands, only the epithelial component is malignant. This malignant component is most commonly adenocarcinoma not otherwise specified, and is recognized as an aggressive clinical entity with propensity for metastasis.

Whether CExPA represents a de novo malignancy or stems from transformation of a benign PA is unclear. Diagnostic criteria include the presence of some histologically benign tissue or history of an excised benign mixed tumor. Diagnosis can be difficult because of the variable size of the malignant component, which may result in biopsy sampling errors. CExPAs are most common in the parotid, followed by the submandibular gland and minor salivary glands.

Malignant transformation is related to the duration of the preexisting benign tumor (Fig. 4). The incidence of transformation is nearly 10% in untreated tumors present for 15 or more years. Among cases reviewed at the AFIP, CExPA occurred an average of 13 years later than their benign counterpart (60 versus 47 years) [41]. Malignant transformation is also seen in with recurrent PAs, with rates ranging from 5% to 7%.

Clinical behavior largely depends on the underlying nature of the malignant component of the tumor; high-grade tumors (adenocarcinoma and ductal carcinoma) are associated with higher rates of regional metastasis. The presence of regional metastasis portends a poor clinical outcome; 5-year survival decreased from 67% to 16% in one study [42]. In a review of 73 patients who had CExPA, Olsen and Lewis [43] reported that 33% had clinically evidence of cervical metastasis at presentation and 16% had occult metastasis after neck dissection.

In a comprehensive review of malignant parotid tumors by Lima and colleagues [44], all cases of CExPA were high-grade tumors. Moreover, grade was a factor in development of metastases and survival.

Cervical lymphadenopathy in the setting of a biopsy-proven CExPA should mandate a neck dissection. Neck dissection confers a survival benefit when performed therapeutically. The value of an elective neck dissection is still debated, although it seems prudent for staging purposes and clearance of occult metastasis. The type of neck dissection for N+ disease (selective versus comprehensive/radical) has not been determined because of the limited number of cases in the literature [45].

Carcinosarcomas are biphasic tumors, with the malignant component comprised of epithelial and mesenchymal tissues. They are rarer than CExPA, representing less than 0.1% of salivary gland tumors. The limited number of cases (8) in the AFIP files confirms their rarity [41].

The major salivary glands are the most common site for carcinosarcomas (80%), although they have been reported in minor salivary glands. Whether they arise de novo or from a preexisting PA, or whether the epithelial and mesenchymal components simultaneously transform is currently debated. Approximately 30% occur in the setting of an existing PA [46]; some experts believe they represent variants of carcinomas.

The prognosis of patients who have salivary carcinosarcomas is extremely poor. A correlation exists between the most abundant malignant histologic component and clinical behavior. The carcinomatous component is typically

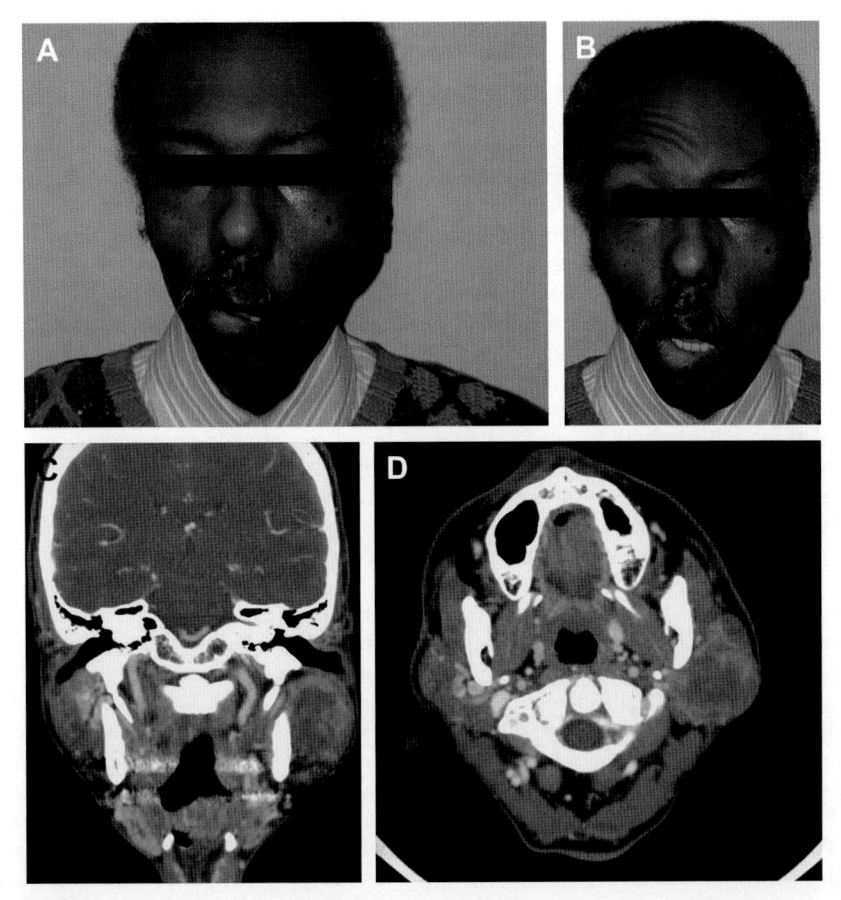

Fig. 4. (A, B) 57-year-old man who has a 10-year history of progressive preauricular swelling. He presented with a complete ipsilateral facial nerve palsy and pain. (C, D) CT scan showing extensive tumor infiltration with a central cystic space; the borders of the tumor are ill-defined.

adenocarcinoma, undifferentiated carcinoma, or squamous cell carcinoma, whereas the sarcomatous tissue is predominantly chondrosarcoma and osteosarcoma [46].

Regional metastasis is uncommon and most metastases are hematogenous rather than lymphatic. The lung is the most common site of metastasis [41]. Regional metastasis mandates a radical neck dissection.

Submandibular gland tumors

The submandibular triangle of the neck (level I) contains the submandibular gland and several first-echelon lymph nodes that drain the oral cavity. Any swelling in this region may indicate a possible neoplasm. Most pathologic processes in the submandibular triangle, however, are nonneoplastic. Approximately three quarters of patients in a survey review of submandibular triangle pathology had either sialadenitis or sialolithiasis. The remainder of the cases were neoplasms; 12% benign and 11% malignant [47].

An estimated 10% to 15% of salivary gland tumors occur in the submandibular gland. The distribution of benign and malignant neoplasms is nearly equal. Most benign tumors are PAs and Warthin's tumors. Adenoid cystic carcinoma (ACC) is the most common malignant neoplasm of the submandibular gland, followed by mucoepidermoid carcinoma (MEC) and malignant mixed tumors. Several rarer tumors have been reported, including acinic cell carcinoma, salivary duct carcinoma, epimyoepithelial carcinoma, carcinosarcoma, oncocytic carcinoma, and primary squamous cell carcinoma.

In the submandibular gland, PA accounts for 40% to 60% of all neoplasia, and 75% of all benign tumors. They occur over a broad age range, from the third to fifth decade [47,48].

Overall, benign tumors have a slight female predilection; the male:female ratio is 2:3 [47]. Malignant submandibular tumors are common later in life (sixth decade) and the gender ratio favors men [49].

Tumors clinically manifest as painless discrete, hard, mobile masses below the inferior border of the mandible. Little correlation is seen between tumor size and symptom duration. Pain is a clinical feature in a minority of patients whose tumors are benign, and is experienced by up to 30% of those whose tumors are malignant [50].

Benign masses of the submandibular gland are difficult to clinically distinguish from those that are malignant, although these tend to be larger and may have faster clinical doubling times [51]. Misdiagnosis and delays are not uncommon, because many patients are preliminary diagnosed with inflammatory or obstructive salivary disorders.

Inflammatory disease is clinically characterized by pain and intermittent swelling, frequently exacerbated with eating. Fixation to the overlying skin and limited mobility are indicative of malignancy, present in only 3% of submandibular tumors [52]. Ipsilateral weakness of the marginal mandibular branch of the facial or hypoglossal nerve, or lingual nerve hypesthesia indicate perineural invasion; they are uncommon late clinical signs almost exclusive to malignancy.

Differential diagnosis of a submandibular mass that has no features of malignancy should include lymphadenopathy, vascular malformation, developmental cysts, and plunging ranula. Hematologic malignancies, including Hodgkin and non-Hodgkin's lymphoma, may manifest as submandibular swellings. Infectious and noninfectious granulomatous disease, such as sarcoidosis and tuberculosis, may also present with swelling and mass in the submandibular region [53]. Bimanual palpation of the gland helps distinguish it from lymphadenopathy. The indolent growth of benign and malignant tumors may lead to erroneous diagnosis and treatment. Many cases are referred to tertiary care centers for management after gland excision [49].

Radiologic evaluation of a submandibular mass is indicated after a thorough history and examination. CT, ultrasound, and MRI can be used to evaluate neck masses. Ultrasound is advocated as an initial noninvasive modality that can assist in determining benign from malignant pathology. It can also be used to guide diagnostic procedures such as FNAB and can help analyze superficial salivary gland lesions with the same precision as CT and MRI [54].

Using ultrasound tumor margin delineation as a decisive tool in distinguishing benign from malignant tumors, Gritzmann [55] showed 90% sensitivity. Ultrasound is a technique-sensitive tool that is underutilized in the United States, where CT and MRI are first-line investigations. Although MRI is widely considered superior in tumor margin determination, Koyuncu and colleagues [56] showed the sensitivity and specificity of CT and MRI were nearly the same for tumor location, tumor margin, and tumor infiltration. Furthermore, they concluded that both modalities provide equivalent diagnostic information for treatment planning purposes. CT may have some benefit in detecting early cortical erosion of the mandible and identifying regional metastatic disease.

In determining the exact anatomic location of submandibular masses (intraglandular versus extraglandular) Chikui and colleagues [57] reported slightly higher accuracy rates with MRI than with contrast-enhanced CT (Fig. 5). Although CT, MRI, and ultrasound enable diagnosis of a submandibular mass, neither seems to safely predict the underlying histology [58]. PET and PET/CT scans have not been shown to predictably differentiate between benign and malignant parotid tumors [59]. In the preoperative evaluation of high-grade salivary gland tumors, however, PET/CT has shown superiority to CT alone in both diagnosis and staging [60].

Preoperative cytologic diagnosis may be obtained through an FNAB. Open biopsy is

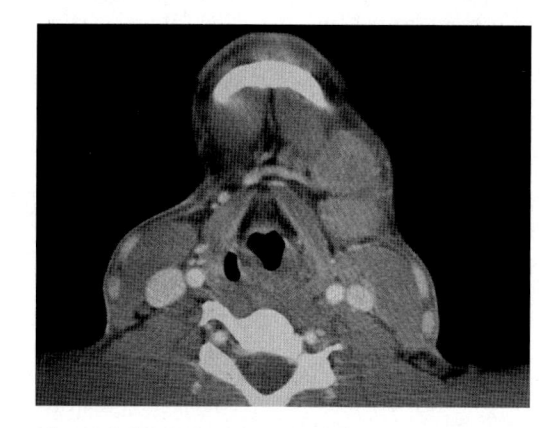

Fig. 5. Axial CT showing a level IB metastatic lymph node from a high-grade mucoepidermoid carcinoma. The tissue plane between the submandibular gland and the level IB lymph node is ill-defined.

generally contraindicated because of potential for tumor seeding and increased risk for local recurrence.

The diagnostic value of FNAB in salivary gland tumors is controversial. FNAB was shown to have a sensitivity and specificity of 73% and 91%, respectively, for distinguishing a benign tumor from a malignancy [61]. Cohen and colleagues [62] concluded that an FNAB positive for malignancy was predictive of the final histologic diagnosis, whereas the predictive value of a negative FNAB was low. Misinterpretation between benign and malignant tumors has been documented, emphasizing that final treatment decisions should not be based on cytologic data alone [47].

Surgery is the primary treatment modality for most if not all salivary gland tumors. Tumors that are preoperatively confirmed as benign can be removed with extracapsular gland dissection. Some authors advocate a more generous resection for PA to include a cuff of normal tissue, because the capsule may be thinner in the submandibular gland [63].

Enucleation is not advocated, because higher rates of local recurrence are seen. PAs are found in proximity to the gland surface in 20% of cases (Fig. 6A) [64]. Extirpation of superficial tumors should involve a margin of connective tissue or platysma, which may mandate isolation and transposition of the marginal mandibular branch of the facial nerve (Fig. 6B).

Although recurrence is less well documented in the submandibular gland, multicentric/multinodular tumors without a pseudocapsule are present in 75% to 98% of recurrent parotid tumors [65,66]. Recurrence is complicated by detection of finite tumor implants. Excising the scar with a margin of the surrounding skin is recommended as part of the en bloc excision [64].

An en bloc resection of level I of the neck is advocated when the diagnosis cannot be confirmed or the tumor is known to be a low-grade malignancy. Some authors have suggested that the initial procedure for all submandibular masses should be a regional dissection. This approach ensures safe removal of benign tumors and simultaneous staging of first-echelon nodes in the case of malignancy [67]. With this approach, low-grade malignancies confined to the gland do not require further treatment after a level I dissection.

A completion selective neck dissection (I–III/IV) is recommended for high-grade tumors. Simple gland excision is often inadequate to treat malignant tumors, which is reflected in lower survival rates [67]. Extraglandular extension requires resection of adjacent tissue to achieve surgical margins. Tumor clearance frequently involves excision of the mylohyoid and digastric muscles and the lingual and hypoglossal nerves [49].

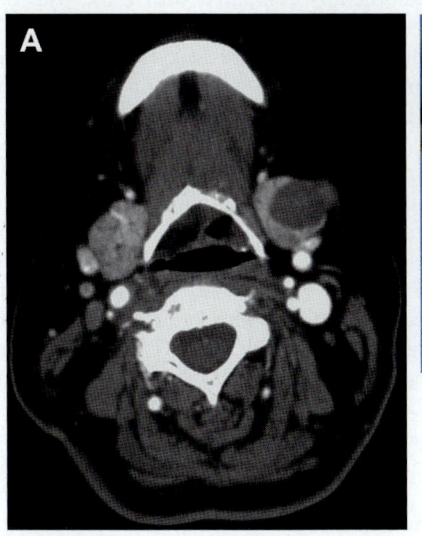

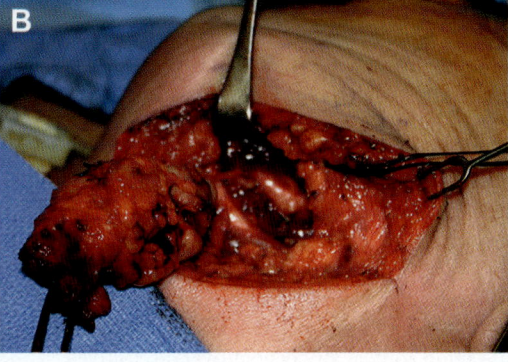

Fig. 6. (*A*) Contrast-enhanced axial CT showing a distinct soft tissue mass in the superficial portion of the left submandibular gland. The mass approximates the platysma. Fine needle aspiration biopsy suggested pleomorphic adenoma. (*B*) Surgical resection of the entire gland with a cuff of platysma muscle as the superficial surgical margin. The final pathology was pleomorphic adenoma. (*From* Carlson E, Ord R. Textbook and color atlas of salivary gland pathology. Oxford: Wiley-Blackwell, 2008; with permission.)

The presence of cervical metastasis and knowledge of a high-grade tumor dictate a systematic approach based on tumor behavior. The likelihood of regional metastasis is partly determined by tumor histology. Patient age, histologic grade, facial nerve involvement, extraglandular extension, and tumor size have been shown to be clinical predictors of nodal metastasis [68].

Tumors with higher rates of cervical metastasis include high-grade MEC, high-grade and anaplastic adenocarcinoma, and salivary duct carcinoma. Spiro [51] reported more frequent metastases with submandibular MEC than from other sites. A strong relationship exists between tumor grade and metastasis. In a clinicopathologic study of patients who had MEC, 33% developed regional metastases, of which 85% had high-grade tumors [69]. ACC infrequently metastasizes to the cervical lymph nodes, and distant metastases are far more common.

The reported rate for clinical lymph node metastasis from malignant submandibular tumors is 8% to 20% [49,70]. The overall rate of cervical metastasis from submandibular tumors, including those harvested during neck dissection, is as high as 41% [71]. The most frequently involved nodes for submandibular malignancies are level II, I, III, IV, and V (in descending order) [72].

An elective neck dissection in an N0 neck is commonly performed when the risk for metastasis is greater than 20%, although its benefit has not been established. This procedure is recommended for high-grade tumors, extracapsular extension, and larger tumors (>4 cm) [73]. Intraoperative frozen section analysis has been used to determine whether to perform an elective neck dissection.

Postoperative radiation has been suggested as an alternative to elective neck dissection [74]. The treatment of the N0 neck in salivary gland cancer has not been evaluated in a prospective controlled manner. A radical neck dissection is indicated with clinical evidence of regional metastasis; however, limited data indicate that a comprehensive neck dissection confers any benefit over a selective neck dissection (I–III or I–IV).

Prognosis largely depends on the histologic grade and stage. Camilleri and colleagues [49] reported that clinical stage at presentation was the most powerful prognosticator; the 5-year survival rates were 85% and 20% in stage I and IV disease, respectively. Hocwald and colleagues [73] stated that the only predictor of clinical outcome on multivariate analysis was histologic evidence of cervical node involvement.

The presence of regional metastases decreases mean survival by greater than 50% [68]. Advanced age and male gender have also been shown to confer a poor prognosis. Although ACC is the most common malignancy, patients who have intermediate- and high-grade MEC have a worse prognosis. Rinaldo and colleagues [75] reported 10-year relative survival rates of 73%, 62%, and 53% for submandibular ACC, CExPA, and MEC, respectively.

Distant metastases occurs in 5% to 50% of patients who have ACC, most commonly the lung, and has been shown to occur years after treatment of the primary, even in the setting of local and regional control [76]. Regional metastasis from submandibular ACC is more common than in the other major salivary glands, presumably because of the proximity of the draining lymph nodes [75].

Traditionally, salivary gland carcinomas were considered radioresistant. Recent reports suggest that radiation may provide some degree of locoregional control. Adjuvant therapy is reserved for patients who have advanced-stage disease (III/IV), inadequate surgical margins, high tumor grade, and high-risk histologic features (perineural/perivascular invasion) [51].

Armstrong and colleagues [70] showed improved local control in patients who had advanced-stage disease who underwent postoperative radiotherapy compared with those who did not (69% versus 40%). Storey and colleagues [77] reported 2-, 5-, and 10-year actuarial locoregional control rates of 90%, 88%, and 88%, respectively, in a cohort involving postoperative radiotherapy.

Mendenhall and colleagues [78] showed improved 10-year locoregional control rates between radiation alone and adjuvant radiotherapy in early- and advanced-stage disease. The overall benefit in locoregional control was also remarkable (81% versus 40%). As a sole treatment modality in patients who had stage I to III disease, radiation provided 10-year overall survival and local control rates of 65% and 75%, respectively. The response rates in these patient may be dose-related, because doses greater than 70 Gy resulted in improved outcomes, particularly with ACC.

Radiation fields, including the tract of invaded named nerves to the skull base, confer a greater degree of local control. Radiation alone is reserved for patients who have advanced-staged disease or those who have severe medical comorbidities. Most patients undergoing radiation alone for curative intent have advanced-stage disease and poor prognosis. Only an estimated 20% of patients who have stage IV disease will be cured with radiation alone [78].

Treatment failures are caused by recurrent or residual primary disease and regional and distant metastasis. Hocwald and colleagues [73] showed that distant failure was more common than locoregional failure (28% versus 19%). Locoregional control provides some survival benefit. Recurrence is related to the number of positive lymph nodes, male gender, named nerve involvement, and extraglandular extension of tumor [78]. The impact of local recurrence on survival depends on stage and tumor grade. The 5- and 10-year determinate survival rates among patients who have recurrent high-grade tumors are 40% and 29% [75]; the 10-year overall survival is 55% to 60% [77,78]. Locally recurrent disease is managed with surgery if possible, followed by radiation.

Conventional postoperative radiotherapy offers limited benefit in the presence of gross residual disease, with locoregional control rates ranging from 20% to 30%. Fast neutron radiotherapy (FNRT) has proven benefit in patients who have gross residual disease. Douglas and colleagues [79] achieved a 6-year actuarial survival rate of 59% using FNRT.

A smaller study comparing FNRT and conventional radiotherapy for inoperable or recurrent salivary gland carcinoma clearly showed the advantages of FRNT, with a locoregional control at 10-years of 56% versus 17% with statistical significance. A modest, statistically insignificant benefit in survival was seen: 25% versus 15% [80]. Severe and life-threatening complications from FNRT are nearly double those of conventional radiotherapy.

Parotid carcinoma and the neck

Parotid carcinomas are uncommon, constituting 14% to 25% of all parotid tumors [51,81]. Zbaren and colleagues [82] stratified patients into high- and low-grade malignancies with near-equal distribution. The most common high-grade tumors were adenocarcinoma, CExPA, squamous cell carcinoma, MEC, and ACC.

Prognosis and management of parotid malignancies are related to the staging and histologic grading of the tumor. Significant prognostic factors also include extraglandular extension, nodal status, perineural invasion, and facial nerve dysfunction [44,68,73]. Advanced age is also considered a poor prognosticator.

Luukkaa and colleagues [83] reported 5-year survival rates of 78%, 25%, 21%, and 23%, respectively, according to stage (I–IV). The presence of nodal metastasis has been shown to affect overall survival [84]. The overall 5-year survival in parotid cancer with and without nodal metastasis is 10% and 75%, respectively [85].

Kaplan and Johns [86] stratified the treatment of parotid malignancies. Early-stage low-grade malignancies (T1 and T2) are addressed with a parotidectomy. Similarly staged high-grade tumors are treated with parotidectomy and selective neck dissection followed by radiotherapy. Recurrent tumors and those with clinical evidence of nodal metastasis are addressed with a nerve-sacrificing parotidectomy and radial neck dissection followed by postoperative radiotherapy.

Significant controversy surrounds the benefit of radiotherapy and neck dissection in managing parotid malignancies. Nodal metastasis in parotid cancer is variable; 16% to 20% of patients have evidence of pathologically involved nodes at presentation [82,84], and the incidence of occult metastasis is approximately 20% [82,87].

Risk for nodal involvement is related to tumor stage and histologic grade. Frankenthaler and colleagues [88] reported that tumor grade, patient age, lymphatic invasion, and extraparotid tumor extension were predictive of occult cervical metastasis. The indications for elective neck dissection have become better defined. Medina [74] recommends elective neck dissection in the following circumstances: high-grade tumor, T3/T4 tumors, facial nerve paralysis, age older than 54 years, extraglandular extension, and perilymphatic invasion.

An observational study of the value of elective neck dissection for parotid malignancies showed a 5-year disease-free survival rate of 86% among patients who underwent this procedure compared with 69% for those who did not. The same study showed a 5-year survival rate of 80% for patients who had an N0 neck, and no difference in survival based on treatment [87]. Armstrong and colleagues [70] suggested that patients at high risk undergo neck dissection involving at least levels I, II, and III.

In reviewing the use of postoperative radiotherapy in managing the N0 neck, Chen and colleagues [89] showed that the use of elective neck irradiation did not confer a statistically significant survival benefit. However, the 5- and 10-year estimated rate of disease-free survival was 81% and 63%, respectively. No patients who underwent elective neck dissection experienced nodal relapse, compared with 24 of 120 who did not have this procedure. Nodal relapse was most common with squamous cell carcinoma, adenocarcinoma, and MEC.

References

[1] Downs-Kelly E, Hoschar AP, Prayson RA. Salivary gland heterotopia in the rectum. Ann Diagn Pathol 2003;7(2):124–6.

[2] Lassaletta-Atienza L, Lopez-Rios F, Martin G, et al. Salivary gland heterotopia in the lower neck: a report of five cases. Int J Pediatr Otorhinolaryngol 1998; 43(2):153–61.

[3] Daniel E, McGuirt WF Sr. Neck masses secondary to heterotopic salivary gland tissue: a 25-year experience. Am J Otolaryngol 2005;26(2):96–100.

[4] Joseph MP, Goodman ML, Pilch BZ, et al. Heterotopic cervical salivary gland tissue in a family with probable branchio-otorenal syndrome. Head Neck Surg 1986;8(6):456–62.

[5] Stingle WH, Priebe CJ Jr. Ectopic salivary gland and sinus in the lower neck. Ann Otol Rhinol Laryngol 1974;83(3):379–81.

[6] Gudbrandsson FK, Liston SL, Maisel RA. Heterotopic salivary tissue in the neck. Otolaryngol Head Neck Surg 1982;90(3 Pt 1):279–82.

[7] Ferlito A, Bertino G, Rinaldo A, et al. A review of heterotopia and associated salivary gland neoplasms of the head and neck. J Laryngol Otol 1999;113(4): 299–303.

[8] McGurk M. The surgical management of salivary gland disease of the sublingual gland and floor of mouth. Atlas Oral Maxillofac Surg Clin North Am 1998;6(1):51–74.

[9] Zhao YF, Jia Y, Chen XM, et al. Clinical review of 580 ranulas. Oral Surg Oral Med Oral Pathol Oral Radiol Endod 2004;98(3):281–7.

[10] Coit WE, Harnsberger HR, Osborn AG, et al. Ranulas and their mimics: CT evaluation. Radiology 1987;163(1):211–6.

[11] Davison MJ, Morton RP, McIvor NP. Plunging ranula: clinical observations. Head Neck 1998; 20(1):63–8.

[12] Mair IW, Schewitsch I, Svendsen E, et al. Cervical ranula. J Laryngol Otol 1979;93(6):623–8.

[13] Yates C. A surgical approach to the sublingual salivary gland. Ann R Coll Surg Engl 1994;76(2): 108–9.

[14] Gnepp DR, editor. Diagnostic surgical pathology of the head and neck. Philadelphia: W.B. Saunders Company; 2001.

[15] Anastassov GE, Haiavy J, Solodnik P, et al. Submandibular gland mucocele: diagnosis and management. Oral Surg Oral Med Oral Pathol Oral Radiol Endod 2000;89(2):159–63.

[16] Crysdale WS, Mendelsohn JD, Conley S. Ranulas—mucoceles of the oral cavity: experience in 26 children. Laryngoscope 1988;98(3):296–8.

[17] Parekh D, Stewart M, Joseph C, et al. Plunging ranula: a report of three cases and review of the literature. Br J Surg 1987;74(4):307–9.

[18] Mahadevan M, Vasan N. Management of pediatric plunging ranula. Int J Pediatr Otorhinolaryngol 2006;70(6):1049–54.

[19] Rho MH, Kim DW, Kwon JS, et al. OK-432 sclerotherapy of plunging ranula in 21 patients: it can be a substitute for surgery. AJNR Am J Neuroradiol 2006;27(5):1090–5.

[20] Fukase S, Ohta N, Inamura K, et al. Treatment of ranula with intracystic injection of the streptococcal preparation OK-432. Ann Otol Rhinol Laryngol 2003;112(3):214–20.

[21] Chow TL, Chan SW, Lam SH. Ranula successfully treated by botulinum toxin type A: report of 3 cases. Oral Surg Oral Med Oral Pathol Oral Radiol Endod 2008;105:1:41–2. Epub 2007 Aug 30.

[22] Lamelas J, Terry JH Jr, Alfonso AE. Warthin's tumor: multicentricity and increasing incidence in women. Am J Surg 1987;154(4):347–51.

[23] Peter Klussmann J, Wittekindt C, Florian Preuss S, et al. High risk for bilateral Warthin tumor in heavy smokers—review of 185 cases. Acta Otolaryngol 2006;126(11):1213–7.

[24] Astor FC, Hanft KL, Rooney P, et al. Extraparotid Warthin's tumor: clinical manifestations, challenges, and controversies. Otolaryngol Head Neck Surg 1996;114(6):732–5.

[25] Snyderman C, Johnson JT, Barnes EL. Extraparotid Warthin's tumor. Otolaryngol Head Neck Surg 1986;94(2):169–75.

[26] Motoori K, Ueda T, Uchida Y, et al. Identification of Warthin tumor: magnetic resonance imaging versus salivary scintigraphy with technetium-99m pertechnetate. J Comput Assist Tomogr 2005;29(4): 506–12.

[27] Raymond MR, Yoo JH, Heathcote JG, et al. Accuracy of fine-needle aspiration biopsy for Warthin's tumours. J Otolaryngol 2002;31(5):263–70.

[28] Parwani AV, Ali SZ. Diagnostic accuracy and pitfalls in fine-needle aspiration interpretation of Warthin tumor. Cancer 2003;99(3):166–71.

[29] McGurk M, Thomas BL, Renehan AG. Extracapsular dissection for clinically benign parotid lumps: reduced morbidity without oncological compromise. Br J Cancer 2003;89(9):1610–3.

[30] McKean ME, Lee K, McGregor IA. The distribution of lymph nodes in and around the parotid gland: an anatomical study. Br J Plast Surg 1985; 38(1):1–5.

[31] Hamilton BE, Salzman KL, Wiggins RH 3rd, et al. Earring lesions of the parotid tail. AJNR Am J Neuroradiol 2003;24(9):1757–64.

[32] Witt RL. The significance of the margin in parotid surgery for pleomorphic adenoma. Laryngoscope 2002;112(12):2141–54.

[33] Natvig K, Soberg R. Relationship of intraoperative rupture of pleomorphic adenomas to recurrence: an

[33] ... 11-25 year follow-up study. Head Neck 1994;16(3): 213–7.
[34] el-Naggar A, Batsakis JG, Kessler S. Benign metastatic mixed tumours or unrecognized salivary carcinomas? J Laryngol Otol 1988;102(9):810–2.
[35] Nouraei SA, Ferguson MS, Clarke PM, et al. Metastasizing pleomorphic salivary adenoma. Arch Otolaryngol Head Neck Surg 2006;132(7):788–93.
[36] Marioni G, Marino F, Stramare R, et al. Benign metastasizing pleomorphic adenoma of the parotid gland: a clinicopathologic puzzle. Head Neck 2003; 25(12):1071–6.
[37] Raja V, China C, Masaki KH, et al. Unusual presentations of uncommon tumors: case 1. Benign metastasizing pleomorphic adenoma. J Clin Oncol 2002;20(9):2400–3.
[38] Wenig BM, Hitchcock CL, Ellis GL, et al. Metastasizing mixed tumor of salivary glands. A clinicopathologic and flow cytometric analysis. Am J Surg Pathol 1992;16(9):845–58.
[39] Bradley PJ. 'Metastasizing pleomorphic salivary adenoma' should now be considered a low-grade malignancy with a lethal potential. Curr Opin Otolaryngol Head Neck Surg 2005;13(2):123–6.
[40] Gnepp DR. Malignant mixed tumors of the salivary glands: a review. Pathol Annu 1993;(28 Pt 1): 279–328.
[41] Ellis GL, Auclair PL. Tumors of the salivary glands. In: Rosai J, Sobin L, editors. Armed Forces Institute of Pathology; 1996.
[42] Chen AM, Garcia J, Bucci MK, et al. The role of postoperative radiation therapy in carcinoma ex pleomorphic adenoma of the parotid gland. Int J Radiat Oncol Biol Phys 2007;67(1):138–43.
[43] Olsen KD, Lewis JE. Carcinoma ex pleomorphic adenoma: a clinicopathologic review. Head Neck 2001; 23(9):705–12.
[44] Lima RA, Tavares MR, Dias FL, et al. Clinical prognostic factors in malignant parotid gland tumors. Otolaryngol Head Neck Surg 2005;133(5): 702–8.
[45] Nouraei SA, Hope KL, Kelly CG, et al. Carcinoma ex benign pleomorphic adenoma of the parotid gland. Plast Reconstr Surg 2005;116(5):1206–13.
[46] Tanahashi J, Daa T, Kashima K, et al. Carcinosarcoma ex recurrent pleomorphic adenoma of the submandibular gland. APMIS 2007;115(6):789–94.
[47] Munir N, Bradley PJ. Diagnosis and management of neoplastic lesions of the submandibular triangle. Oral Oncol 2008;44(3):251–60. Epub 2007 Apr 27.
[48] Alves FA, Perez DE, Almeida OP, et al. Pleomorphic adenoma of the submandibular gland: clinicopathological and immunohistochemical features of 60 cases in Brazil. Arch Otolaryngol Head Neck Surg 2002;128(12):1400–3.
[49] Camilleri IG, Malata CM, McLean NR, et al. Malignant tumours of the submandibular salivary gland: a 15-year review. Br J Plast Surg 1998;51(3): 181–5.
[50] Spiro J, Spiro RH. The neck: diagnosis and surgery. St. Louis: Mosby; 1994 295–306.
[51] Spiro RH. Salivary neoplasms: overview of a 35-year experience with 2,807 patients. Head Neck Surg 1986;8(3):177–84.
[52] Terhaard CH, Lubsen H, Van der Tweel I, et al. Salivary gland carcinoma: independent prognostic factors for locoregional control, distant metastases, and overall survival: results of the Dutch head and neck oncology cooperative group. Head Neck 2004;26(8):681–92 [discussion 692–93].
[53] Rapidis AD, Stavrianos S, Lagogiannis G, et al. Tumors of the submandibular gland: clinicopathologic analysis of 23 patients. J Oral Maxillofac Surg 2004; 62(10):1203–8.
[54] Yousem DM, Kraut MA, Chalian AA. Major salivary gland imaging. Radiology 2000;216(1):19–29.
[55] Gritzmann N. Sonography of the salivary glands. AJR Am J Roentgenol 1989;153(1):161–6.
[56] Koyuncu M, Sesen T, Akan H, et al. Comparison of computed tomography and magnetic resonance imaging in the diagnosis of parotid tumors. Otolaryngol Head Neck Surg 2003;129(6):726–32.
[57] Chikui T, Shimizu M, Goto TK, et al. Interpretation of the origin of a submandibular mass by CT and MRI imaging. Oral Surg Oral Med Oral Pathol Oral Radiol Endod 2004;98(6):721–9.
[58] Rudack C, Jorg S, Kloska S, et al. Neither MRI, CT nor US is superior to diagnose tumors in the salivary glands—an extended case study. Head Face Med 2007;3:1–8.
[59] Rubello D, Nanni C, Castellucci P, et al. Does 18F-FDG PET/CT play a role in the differential diagnosis of parotid masses. Panminerva Med 2005;47(3): 187–9.
[60] Jeong HS, Chung MK, Son YI, et al. Role of 18F-FDG PET/CT in management of high-grade salivary gland malignancies. J Nucl Med 2007; 48(8):1237–44.
[61] Hughes JH, Volk EE, Wilbur DC. Pitfalls in salivary gland fine-needle aspiration cytology: lessons from the college of American pathologists interlaboratory comparison program in nongynecologic cytology. Arch Pathol Lab Med 2005;129(1):26–31.
[62] Cohen EG, Patel SG, Lin O, et al. Fine-needle aspiration biopsy of salivary gland lesions in a selected patient population. Arch Otolaryngol Head Neck Surg 2004;130(6):773–8.
[63] Webb AJ, Eveson JW. Pleomorphic adenomas of the major salivary glands: a study of the capsular form in relation to surgical management. Clin Otolaryngol Allied Sci 2001;26(2):134–42.
[64] Laskawi R, Ellies M, Arglebe C, et al. Surgical management of benign tumors of the submandibular gland: a follow-up study. J Oral Maxillofac Surg 1995;53(5):506–8 [discussion 509].
[65] Zbaren P, Tschumi I, Nuyens M, et al. Recurrent pleomorphic adenoma of the parotid gland. Am J Surg 2005;189(2):203–7.

[66] Glas AS, Vermey A, Hollema H, et al. Surgical treatment of recurrent pleomorphic adenoma of the parotid gland: a clinical analysis of 52 patients. Head Neck 2001;23(4):311–6.
[67] Weber RS, Byers RM, Petit B, et al. Submandibular gland tumors. Adverse histologic factors and therapeutic implications. Arch Otolaryngol Head Neck Surg 1990;116(9):1055–60.
[68] Bhattacharyya N, Fried MP. Nodal metastasis in major salivary gland cancer: predictive factors and effects on survival. Arch Otolaryngol Head Neck Surg 2002;128(8):904–8.
[69] Brandwein MS, Ivanov K, Wallace DI, et al. Mucoepidermoid carcinoma: a clinicopathologic study of 80 patients with special reference to histological grading. Am J Surg Pathol 2001;25(7):835–45.
[70] Armstrong JG, Harrison LB, Thaler HT, et al. The indications for elective treatment of the neck in cancer of the major salivary glands. Cancer 1992; 69(3):615–9.
[71] Terhaard CH. Postoperative and primary radiotherapy for salivary gland carcinomas: indications, techniques, and results. Int J Radiat Oncol Biol Phys 2007;69(2 Suppl):S52–5.
[72] Terhaard CH, Lubsen H, Rasch CR, et al. The role of radiotherapy in the treatment of malignant salivary gland tumors. Int J Radiat Oncol Biol Phys 2005;61(1):103–11.
[73] Hocwald E, Korkmaz H, Yoo GH, et al. Prognostic factors in major salivary gland cancer. Laryngoscope 2001;111(8):1434–9.
[74] Medina JE. Neck dissection in the treatment of cancer of major salivary glands. Otolaryngol Clin North Am 1998;31(5):815–22.
[75] Rinaldo A, Ferlito A, Pellitteri PK, et al. Management of malignant submandibular gland tumors. Acta Otolaryngol 2003;123(8):896–904.
[76] Cohen AN, Damrose EJ, Huang RY, et al. Adenoid cystic carcinoma of the submandibular gland: a 35-year review. Otolaryngol Head Neck Surg 2004; 131(6):994–1000.
[77] Storey MR, Garden AS, Morrison WH, et al. Postoperative radiotherapy for malignant tumors of the submandibular gland. Int J Radiat Oncol Biol Phys 2001;51(4):952–8.
[78] Mendenhall WM, Morris CG, Amdur RJ, et al. Radiotherapy alone or combined with surgery for salivary gland carcinoma. Cancer 2005;103(12): 2544–50.
[79] Douglas JG, Koh WJ, Austin-Seymour M, et al. Treatment of salivary gland neoplasms with fast neutron radiotherapy. Arch Otolaryngol Head Neck Surg 2003;129(9):944–8.
[80] Laramore GE, Krall JM, Griffin TW, et al. Neutron versus photon irradiation for unresectable salivary gland tumors: final report of an RTOG-MRC randomized clinical trial. Radiation Therapy Oncology Group. Medical Research Council. Int J Radiat Oncol Biol Phys 1993;27(2):235–40.
[81] Gallo O, Franchi A, Bottai GV, et al. Risk factors for distant metastases from carcinoma of the parotid gland. Cancer 1997;80(5):844–51.
[82] Zbaren P, Schupbach J, Nuyens M, et al. Carcinoma of the parotid gland. Am J Surg 2003; 186(1):57–62.
[83] Luukkaa H, Klemi P, Leivo I, et al. Salivary gland cancer in Finland 1991–96: an evaluation of 237 cases. Acta Otolaryngol 2005;125(2):207–14.
[84] Kelley DJ, Spiro RH. Management of the neck in parotid carcinoma. Am J Surg 1996;172(6): 695–7.
[85] Spiro RH, Huvos AG, Strong EW. Cancer of the parotid gland. A clinicopathologic study of 288 primary cases. Am J Surg 1975;130(4):452–9.
[86] Kaplan MJ, Johns ME. Salivary gland cancer. Clin Oncol 1986;5(3):525–47.
[87] Zbaren P, Schupbach J, Nuyens M, et al. Elective neck dissection versus observation in primary parotid carcinoma. Otolaryngol Head Neck Surg 2005;132(3):387–91.
[88] Frankenthaler RA, Byers RM, Luna MA, et al. Predicting occult lymph node metastasis in parotid cancer. Arch Otolaryngol Head Neck Surg 1993; 119(5):517–20.
[89] Chen AM, Garcia J, Lee NY, et al. Patterns of nodal relapse after surgery and postoperative radiation therapy for carcinomas of the major and minor salivary glands: what is the role of elective neck irradiation? Int J Radiat Oncol Biol Phys 2007;67(4): 988–94.

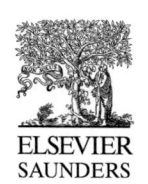

Neck Dissection: Nomenclature, Classification, and Technique
Jon D. Holmes, DMD, MD, FACS[a,b]

[a]Oral and Facial Surgery of Alabama, 1500 19th Street South, Birmingham, AL 35205, USA
[b]University of Alabama at Birmingham, Birmingham, AL, USA

The ability of a cancer to metastasize most commonly manifests itself by growth in regional lymph nodes. Lymph node status is the single most important prognostic factor in head and neck cancer because lymph node involvement basically decreases overall survival by 50%. Unfortunately, approximately 40% of patients with oral cancer will harbor cervical lymph node metastasis at presentation [1]. Appropriate management of the regional lymphatics, therefore, plays a central role in the treatment of the head and neck cancer patients. Removal of the at-risk lymphatic basins serves two important purposes. First, it allows the removal and identification of occult metastasis in patients in whom cervical metastasis are a risk, which is referred to as an elective neck dissection. Secondly, it allows the removal of disease in patients in whom metastasis are highly suspected based on imaging, clinical examination or fine needle aspiration, which is referred to as a therapeutic neck dissection. (Note that the term "prophylactic neck dissection" should be avoided and replaced with the more accurate term "elective neck dissection," when discussing removal of at-risk lymphatic basins in the absence of clinical evidence of metastasis.) Performing an appropriate neck dissection results in minimal morbidity for the patient, provides invaluable data to accurately stage the patient, and guides the need for further therapy. It is especially indicated in almost all cases of oral cavity cancer, for which the treatment of choice for the primary remains surgery in most cases.

The purpose of this article is to present the history and evolution of neck dissections, including an update on the current state of nomenclature and current neck dissection classification, describe the technique of the most common neck dissection applicable to oral cavity cancers, and discuss some of the complications associated with neck dissection. Finally, a brief review of sentinel lymph node biopsy will be presented. Indications for the various neck dissections are discussed in other articles in this issue and in other excellent reviews [2].

Lymph node levels: anatomy and nomenclature

The head and neck are drained by a rich network of interconnected lymphatics. Knowledge of regional lymph flow and cervical lymph node anatomy is necessary for staging and guiding therapy, whether surgery for occult metastasis or designing an appropriate radiation treatment plan.

Rouviere [3] demonstrated that the lymph drainage from mucosal sites within the head and neck occurred in a predictable pattern leading to one or more of the approximately 300 lymph nodes located above the clavicle. Lindberg [4] subsequently found that cancers of the head and neck metastasize in a consistent manner to first echelon lymph nodes. In areas disturbed by previous surgery, radiation or bulky tumors, lymph flow can completely bypass first echelon nodes because of increased hydrostatic pressure within the node [5]. Building upon the work of Rouviere and Lindberg, Shah and others demonstrated the efficacy of modifications of the standard neck dissection

E-mail address: j-holmes@mindspring.com

and selective removal of nodes at highest risk (see discussion below on selective neck dissection). Important to communication among researchers and clinicians, a division of cervical lymph nodes into levels defined by clinical and radiographic landmarks was proposed by clinicians at Memorial Sloan-Kettering Cancer Center. Subsequent modifications suggested by the Head and Neck Service at M.D. Anderson resulted in the generally accepted levels endorsed by the American Head and Neck Society and the American Academy of Otolaryngology and defined below [6–8]. The most important aspect of the current subdivisions is the correlation between radiographic landmarks used by radiologists and radiation oncologists; and surgical landmarks to describe accurately which lymph node basins are excised (Fig. 1).

Level I

Level I includes the submandibular and submental nodes. It extends from the inferior border of the mandible superiorly to the hyoid inferiorly, and is bounded by the digastric muscle. It may be subdivided:

- Level I a: The submental group. Lies between the anterior bellies of the digastric muscles. Bounded superiorly by the symphysis and inferiorly by the hyoid;
- Level I b: The submandibular group. Bounded by the body of the mandible superiorly, the posterior belly of the digastric muscle inferiorly, the stylohyoid muscle posteriorly, and the anterior belly of the digastric anteriorly. It includes the pre- and postvascular nodes that are related to the facial artery.

Lymph nodes contained within level I are at highest risk in oral cancers involving the skin of the chin, lower lip, tip of the tongue, and floor of the mouth [3,4].

Level II

Level II contains the upper jugular lymph nodes that surround the upper third of the internal jugular vein and the spinal accessory nerve. It includes the jugulodigastric node (also known as the principle node of Kuttner) which is the most common node containing metastases in oral cancer. It is also frequently subdivided based on the course of the spinal accessory nerve.

- Level II a: Bounded superiorly by the skull base, inferiorly by the hyoid bone radiographically and the carotid bifurcation surgically, anteriorly by the stylohyoid muscle and posteriorly by a vertical plane defined by the spinal accessory nerve.
- Level II b: Bounded superiorly by the skull base, inferiorly by the hyoid bone radiographically and the carotid bifurcation surgically, anteriorly by a vertical plane defined by the spinal accessory nerve and posteriorly by the lateral aspect of the sternocleidomastoid muscle.

Nodal tissue within level II receives efferent lymphatics the parotid, submandibular, submental, and retropharyngeal nodal groups. It also is at risk for metastases from cancers arising in many oral and extra-oral sites, including, the nasal cavity, pharynx, middle ear, tongue, hard and soft palate, and tonsils [3,4].

Level III

Level III encompasses node-bearing tissue surrounding the middle third of the internal jugular vein. It is bounded superiorly by the inferior border of level II (hyoid radiographically and carotid bifurcation surgically), inferiorly by the omohyoid muscle surgically and the cricoid cartilage radiographically, anteriorly by the sternohyoid muscle and posteriorly by the lateral border of the sternocleidomastoid muscle. Level III contains the dominant omohyoid node and receives lymphatic drainage from level II and level V. In addition, it can receive efferent lymphatics

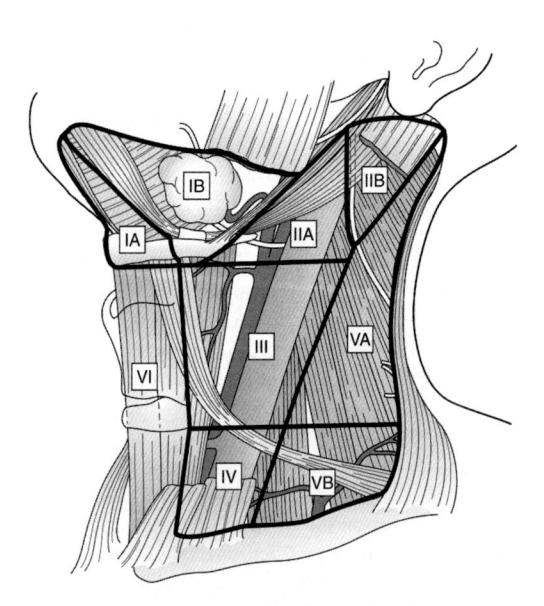

Fig. 1. Current lymph node levels.

from the retropharyngeal, pretracheal, tongue base, and tonsils.

Level IV

Level IV contains the nodal tissue surrounding the inferior third of the internal jugular vein. It extends from the inferior border of level III to the clavicle. Anteriorly, it is bounded by the lateral border of the sternohyoid muscle; and posteriorly, by the lateral border of the sternocleidomastoid muscle. It contains a variable number of nodes that receive efferent flow primarily from levels III and IV. The retropharyngeal, pretracheal, hypopharyngeal, laryngeal and thyroid lymphatics also make a contribution. Only rarely is level IV involved with metastatic cancer from the oral cavity without involvement of one of the higher levels.

Level V

Level V makes up the posterior triangle. Similar to levels I and II, level V may be subdivided.

- Level V a: Begins at the apex formed by the intersection of the sternocleidomastoid and the trapezius. The inferior border is established by a horizontal line defined by the lower edge of the cricoid cartilage. Medially, the posterior edge of the sternocleidomastoid forms the anterior edge and the anterior border of the trapezius forms the posterior (lateral) border.
- Level V b: Begins at a line defined by the inferior edge of the cricoid cartilage and extends to the clavicle. It shares the same medial and lateral borders as level Va.

Level V receives efferent flow from the occipital and post auricular nodes. Its importance in primary oral cavity cancers is limited except when lymph flow is redirected by metastases in the higher levels. Oropharyngeal cancers, however, such as tongue base and tonsillar primaries can spread to level V nodes.

Level VI

The anterior compartment lymph node group is of minimal importance in primaries originating in the oral cavity. It is made up of the lymph node bearing tissue occupying the visceral space. It begins at the hyoid bone, extends inferior to the suprasternal notch, and laterally is bound by the common carotid arteries.

Evolution of neck dissection in the management of head and neck cancer

While both Chelius and Kocher seperately recommended removal of regional lymph nodes in the treatment of head and neck cancer as early as the mid-nineteenth century, it is George Crile, Sr., who receives credit for his systematic description of management of cervical lymphatics in cancers of the head and neck [9]. His oft-quoted 1906 article, published in *JAMA*, recapitulated and expanded upon his less well-known 1905 article published in *The Transactions of the Southern Surgical and Gynecological Association*. Both articles presented his justification of and technique for addressing the cervical lymphatics in a systematic fashion in cancers of the head and neck; he championed their removal in surgical treatment of head and neck cancer. Crile [10–12] was strongly influenced by Halsted's work in breast cancer, and he drew parallels to the management of head and neck cancers recommending the en bloc removal of non-lymphatic structures along with the regional lymphatics similar to the method of mastectomy of the day (ie, the sternocleidomastoid muscle was removed similar to the pectoralis muscle and the internal jugular vein was sacrificed similar to the axillary vein). It is interesting to note that although Crile suggested in these early publications that the spinal accessory nerve could be preserved if not directly involved with cancer, later surgeons purporting to follow his example recommended its removal in all cases. Martin and colleagues [13] stated that any attempt to preserve the spinal accessory nerve should be "condemned unequivocally." Other structures, such as the submandibular gland were also preserved in some cases presented by Crile. Careful study of Crile's original article text and illustrations reveals that only a portion of the patients, primarily those with evidence of cervical metastasis, underwent what would come to be known as his greatest contribution to head and neck surgery: the radical neck dissection.

Crile's contribution was further expanded during the Hayes/Martin era at Memorial Hospital in New York City. Other authors had published on the utility of neck dissection in the management of head and neck cancer, including descriptions of composite resections combining neck dissection with removal of the primary and mandible in bloc; however, it was Martin's comprehensive treatise published in 1951 that summarized his indications, technique, and outcomes with the radical neck dissection; and cemented his place in head and neck surgical history [13,14]. In his treatise, Martin promoted a radical neck dissection with removal of the lymphatic structures from the inferior border of the mandible superiorly to the clavicle inferiorly, and the midline of the neck anteriorly to the anterior edge of the trapezius muscle posteriorly. In addition, the en bloc removal included the removal of three defining, non-lymphatic structures: the sternocleidomastoid muscle; the internal jugular vein; and the spinal accessory nerve. Martin acknowledged some surgeons' preference for "a more limited dissection" in some circumstances; he recommended these more limited operations be termed "partial neck dissection." In general, however, he condemned these more limited removals, making special reference to the "supraomohyoid neck dissection." Understanding the morbidity associated with the radical neck dissection, Martin's indications were precise and included: the presence of known cervical metastasis (ie, therapeutic neck dissection); plan for control of the primary; no evidence of distant metastasis; reasonable chance of removal of the cervical metastasis; and finally, that the neck dissection should offer a more certain chance of cure than radiation therapy [13]. Martin's profound influence on a generation of surgeons trained in head and neck surgery led to the radical neck dissection becoming *the* operation for management of the cervical lymph nodes in head and neck cancer. Despite an evolution and narrowing of the indications for the radical neck dissection, it remains, in the minds of most head and neck surgeons, the standard operation upon which all variations are compared both in technique and outcomes (see classifications below).

As the field of head and neck surgery evolved, surgeons began to question the dogma promulgated from Memorial Hospital. This questioning was especially prevalent among surgeons from different specialties and abroad. In many ways, fragmentation among head and neck surgeons of different backgrounds and specialties led to different opinions and ideas regarding the indications and technique of neck dissection. Surgeons began to question the wisdom of limiting neck dissection to those with proven cervical metastasis, and they explored ways of limiting morbidity if one were to apply elective neck dissection more liberally. In 1967, Bocca and Gavilian, following the lead of Suarez, published the technique of "functional neck dissection" which preserved non-lymphatic cervical structures, including the spinal accessory nerve, internal jugular vein, sternocleidomastoid muscle, and in cases without direct involvement, the submandibular gland, thereby sparing morbidity without sacrificing loco-regional control. The dissection was based on the concept that the fibro-adipose lymph node-bearing tissue could be removed en bloc by careful dissection of the fascia from non-lymphatic structures. It should be noted that the authors recommended preservation of these structures only when they were not in contact with suspected involved lymph nodes [15–17]. Although properly considered one of the earliest proponents of functional neck dissection, Suarez's [18] previous publications had not been in English and therefore, they had escaped the notice of many European and American surgeons. Subsequent to the publications by Bocca, Calearo, and Gavilian, there was an explosion in interest in more limited neck dissections; publications describing a variety of modifications to the accepted technique of radical neck dissection began to appear. These numerous publications often used a variety of terms often describing the same technique; the variation in terms led to an enormous amount of confusion among clinicians and consternation among trainees who tried to decipher a variety of overlapping terms and the indications for each type of named dissection. The resultant, often misused, terminology of neck dissection was standardized by the American Academy of Otolaryngology's Committee for Head and Neck Surgery and Oncology in 1991 [19].

The goals of the committee were: to develop a standardized system of neck dissection terminology that preserved traditional terms (such as radial neck dissection and modified neck dissection), while avoiding eponyms and acronyms; to define the lymph node levels and non-lymphatic structures removed in each type of neck dissection; and, to standardize the clinical and surgical boundaries of the lymph node levels (see discussion above). An update, published in 2002, attempted to answer some of the criticisms of the original system and take into account advances in clinical practice. These revisions, proposed in 2001, sought to improve communication with radiologists and other clinicians [8]. These proposed changes were primarily in regard to the selective neck dissections and specific names, such as supraomohyoid neck dissection; such names were eliminated in favor of the phrase "selective neck dissection" followed in parentheses by the levels removed (see discussion of classifications below) (Table 1). Although not universally accepted initially (ie, other classifications exist), the standard suggested by the committee has led to improved communication among clinicians across surgical and non-surgical specialties who treat head and neck patients [20].

Classification of neck dissections

Neck dissections can be broadly classified as comprehensive or selective. Comprehensive neck dissections include all of the lymph node levels removed in a standard radical neck dissection (levels I–V), and include radical neck dissection and modified radical neck dissection. A dissection that leaves in place one or more of these levels is considered a selective neck dissection. Likewise, any dissection that removes additional lymph node levels or non-lymphatic structure is termed an extended neck dissection. Specific definitions are outlined below:

Radical neck dissection (RND):
Refers to the removal of all ipsilateral cervical lymph node groups extending from the inferior border of the mandible to the clavicle, from the lateral border of the sternohyoid muscle, hyoid bone, and contralateral anterior belly of the digastric muscle medially, to the anterior border of the trapezius. Included are levels I–V. This entails the removal of three important, non-lymphatic structures: the internal jugular vein, the sternocleidomastoid muscle, and the spinal accessory nerve (Fig. 2).

Modified radical neck dissection (MRND):
Refers to removal of the same lymph node levels (I–V) as the radical neck dissection, but with preservation of the spinal accessory nerve, the internal jugular vein, or the sternocleidomastoid muscle. The structures preserved should be named. Some authors propose subdividing the modified neck dissection into three types: type I preserves the spinal accessory nerve; type II preserves the spinal accessory nerve and the sternocleidomastoid muscle; and type III preserves the spinal accessory nerve, the sternocleidomastoid muscle, and the internal jugular vein; but the standard is to name the preserved structure following the MRND abbreviation, instead of using subtypes.

Selective neck dissection (SND)
Refers to the preservation of one or more lymph node groups normally removed in a radical neck dissection. In the 1991 classification scheme, there were several "named" selective neck dissections. For example, the supraomohyoid neck dissection removed the lymph nodes from levels I–III. The subsequent proposed modification in 2001 sought to eliminate these named dissections. The committee proposed that selective neck dissections be named for the cancer that

Table 1
Comparison of 1991 and 2002 neck dissection classification

1991 classification	2001 classification
Radical neck dissection	Radical neck dissection
Modified radical neck dissection	Modified radical neck dissection
Selective neck dissection a. Supraomohyoid b. Lateral c. Posterolateral d. Anterior	Selective neck dissection: avoid named neck dissection. Instead each variation should be denoted SND followed by parenthesis containing designations for the nodal levels or sublevels removed
Extended neck dissection	Extended neck dissection

From Robbins KT, Clayman G, et al. Neck dissection classification update. Arch Otolaryngol Head Neck Surg 2002;128:751–8; with permission.

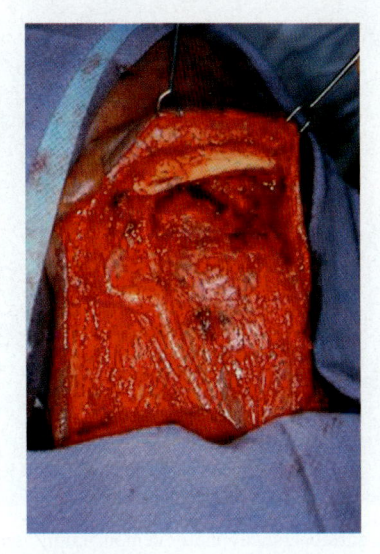

Fig. 2. Intraoperative photo following radical neck dissection with sacrifice of internal jugular vein, spinal accessory nerve, and sternocleidomastoid muscle.

the surgeon was treating and to name the node groups removed. For example, a selective neck dissection for most oral cavity cancers would encompass those node groups most at risk (levels I–III) and be referred to as a SND (I–III) (Fig. 3).

Extended neck dissection

The term extended neck dissection refers to the removal of one or more additional lymph node groups, non-lymphatic structures or both, not encompassed by a radical neck dissection, for example, mediastinal nodes or non-lymphatic structures, such as the carotid artery and hypoglossal nerve (Fig. 4).

It is important to remember that classification schemes are continually changing; as science evolves, the indications for different dissections will certainly change. For example, in the case of an oral cavity primary without evidence of lymph node metastases, a selective neck dissection, removing lymph nodes from levels I–III is the generally accepted procedure of choice. Shah and others demonstrated that a supraomohyoid neck dissection eradicates occult metastatic disease in 95% of patients [21]. Some surgeons, however, advocate including level IV (extended supraomohyoid neck dissection) to decrease the risk, however small, of missed occult metastases. The strength of the current classification system lies in its specificity regarding lymph node basins

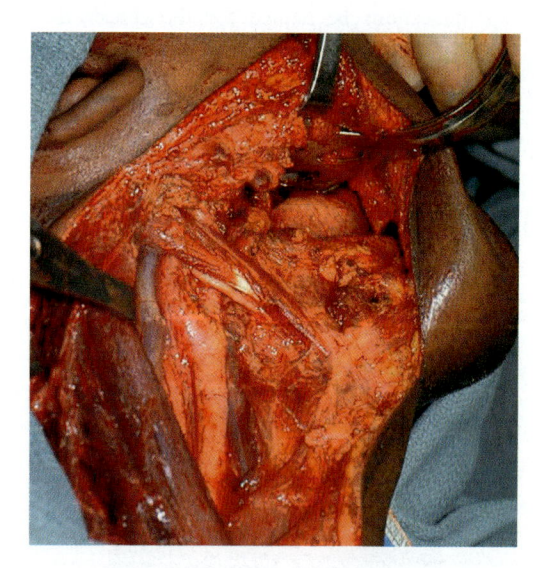

Fig. 3. Intraoperative photo demonstrating selective neck dissection of levels I–III, previously known as supraomohyoid neck dissection, but described as SND (I–III) in current nomenclature.

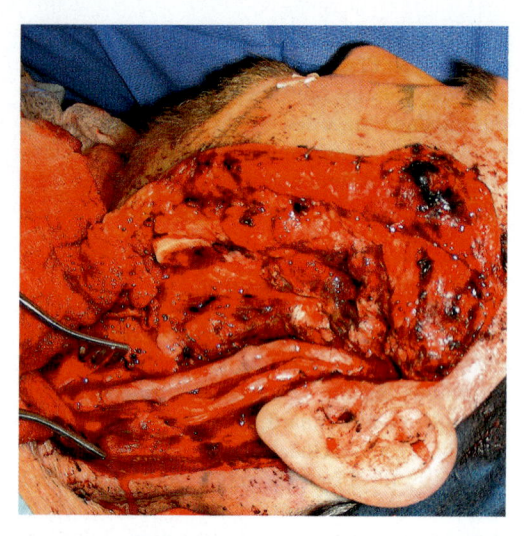

Fig. 4. Extended neck dissection demonstrating sacrifice of carotid artery and reconstruction using a vein graft.

treated and avoidance of named dissections, which may not reflect differences in technique amongst different surgeons.

Brief mention should also be made regarding another controversy in the evolution of neck dissection: the concept of in-continuity versus discontinuity neck dissections. In the past, it was considered mandatory to remove the primary tumor in direct continuity with the neck dissection, in one specimen [13,14]. Work by Spiro and Strong [22] found no adverse impact on survival when neck dissection was performed in a discontinuous manner. Bias might have occurred, however, as smaller lesions were in the discontinuity group. A study by Leeman and colleagues [23] found worse outcome in stage II cancer of the tongue with discontinuity neck dissection with local recurrence rates (19.1% versus 5.3%) and 5-year survival (63% versus 80%). At this time most surgeons prefer an in-continuity approach if technically feasible, without the resection of obviously uninvolved structures such as the mandible.

Technique

Many excellent surgical atlases are available that offer complete descriptions of the technique of the various neck dissections [24]. The technique of modified neck dissection (MRND) is described, here, and it is easily adapted to performance of selective neck dissection (SND) and radical neck dissection (RND), with exceptions noted.

Positioning the patient with a shoulder roll or on a Mayfield headholder with slight extension makes dissection easier. A myriad of incisions have been described for access to various neck dissections, including very limited incisions, which are combined with good retraction for selective neck dissections [25]. The choice of incision design in MRND is guided by the need for access to the cervical lymphatic basins contained in levels I–V. In addition, the need for access to the oral cavity in combined approaches, ie, lip splitting, should be considered. It should be noted here that there are two approaches classically taught for the MRND: the original anterior-posterior approach of Suerez, which was popularized by Bocca, and the Suen approach, which is an anterior approach popular in the United States. The later requires good retraction of the SCM laterally to access the posterior neck, and yet access may still be limited [26–28]. For an anterior approach to the MRND, an oblique incision extending from the mastoid inferiorly and crossing the sternocleidomastoid muscle then extending across the neck in a natural neck crease at approximately the level of the cricoid cartilage allows adequate access in most cases (the so-called "hockey stick" incision). For access to level I, the incision must be carried across the midline enough to allow retraction superiorly. Alternatively, an apron type flap with the horizontal component placed higher combined with a releasing incision trailing posterior-inferior (Schobinger) [29] can be used. If needed, the author of this article prefers a modification with the trifurcation placed lower in the neck (Lahey) [30], which is more important in cases of RND where the sternocleidomastoid muscle is sacrificed and the carotid at increased risk (Fig. 5).

Elevation of superior and inferior flaps in a subplatysmal plane above the superficial layer of the deep cervical fascia is accomplished to the level of the inferior border of the mandible and clavicle respectively (Fig. 6). The platysma terminates posteriorly, and in this area, the dissection will be in a subcutaneous plane. The external jugular vein serves as an excellent guide to keep this dissection at the appropriate level because the dissection should be superficial to it. A good tip is to keep the flaps under good tension perpendicular to the neck to aid in their elevation. The spinal accessory nerve courses in a subcutaneous plane as it exits from the posterior aspect of the SCM, and care must be taken to identify and protect this nerve as flaps are developed here in the anterior-posterior approach. This author's preference

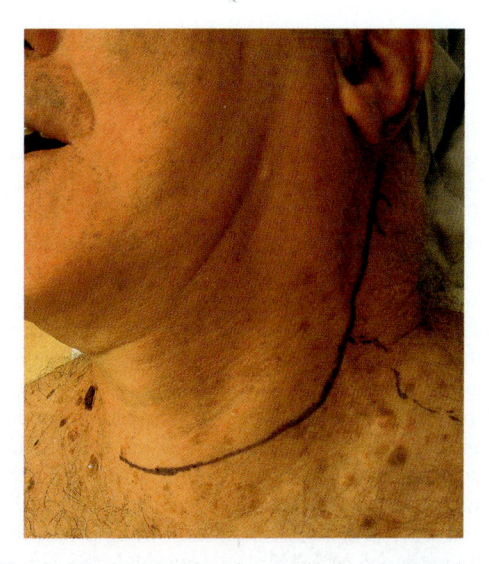

Fig. 5. Standard incision for modified neck dissection. Posterior extension (dotted) can be performed to allow improved access to posterior triangle (level V).

is an anterior approach in most cases: the nerve will be identified early in the dissection and followed posterior and inferior through the posterior triangle.

At this point in the procedure, it is helpful to think of the neck dissection as an exercise in dissecting and preserving four nerves: the marginal mandibularis; the spinal accessory; the hypoglossal; and the lingual nerve, all of which serve as landmarks along the pathway to

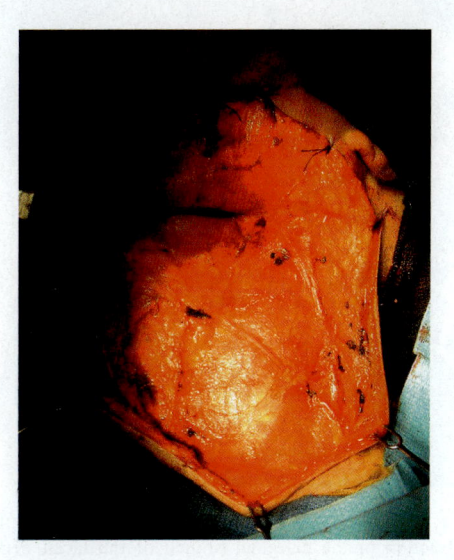

Fig. 6. Elevation of subplatysmal flaps exposes the superficial layer of the deep cervical fascia.

completion of the neck dissection. First, the marginal mandibular nerve is protected. Often it can be identified along its course through the superficial layer of the deep cervical fascia following elevation of the subplatysmal flaps. Otherwise, it can be preserved by dividing the superficial layer of the deep cervical fascia two centimeters below the inferior border of the mandible. The facial vein can be divided and retracted superiorly to protect the nerve as the fascia over the submandibular gland is dissected. The vein can be sutured superiorly to retract and protect the nerve during the remaining dissection (Figs. 7 and 8). This author's preference is to dissect the nodes associated with the facial vessels (ie, prevascular nodes) in most cases at this point. It is often difficult to keep these nodes in continuity with the remainder of the neck dissection while protecting the marginal nerve, and if separated, the nerves should be labeled and submitted separately so that they are not lost. Dissection then frees the attachments along the length of the inferior border of the mandible. Subsequently, attention is directed to identifying the spinal accessory nerve, the defining point of the modified neck dissection.

An incision is made through fascia along the anterior edge of the SCM. The external jugular vein will be ligated at this point. Authors disagree on the need for removal of the fascia overlying the lateral aspect of the SCM, with some authors reporting less morbidity if it is preserved. This author's preference in most cases is to incise the fascia approximately 1 cm posterior to the anterior edge, and then elevate it around the edge and onto the medial surface. Alternatively, the entire fascia can be elevated from the SCM. Dissection then proceeds along a broad front along the medial surface of the SCM. Attempting to dissect directly to the spinal accessory nerve at this time should be avoided as there is a tendency to be working within a hole, and injury to small vessels associated with the nerve can make visibility difficult. Instead, dissecting along a broad front allows improved visibility. The dissection is carried down to the level of the posterior belly of the digastric, which can be retracted superiorly with a right angle retractor. An assistant using right angle retractors at right angles to each other can effectively retract the SCM laterally and the posterior belly of the digastric superiorly, offering an excellent view of the operative field. The spinal accessory nerve will become visible with careful dissection, spreading in the direction of the nerve's course anterior-superior to posterior-inferior. Once identified, a decision must be made regarding level IIb (submuscular recess), which in many cases can be left (see discussion of nerve injuries in complications below). If it is to be removed, the spinal accessory must be mobilized by splitting the fibroadipose node-bearing tissue above it and dissecting it free. The nerve should be handled carefully since manipulation alone can lead to long-term dysfunction. Using a vein retractor to protect the nerve, cautery and blunt dissection are used to dissect the node-bearing tissue from level IIB. The deep cervical fascia overlying the splenius capitus, levator scapulae, and scalene muscles should be preserved. Also, care must be taken not to injure the internal jugular vein at this level as control of the subsequent bleeding can be troublesome. The fibroadipose node-bearing tissue is then passed under the spinal accessory nerve and kept in continuity with the remainder of the neck dissection. This maneuver, which defines the modified neck dissection, was the subject of the most vocal criticisms of the technique, as it appeared to break with the en bloc concept of removal that was championed for so many years.

Dissection then proceeds posteriorly while keeping the spinal accessory nerve in view. The posterior limit of the dissection is usually the cervical plexus rootlets coursing from the posterior edge of the SCM. Although they can be

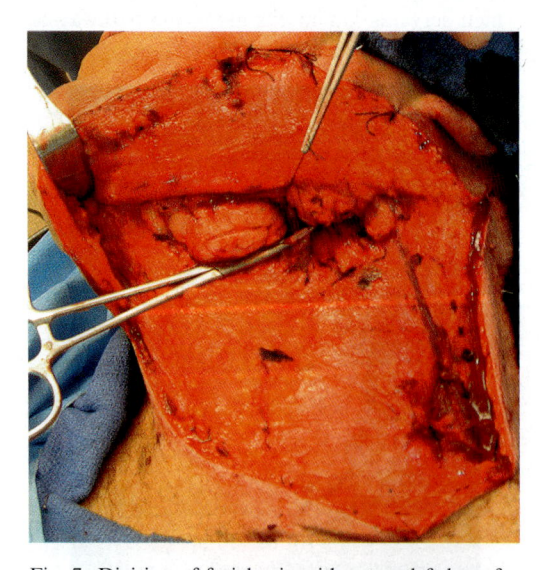

Fig. 7. Division of facial vein with suture left long for retraction of the marginal branch of the facial nerve. Note the fascia has been elevated off the submandibular gland.

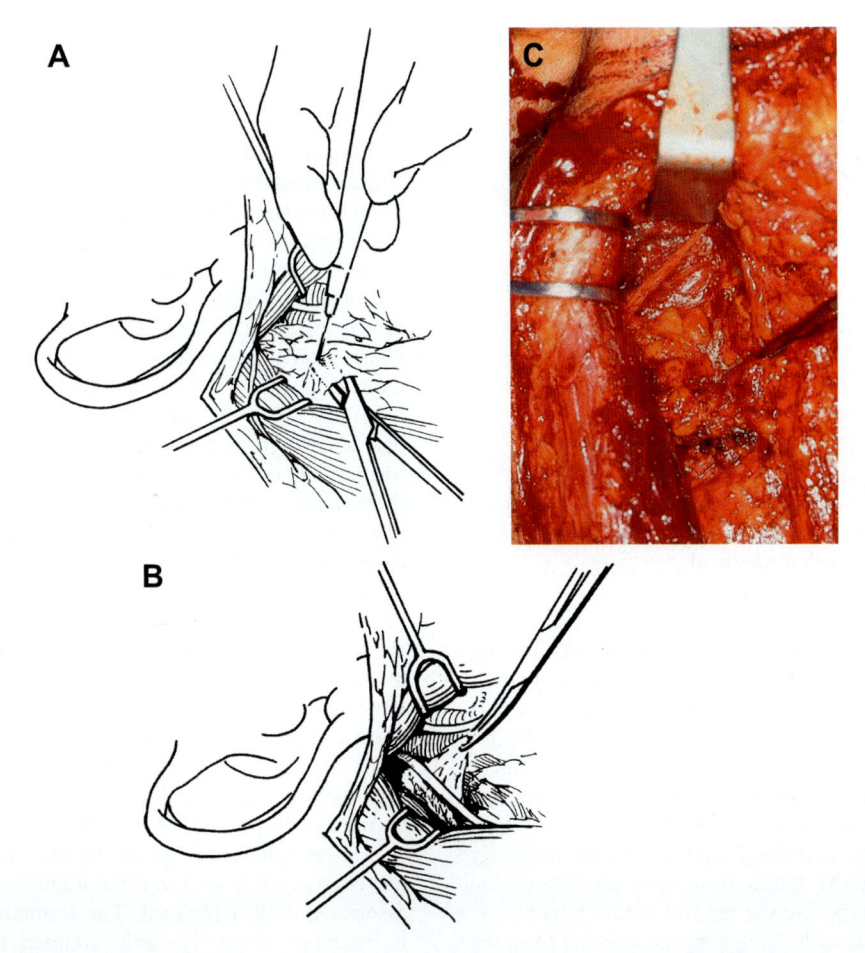

Fig. 8. (*A*) Incising node bearing tissue over spinal accessory nerve. (*From* Lore JM, Medina J. An atlas of head and neck surgery. 4th edition. Philadelphia: Saunders; 2004. p. 809; with permission.) (*B*) passing node bearing tissue from level IIb under nerve. (*From* Lore JM, Medina J. An atlas of head and neck surgery. 4th edition. Philadelphia: Saunders; 2004. p. 809; with permission.) (*C*) Intraoperative photo demonstrating passing tissue under nerve following dissection on submuscular recess (level IIb). Note right angle retraction of posterior belly of digastric and sternocleidomastoid muscle).

sacrificed without undue sequelae, they are preserved unless there is known nodal disease in this area. The posterior limit of the dissection superiorly usually corresponds to the posterior edge of the SCM. Inferiorly, the spinal accessory nerve is identified as it exits the posterior edge of the SCM. Using an anterior approach, retraction for dissection of the posterior triangle can be difficult. If an anterior-posterior approach is used with a releasing incision (Schobinger or Lahey) [30], the spinal accessory nerve can be identified exiting the posterior edge of the SCM, and then the skin flaps can be elevated keeping the nerve in view (Fig. 9). This approach allows a more comprehensive removal of level V in most cases and it is more likely to be used in the presence of bulky, clinical neck disease. Again, dissection of the posterior triangle should be kept superficial to the deep cervical fascia. Often, blunt dissection with a finger covered with gauze can aid sweeping the node-bearing tissue in this area.

Subsequently, the nodal contents are brought underneath the SCM while retracting it superiorly (Fig. 10A, B) Retracting the contents anteriorly, the contents are then sharply dissected across the internal jugular vein. Blade dissection combined with good traction on the specimen and counter-traction on the vein is helpful here. (Fig. 11A, B) Alternatively, blunt dissection with a fine hemostat combined with cautery can be

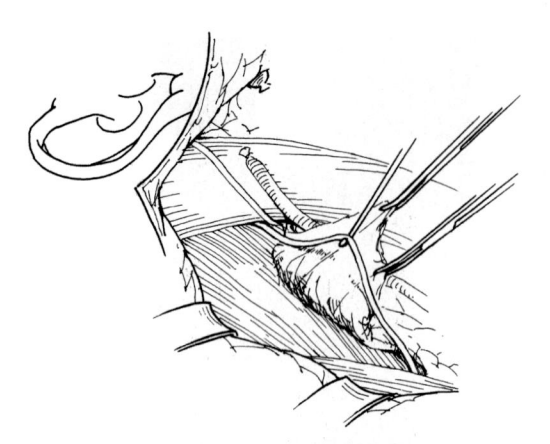

Fig. 9. Nodal contents of posterior triangle brought underneath the spinal accessory nerve in the posterior triangle. (*From* Lore JM, Medina J. An atlas of head and neck surgery. 4th edition. Philadelphia: Saunders; 2004. p. 810; with permission.)

used. Tributaries to the internal jugular vein are ligated and divided. Rarely, the internal jugular vein will be entered accidentally during this part of the operation. If so, the opening should be immediately occluded to prevent air entrainment into the vein. A helpful maneuver is to place one finger above the rent and one below, and then retract one superiorly and the other inferiorly expressing the blood from that portion of the vein and exposing the rent for suture repair.

As the node bearing tissue is dissected from the inferior portion of the vein, the omohyoid muscle will typically be divided. Dissection continues across the carotid artery. The hypoglossal nerve is identified typically 1–2 cm above the carotid bifurcation. Once the hypoglossal nerve has been identified, dissection can proceed anteriorly up to the submental area following the anterior belly of the omohyoid to the hyoid then clearing the nodal tissue along the anterior belly of the digastric. Level I is cleared by dissecting to the level of the mylohyoid. This is best performed with cautery to control troublesome bleeding from the arterial branch to the mylohyoid muscle. Once the posterior edge of the mylohyoid is identified, a right angle retractor is placed and the muscle is distracted anteriorly exposing the lingual nerve as the contents of the submandibular triangle, whose attachments were previously freed from the inferior border of the mandible are distracted inferiorly (Fig. 12). The submandibular duct is ligated and transected. The attachments of the lingual nerve to the submandibular gland are then divided. Finally, the facial artery is encountered again and divided which allows the specimen to be delivered (Fig. 13A, B).

Variations to the technique described above are numerous. In addition to surgeon preferences, the techniques are adapted to the oncologic goals of the particular case. For example, the selective removal of levels I–III, which in the past was known as the supraomohyoid neck dissection, is the most commonly performed neck dissection for oral cavity cancer. Some authors [31,32], however, encourage the removal of level IV in certain cases, such as tongue cancer, given the 9% rate of skip metastasis to this level and the limited morbidity associated with it removal. The technique which is described above is easily adapted for these variations, and the principles remain the same. It is important in the current classification scheme to note which levels were addressed in the dissection, in addition to the type of dissection, so that proper communication with other clinicians is possible.

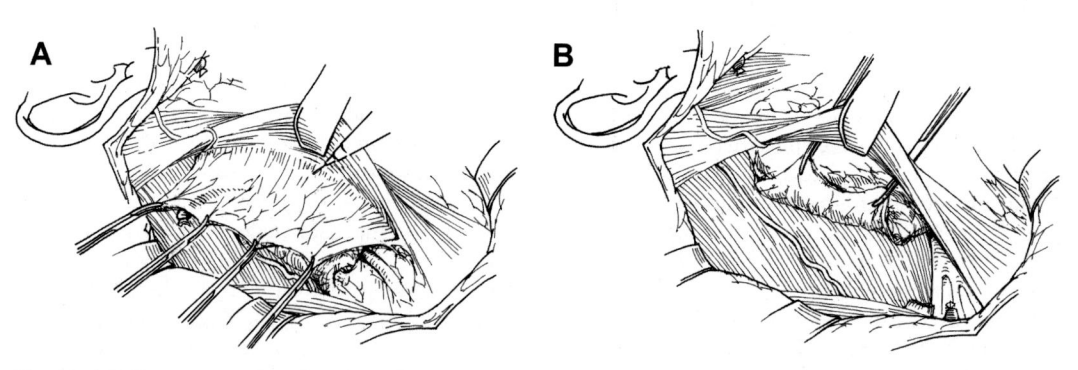

Fig. 10. (*A, B*) Demonstrating dissection of posterior triangle passing underneath the SCM in the anterior-posterior approach. (*From* Lore JM, Medina J. An atlas of head and neck surgery. 4th edition. Philadelphia: Saunders; 2004. p. 810; with permission.)

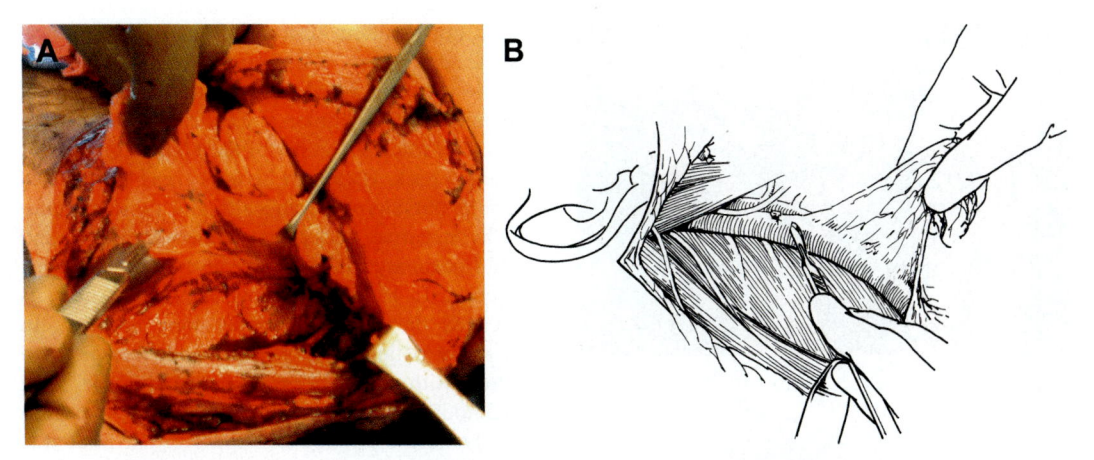

Fig. 11. (*A, B*) Blade dissection along the internal jugular vein. (*From* Lore JM, Medina J. An atlas of head and neck surgery. 4th edition. Philadelphia: Saunders; 2004. p. 813; with permission.)

Sentinel node biopsy

As surgeons pursue less invasive surgical modalities, dissection of the N0 neck (staging neck dissection or elective neck dissection) is becoming increasingly limited through the use of selective neck dissections; their goal, as noted above, is to remove those nodal basins at highest risk for harboring occult metastases based on the site of the primary. Perhaps the ultimate evolution of selective neck dissection is the sentinel node biopsy (SNB). The sentinel node technique, first popularized for melanoma, has been investigated for use in head and neck cancer [33,34]. In theory, it allows the identification and removal of the lymph node ("sentinel node") that would first receive metastases from a given site. An excellent review of the indications and technique was presented by Shellenberger [35]. Briefly, the technique involves injecting the area surrounding the primary site with a radioactive-labeled colloid: 99mTc-sulfur colloid. (Various molecular weights can be chosen depending on the transit time desired.) A radiograph can be taken to localize the sentinel node, which is the first node that receives lymph flow from the area of the tumor. The patient is then taken to the operating room where the surgeon may inject isosulfan blue, a dye, around the tumor. This will also drain to the first echelon node and stain it blue, assisting the surgeon in its identification during surgery. Also, the surgeon will use a gamma detection probe counter probe to identify the node with the highest concentration of radioactive colloid. The node is then removed and if it is histologically positive, further treatment such as completion of neck dissection and/or radiation may be indicated. In melanoma, sentinel node biopsy has a reported sensitivity of 82%–100%, and very few false negatives [36,37]. It should be noted that the lymph nodes removed via the sentinel node technique are subjected to much closer pathologic scrutiny, including analysis of more sections through the node and immunohistochemical analysis in some cases.

The technique of sentinel node biopsy has been investigated in the head and neck with varying results. Problems with applying the sentinel node technique to the oral cavity relate to the rich lymphatic drainage pattern with possible bilateral drainage, and the complex anatomy in the cervical region, which can lead to difficulty in dissecting a single node from the neck. In addition, close

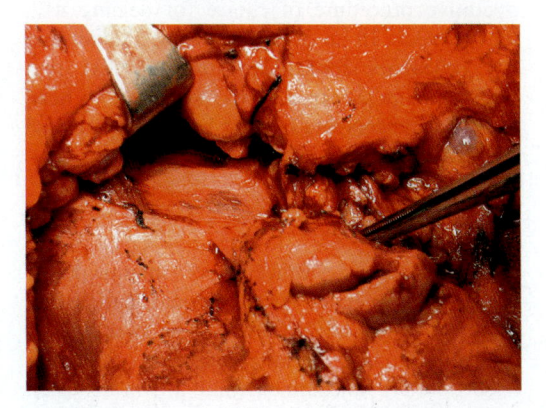

Fig. 12. Retraction of the posterior edge of the mylohyoid muscle anteriorly and of the submandibular triangle contents inferiorly brings the lingual nerve into view.

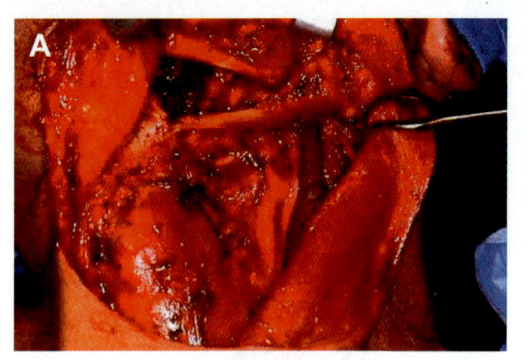

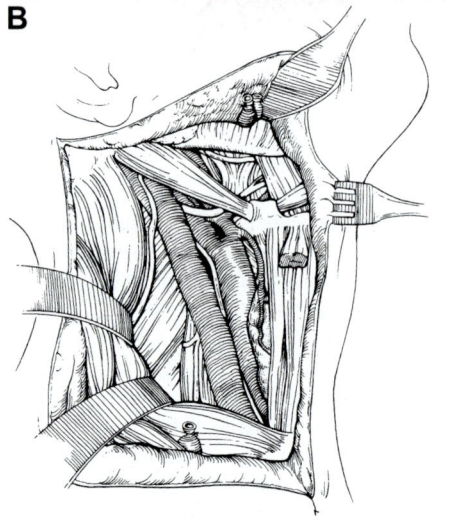

Fig. 13. Photo (*A*) and schematic (*B*) demonstrating completed dissection. (*From* Thawley SE, Panje WR, Batsakis JG, et al. Comprehensive management of head and neck tumors, volume 2. 2nd edition. Philadelphia: Saunders; 1999. p. 1410; with permission.)

proximity of the sentinel node to the primary, for example, a FOM primary and submental node, can lead to the accumulation of colloid around the primary which can obscure the sentinel node. The rich lymphovascular network can also lead to drainage to several nodes. Civantos and his colleagues [38] used the sentinel node technique in 18 oral cavity cancers with N0 necks. They compared sentinel node biopsy to CT scan and PET scan by obtaining a CT and PET followed by SNB and neck dissection. They found 10 true positives: six identified on frozen, two on permanent, two on immunoperoxidase staining for cytokeratin. In six specimens, the sentinel node was the only positive node. They also found seven true negatives and one false negative. In one case, the sentinel node identified by the radioactive colloid did not contain cancer, but another cervical node did. They also found that tumor in the node can lead to obstruction and redirection of lymphatic flow. Pitman and colleagues [39] further demonstrated the utility of the SNB technique for the N0 neck. Hyde and his collegues [40] reported on 19 patients with clinically and radiographically negative necks that underwent SNB and PET scanning followed by conventional neck dissection. In 15 of 19 patients, the sentinel node as well as the remaining nodes were negative. In 3 of 19 patients, the sentinel node was positive along with other nodes. In one patient, the sentinel node was negative, but another node removed in the neck dissection was positive. The node was located close to the primary, which often leads to difficulty discriminating activity due to the tumor and that of adjacent nodes. Interestingly, PET failed to reveal cancer in the four patients with subsequently identified cervical metastasis (see previous discussion on PET scanning). The true contribution of the sentinel node concept may be the information that has been gained from the careful analysis of the lymph nodes, which are subjected to more intense histopathologic evaluation than lymph nodes removed in classic neck dissections. Studies have demonstrated that review of lymph nodes deemed negative by light microscopy were subsequently found to be positive with more numerous node sectioning and/or immunohistochemical analysis. Because it can be assumed that patients with these previously unreported metastases were not irradiated in many cases, the traditional neck dissection may have been therapeutic more often than some believed. In the future, the SNB as the ultimate evolution of selective neck dissection may become the operative procedure of choice for dealing with the N0 neck. In an excellent review, Pitman and her colleagues concluded, however, that that SNB remains an experimental technique in head and neck cancers and has not become a standard of care [41].

Complications

Complications, which are unanticipated, should be separated from normal anticipated sequelae of neck dissection, such as swelling and bruising. Complications associated with neck dissection are uncommon, and are more often related to patient factors rather than the surgeon's technique. For example, a history of chemoradiation therapy is associated with a 26%–35%

complication rate in patients undergoing neck dissections [42,43]. Given the increased (and often questionable) use of neo-adjuvant therapy, surgeons must be prepared for longer, more tedious dissections, and increased complications. Other patient factors, such as tobacco and alcohol abuse, malnutrition, and diabetes can directly affect complication rates. Briefly discussed here are the more common complications: neurologic injury, vascular injury, thoracic duct injury (chyle leak), and wound infection.

Neurologic

Most modifications of neck dissections have been made in an attempt to prevent the morbidity of radical neck dissection. Specifically, the painful shoulder syndrome associated with sacrifice of the spinal accessory nerve lead many (including Crile himself) to preserve the nerve, and paved the way for modified neck dissections (Fig. 14). Interestingly, not all patients in whom the nerve is intentionally sacrificed develop shoulder weakness, and while preservation of the spinal accessory nerve decreases the incidence of painful shoulder syndrome, it does not eliminate it. Extensive skeletonization of the nerve performed during modified neck dissections including level IIB can result in significant dysfunction even if the nerve is preserved. Several studies have suggested that dissection of level IIB (above the nerve) is unnecessary in the clinically node-negative neck because of the low incidence of metastases in this area (1.6%), and is recommended only if bulky disease is present in level IIa [44]. It is this author's practice to exclude extensive dissection of this area in most oral cavity cancers, and the clinically N0 neck. Patients with signs of shoulder dysfunction should be referred for physical therapy.

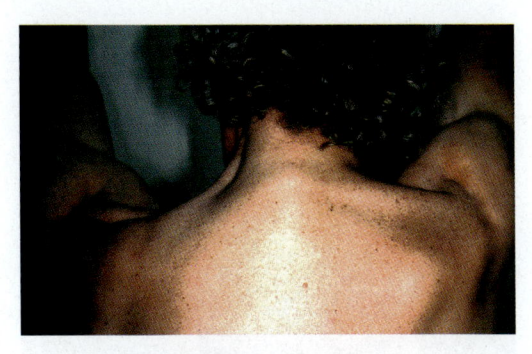

Fig. 14. Shoulder syndrome associated with sacrifice of spinal accessory nerve. (*Courtesy of* Eric Dierks, DMD, MD, FACS, Portland, OR.)

The facial nerve is at some risk during neck dissection. Specifically, injury to the marginal mandibular branch is not uncommon. Retraction can temporarily disrupt function, and patients should be counseled that while most will recover, some will not. Higher dissection in the area of the tail of the parotid in an attempt to clear bulky disease can result in injury to the cervicofacial division of the facial nerve or even the main trunk, but this is rare. Injury recognized intraoperatively or in the early postoperative period should be repaired.

Injury to the hypoglossal nerve is possible during neck dissection. The procedure is especially problematic in the patient who has previously undergone radiation therapy leading to scarring and fibrosis in the neck. A confluence of veins around the nerve just anterior to the carotid artery can lead to troublesome bleeding and inadvertent injury to the nerve. In addition, bulky nodal disease in the area can lead to nerve transection while trying to obtain adequate margins. Immediate repair can be considered, although results are unsatisfying in most cases. Fortunately, unilateral injury to the hypoglossal nerve is fairly well tolerated by most patients.

Phrenic nerve injury in patients undergoing neck dissection has been reported to be as high as 8% by some authors [45]. Fortunately, the true incidence is likely much lower in modified and selective neck dissections. The nerve lies under the deep cervical fascia over the anterior scalene muscles and this fascia should be preserved. Again, difficulty may be encountered dissecting in the postirradiated field or in cases of bulky disease. Injury is usually manifested by elevation of the hemi-diaphragm noted on postoperative chest radiographs; bilateral injury can lead to respiratory failure. Pulmonary complications are usually limited unless the patient has pre-existing pulmonary compromise, a not uncommon co-morbidity among head and neck patients.

Injury to the brachial plexus can similarly occur when dissection is inadvertently performed deep to the prevertebral fascia low in the neck. It is a devastating injury, and early recognition should lead to appropriate consultation and consideration of repair. Unfortunately, repairs are associated with less than satisfactory results in most cases.

Horner's syndrome (ie, ptosis, miosis, and anhydrosis) results from injury to the cervical sympathetic trunk, which lies posterior to the carotid sheath. The cervical sympathetic trunk is at risk when dissection is carried posterior to the carotid, which is rarely indicated.

The vagus nerve is at greatest risk during ligation of the internal jugular vein. Damage results in unilateral vocal cord paralysis, which is manifested by a "breathy," weak voice. If the injury is high in the neck before the branch of the superior laryngeal nerve, then laryngeal sensation is impaired and aspiration becomes a risk. Vocal cord augmentation or medialization procedures may be helpful.

Injury to the lingual nerve can occur during removal of the primary, but the lingual nerve is also at risk when it is distracted along with the contents of the submandibular triangle. This is especially true when the lingual nerve has been mobilized aggressively during the extirpation of the primary. In addition, blind clamping of lingual vessels can lead to its injury. The attachments between the nerve and submandibular gland should be carefully transected while keeping the nerve in view.

Vascular

Vascular injury can be classified as intraoperative or late. Intraoperative complications include carotid sinus sensitivity and vessel laceration, which in this discussion will include thoracic duct injury. Late injuries discussed here include hemorrhage—specifically, hemorrhage in the postoperative setting.

Carotid sinus sensitivity results from manipulation of the carotid body, and it typically manifests as acute bradycardia and decreased cardiac output. Atropine can be given, but the best results are usually obtained by subadventitial administration of a small amount (<1 cc) of plain 1% lidocaine, although this practice has been questioned [46].

Intraoperative hemorrhage is controlled with pressure and appropriate ligature, either suture or clips (see discussion above under technique). In the postradiated setting hemorrhage can become more of an issue as fibrotic tissue prevents the collapse of veins as well as the normal retraction and constriction of arteries. This can make the dissection much more tedious, leading to injury and ligation of unintended vessels, such as the internal carotid artery. Laceration of the common or internal carotid arteries should be promptly repaired if a preoperative assessment to establish the presence of collateral cerebral circulation (carotid occlusion test) has not been done.

Injury to the thoracic duct usually occurs during manipulation of the internal jugular vein deep in the left neck were it lies posterior to the vein. Prevention is the best policy. When dividing the lymphatic tissue low in the left neck, especially in cases were the internal jugular vein is divided, the tissue should be clamped and suture-ligated. Injury is manifested by appearance of milky fluid in the surgical field (Fig. 15). Outcomes are improved if the injury is recognized intraoperatively. If injury is suspected or to confirm the repair, the anesthesiologist can hold a positive pressure breath to increase intrathoracic pressure. Injuries recognized intraoperatively should be managed by oversewing the duct with multiple nonabsorbable sutures under loupe magnification, if possible. Injury in usually heralded in the postoperative setting by unexpectedly high drain output from the left neck or by the appearance of milky fluid in the suction drains It can be confirmed by testing the triglyceride content of the drainage and comparing them to serum values. Many of these leaks can be controlled by conservative measures: medium triglyceride diet (questioned by some authors); pressure; and suction drainage. Surgical exploration is indicated in leaks greater than 300–400 mL/day or leaks persisting more than 4–5 days. Chylous leaks can lead to significant electrolyte disturbances and malnutrition; consideration should be given to total parenteral nutrition (TPN) in the short-term. Surgical exploration of leaks can be a frustrating exercise and requires patience. The patient can be fed a rich milk or cream product preoperatively in an attempt to increase chyle production and aid intraoperative identification of the leak. Discussions with anesthesia staff should be held regarding timing of this as it relates to NPO status. Use of

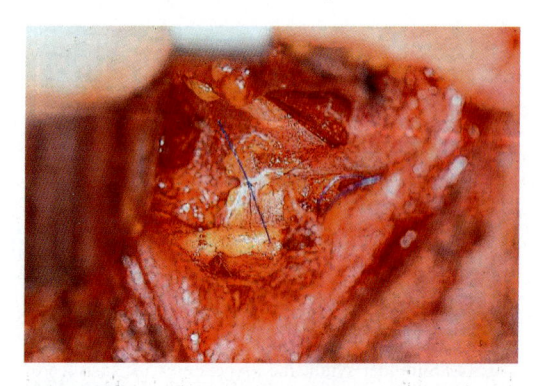

Fig. 15. Intraoperative photo demonstrating chyle leak and suturing.

sclerosing agents, such as doxycycline, or fibrin glue has been advocated. Oversewing the area and consideration of importation of vascularized tissue, such as a myofascial free or pedicled flap, probably offers the best chance at successful resolution.

Late vascular complications typically involve hemorrhage in the form of carotid blowout, and these are almost always a result of previously irradiated tissue breakdown and/or infection. Loss of free tissue transfers with avulsion of the arterial pedicle can also result in late hemorrhage. While some authors have recommended leaving failed flaps in place for a period of time, caution should be exercised as the vascular pedicle can break down resulting in significant hemorrhage [47]. Prevention strategies include: appropriate use of prophylactic antibiotics; importation of vascularized tissue in compromised situations; and optimization of the patient's ability to heal through careful handling of tissues, maximizing nutrition, and confirming adequate thyroid function in the previously irradiated patient.

Operations on the oral cavity are considered "clean-contaminated," and therefore, perioperative antibiotics are indicated. Several well-controlled studies have demonstrated that antibiotics started before the incision and continued for no more that 24 hours serve to minimize perioperative infections and the emergence of resistant strains. Continuation beyond 24 hours should be considered in patients at increased risk or those with ongoing contamination. First generation cephalosporins and clindamycin represent the most commonly used prophylactic antibiotics in oral cancer surgery. Topical antimicrobials, such as chlorhexidine and clindamycin rinses, have also been shown to successfully reduce the incidence of infections [48,49].

Coverage of major vessels with imported tissue should be strongly considered in cases of RND in the postoperative setting. Free tissue transfer or pedicled flaps offer the ability to import non-irradiated tissue into the field.

Summary

Surgical management of cervical lymph node metastasis, both occult and evident, continues to evolve. It is clear that metastases are an indication of aggressiveness, and that they portend a poorer prognosis. Once the cancer has developed the necessary genetic mutations to break free and colonize independent of the primary, the chance of cure with single modality therapy diminishes. In his presidential address to the New England Surgical Society, Blake Cady MD, FACS referred to "lymph node metastases as the speedometers of the oncologic vehicle, not the engine. Indicators, not governors of survival"[50]. Clearly, the role for the radical neck dissection has diminished greatly as less invasive surgical techniques for dealing with the cervical lymphatics have gained popularity. This trend will likely continue, as the role of surgery in the control of metastatic disease is better defined [6,51,52]. As is true in most cases in surgery, what is thought to be new usually means history was not studied closely enough. The concepts of elective neck dissection, modified neck dissection, and selective neck dissection were described by the fathers of head and neck surgery. Indications for the various neck dissections, however, continue to evolve. A comprehensive discussion of the management of cervical lymph nodes in each subsite within the head and neck is beyond the scope of this article. Excellent reviews are available and recommended [2,7,53].

Most importantly, during this time of evolution, clinicians must be able to accurately communicate amongst each other what surgery was performed; what structures were sacrificed and which were preserved; and specifically, what lymph node basins were addressed. Avoidance of nonstandard, named neck dissections and the use of more accurate descriptions are important in this regard. Equally important is the need to educate nonsurgeons in the nomenclature and in the use of more limited dissections. Caution is merited when extrapolating previous research results in which patients may have received more comprehensive neck dissections to patients who may have received more limited dissections, especially in decisions regarding the need for adjuvant therapy.

References

[1] Mendenhall WM, Million RR, Cassisi NJ. Elective neck irradiation in squamous cell carcinoma of the head and neck. Head Neck Surg 1980;3:15–9.

[2] Carlson ER, Miller I. Surgical management of the neck in oral cancer. Oral Maxillofac Surg Clin North Am 2006;18:533–46.

[3] Rouviere H. Anatomy of the human lymphatic system. (Translation by Tobies MJ). Ann Arbor (MI): Edwards Brother; 1938.

[4] Lindberg R. Distribution of cervical lymph node metastases from squamous cell carcinoma of the upper respiratory and digestive tracts. Cancer 1972;29: 1446–9.

[5] Strauli P. The lymphatic system and cancer localization. In: Wiser RW, Ado Tl, Wood S, editors. Endogenous factors influencing host-tumor balance. Chicago: University of Chicago Press; 1967. p. 249–54.
[6] Robbins KT, Atkinson JL, Byers RM, et al. The use and misuse of neck dissection for head and neck cancer. J Am Coll Surg 2001;193:91–102.
[7] Pillsbury HC, Clark M. A rationale for therapy of the N0 neck. Joseph H. Ogura Lecture. Laryngoscope 1997;107:1294–315.
[8] Robbins KT, Clayman G, Levine PA, et al. Neck dissection classification update. Arch Otolaryngol Head Neck Surg 2002;128:751–8.
[9] Shah JP. Foreward. In: Gavilan J, Herranz J, DeSanto LW, editors. Functional and neck dissection. New York: Thieme; 2002. p. vii.
[10] Crile GW. Excision of cancer of the head and neck with special reference to the plan of dissection based upon one hundred thirty-two operations. JAMA 1906;47:1780–6.
[11] Crile GW. On the surgical treatment of cancer of the head and neck. Transactions Southern Surgical Gynecological Association 1905;18:109–27.
[12] Crile GW. Carcinoma of the jaws, tongue, cheek and lips. Surg Gynecol Obstet 1923;36:159–62.
[13] Martin H, Delvalle B, Ehrlich H, et al. Neck dissection. Cancer 1951;4:441–99.
[14] Ward GE, Robben JO. A composite operation for radical neck dissection and removal of cancer of the mouth. Cancer 1951;4:98–109.
[15] Calearo CV, Teatini G. Functional neck dissection: anatomical grounds, surgical technique clinical observations. Ann Otol Rhinol Laryngol 1983;92: 215–22.
[16] Bocca E. Supraglottic laryngectomy and functional neck dissection. J Laryngol Otol 1966;80:831–8.
[17] Gavilan J, Monux A, Herranz J, et al. Functional neck dissection: surgical technique. Operative Techniques in Otolaryngology-Head and Neck Surgery 1993;4:258–65.
[18] Suarez O. El problema de las metastasis linfaticas y alejades del cancer de laringe e hipofaringe. Rev Otorrinolaringol Santiago 1963;23:83–99.
[19] Robbins KT, Medina JE, Wolfe GT, et al. Standardizing neck dissection terminology. Official report of the Academy's Committee for Head and Neck Surgery and Oncology. Arch Otolaryngol Head Neck Surg 1991;117:601–5.
[20] Medina JE. A rational classification of neck dissections. Otolaryngol Head Neck Surg 1989;100:169–76.
[21] Shah JP, Candela FC, Poddar AK. The patterns of cervical lymph node metastases from squamous cell carcinoma of the oral cavity. Cancer 1990;66: 109–13.
[22] Spiro RH, Strong EW. Discontinuous partial glossectomy and radical neck dissection in selected patients with epidermoid carcinoma of the mobile tongue. Am J Surg 1973;126:544–6.
[23] Leemans CR, Tiwari R, Nauta JJ, et al. Discontinuous versus in-continuity neck dissection in carcinoma of the oral cavity. Arch Otolaryngol Head Neck Surg 1991;117:1003–6.
[24] Shah JP. Head and neck surgery and oncology. 3rd edition. New York: Elsivier; 2003.
[25] Kademani D, Dierks EJ. A straight-line incision for neck dissection: technical note. J Oral Maxillofac Surg 2005;63:563–5.
[26] Bocca E, Pignataro O. A conservation technique in radical neck dissection. Ann Oto Rhino Laryngol 1967;76:975–8.
[27] Suen JY. Functional neck dissection. In: Ballantyne JC, Harrison DFN, editors. Rob and Smith's operative surgery. London: Butterworth; 1986. p. 382–90.
[28] Gleich LL. Modified neck dissection. In: Gluckman JL, Johnson JT, editors. Surgical management of neck metastases. London: Martin Dunitz; 2003. p. 59–69.
[29] Yoel J, Linares CA. The Schobinger incision: Its advantages in radical neck dissections. Am J Surg 1964;108:526–8.
[30] Medina JE, Loré JM. The neck. In: Loré JM, Medina JE, editors. An atlas of head and neck surgery. 4th edition. Chapter 24. Philadelphia: Elsevier; 2005. p. 804.
[31] Byers RM, Weber RS, Andrews T, et al. Frequency and therapeutic implications of "skip metastasis" in the neck from squamous carcinoma of the tongue. Head Neck 1997;19:14–9.
[32] Shah JP, Candela FC, Poddar AK. The pattern of cervical lymph node metastases from squamous carcinoma of the oral cavity. Cancer 1990;66:109–13.
[33] Morton DL, Wen DR, Wong JH, et al. Technical details of intraoperative lymphatic mapping for early stage melanoma. Arch Surg 1992;127: 392–9.
[34] Morton DL, Wen DR, Foshag LJ, et al. Intraoperative lymphatic mapping and selective cervical lymphadenectomy for early stage melanomas of the head and neck. J Clin Oncol 1993;11:1751–6.
[35] Schellenberger TD. Sentinal lymph node biopsy in the staging of oral cancer. Oral Maxillofac Surg Clin North Am 2006;18:547–63.
[36] Krag DN, Meijer SJ, Weaver DL, et al. Minimal access surgery for staging of malignant melanoma. Arch Surg 1995;130:654–8.
[37] Glass LF, Messina JL, Cruse W, et al. The use of intraoperative radiolymphoscintigraphy for sentinel node biopsy in patients with malignant melanoma. Dermatol Surg 1996;22:715–20.
[38] Civantos FJ, Gomez C, Duque C, et al. Sentinal node biopsy in oral cavity cancer: correlation with PET scan and immunohistochemistry. Head Neck 2003;25:1–9.
[39] Pitman KT, Johnson JT, Brown ML, et al. Sentinel lymph node biopsy in head and neck squamous cell carcinoma. Laryngoscope 2002;112:2101–13.

[40] Hyde NC, Prvulovich E, Newman L, et al. A new approach to pre-treatment assessment of the N0 neck in oral squamous cell carcinoma: the role of sentinel node biopsy and positron emission tomography. Oral Oncol 2003;39:350–60.

[41] Pitman KT, Ferlito A, Devaney KO, et al. Sentinal lymph node biopsy in head and neck cancer. Oral Oncol 2003;39:343–9.

[42] Anderson PE, Warren F, Spiro J, et al. Results of selective neck dissection in management of the node positive neck. Arch Otolaryngol Head Neck Surg 2002;128:1180–4.

[43] McHam SA, Adelstein DJ, Rybicki LA, et al. Who merits a neck dissection after definitive chemoradiotherapy for N2-N3 sqaumous cell head and neck cancer? Head Neck 2003;25:791–7.

[44] Kraus DH, Rosenberg DB, Davidson BJ, et al. Supraspinal accessory lymph node metastases in supraomohyoid neck dissection. Am J Surg 1996;172:646–9.

[45] de Jong AA, Manni JJ. Phrenic nerve paralysis following neck dissection. Eur Arch Otorhinolaryngol 1991;248:132–4.

[46] Babin RW, Panje WR. The incidence of vasovagal reflex activity during radical neck dissection. Laryngoscope 1980;90:1321–3.

[47] Wheatley MJ, Meltzer TR. The management of unsalvageable free flaps. J Reconstr Microsurg 1996;12:227–9.

[48] Becker GD, Parell GJ. Cefazolin prophylaxis in head and neck cancer surgery. Ann Otol Rhinol Laryngol 1979;88:183–6.

[49] Mombelli G, Coppens L, Dor P, et al. Antibiotic prophylaxis in surgery for head and neck cancer: comparative study of short and prolonged administration of carbencillin. J Antimicrob Chemother 1981;7:665–71.

[50] Cady B. Lymph node metastases: indicators but not governors of survival. Arch Surg 1984;119: 1067–72.

[51] Ferlito A, Rinaldo A, Robbins KT, et al. Changing concepts in the surgical management of cervical node metastasis. Oral Oncol 2003;39:429–35.

[52] Kowalski LP, Magrin J, Waksman F, et al. Supraomohyoid neck dissection in the treatment of head and neck tumors: survival results in 212 cases. Arch Otolaryngol Head Neck Surg 1993;119:958–63.

[53] Ghali GE, Li BDL, Minnard EA. Management of the neck relative to oral malignancy. Selected Readings in Oral and Maxillofacial Surgery 1998;6(2): 1–36.

Management of the N0 Neck in Oral Squamous Cell Carcinoma

Allen Cheng, DDS, Brian L. Schmidt, DDS, MD, PhD, FACS*

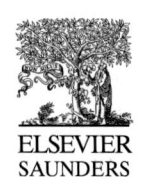

Department of Oral & Maxillofacial Surgery, University of California, 521 Parnassus Avenue, Room C-522, Box 0440, San Francisco, CA 94143-0440, USA

Squamous cell carcinoma (SCC) of the oral cavity has a poor prognosis that has only marginally improved despite the medical, surgical, and biochemical advances of the past 50 years [1–3]. Local recurrence in the oral cavity and metastasis through the lymphatics to regional lymph nodes are the most important causes of this poor prognosis, with regional metastasis halving 5-year survival rates [4–8].

Treatment of primary oral SCC tumors follows clear oncologic principles: resection of tumors with a 1 to 1.5-cm margin of normal tissue [9–16]. Treatment of clinically evident neck metastasis is equally clear: dissection and extirpation of the neck fibroadipose and lymphatic tissues, and removal of associated structures [17–21].

However, management of the neck when metastasis is not clinically evident (N0) is where the greatest ambiguity lies, given the unpredictable propensity of oral SCC for occult neck metastasis and the grave prognosis it portends [22–24]. Reports show rates of occult metastasis for oral SCC ranging from 20% to 45% [22,25–30]. When neck metastasis is detected after initial surgery, a greater surgical resection is required for salvage, with increased morbidity and poorer outcomes; or the tumor is nonresectable [23,31]. However, elective treatment of the N0 neck may prevent these recurrences and the need for more radical surgery, but may also subject a patient to an unnecessary major surgery and its associated risks, particularly the shoulder syndrome described by Nahum and colleagues [5,9,32–34].

The decision regarding the N0 neck has been debated extensively [32,33,35]. Countless studies have been published associating various clinical factors, biomarkers, and radiologic findings with the likelihood of occult metastasis in an effort to elucidate the proper treatment algorithm. This plethora of data and variety of recommendations may be why every oncologic surgeon is, as O'Brien and colleagues [26] described, "guided as much by personal philosophy and local custom as by scientific evidence" on whether and how to treat the N0 neck.

This article presents the controversies surrounding management of the N0 neck, discusses the benefits and pitfalls of different approaches toward its evaluation and management, and attempts to achieve a consensus on the appropriate algorithm for management.

When to treat the N0 neck

The decision to treat the N0 neck is easily reached when patients have a deeply invasive T4 tumor of the retromolar trigone or, in contrast, a superficial T1 tumor of the lip. In the former example, the neck is surgically accessed in the approach to remove the primary tumor and the risk for occult metastasis is high, and therefore the indications for an elective neck dissection are clear. In the latter example, the tumor behaves in a more indolent fashion, similar to a cutaneous SCC. Because the surgical approach does not include the neck and the risk for regional involvement is low, a neck dissection is not required and close observation is appropriate.

The lesions that lie between these two extremes pose a challenge, because the clinical behavior of

* Corresponding author.
E-mail address: brian.schmidt@ucsf.edu (B.L. Schmidt).

oral cavity SCC is capricious and unpredictable based on current clinical, pathologic, or molecular characteristics. The T1 or T2 tumors that are 3 to 4 mm thick trouble surgeons. Every busy oncologic surgeon who treats oral cancer can recall a patient who had a superficial T1 lesion that was resected with widely clear margins, but ultimately returned in 1 year with multiple neck metastases and then eventually died of the disease. This is the patient who is most disturbing and spurs oncologists toward more aggressive management.

Few rigorously designed studies are available to guide surgeons in the management of the N0 neck. A commonly cited study is the Weiss and colleagues [36] decision tree analysis, which proposes that a 20% risk for occult metastasis should be the threshold for treating the neck. This seminal paper is so central to the decision regarding elective treatment of the neck that revisiting this work is essential in any discussion about when to treat the N0 neck.

In their study, Weiss and colleagues [36] performed a computer-assisted mathematical analysis of the decisions and associated outcomes involved in managing the N0 neck, weighting the outcomes with their likelihood of occurrence and relative cost and benefit to patients. They created a decision tree beginning with the decision to operate, irradiate, or closely observe (Fig. 1). Each of these decisions branch out to different possible outcomes and further decisions.

The most distal branches of the decision tree were given probabilities for occurrence based on data from a review of seven clinical series published from 1971 to 1984 [21,37–42]. Each of the outcomes, including cure, death, cure with surgery, cure with radiation, and cure with salvage, were weighted based on desirability. Desirability was determined by three head and neck surgeons using a "time tradeoff method," which refers to how much time of life these surgeons would give up to have better function. For example, if one were willing to trade 4 months of life for better function, and the life expectancy was 120 months with a particular treatment, then the usefulness rating is 97% (116/120). Using this methodology, Weiss and colleagues [36] concluded that the benefits outweigh the costs in prophylactically treating the N0 neck only when the risk for occult metastasis exceeds 20%.

Their threshold of 20% has been used in many studies attempting to identify clinical factors, such as stage, thickness, depth of invasion, and histologic characteristics of the invasive front, as criteria for deciding on management of the neck.

Quality of life and its role in decision making

Analyses such as that of Weiss and colleagues [36] have limitations. Clinical outcomes are difficult to prioritize, and a critical piece of information is missing from their analysis: the reported effects on quality of life and how quality of life compares among types of treatments and between treatment and observation. A patient's perception of quality of life is profoundly individual and often different from the surgeon's perception of success.

The issue in question is whether patients would prefer to undergo an elective neck dissection that may not be necessary or be at risk for developing a recurrence, have a markedly worse prognosis, and face the possibility of a much more disfiguring and morbid surgery in the form of a radical neck dissection (RND) and chemoradiation therapy. To arbitrarily assign values to each of these outcomes based on the opinions (although experienced) of a handful of surgical colleagues is an inaccurate estimate of each outcome's subjective desirability from a patient's perspective [43,44].

Since that publication, the use of the selective neck dissection (SND) has supplanted RND as the preferred elective treatment for the neck [18,19]. Quality of life studies using general wellness and shoulder function-specific assessments have shown that the SND, when restricted to levels I to III, is not a significant detriment to quality of life, with outcomes in patients who underwent neck dissection nearly equal to those who did not [45–49]. In contrast, patients who had undergone RND or modified RND (MRND), similar to those in the series of studies referenced by Weiss and colleagues [36], had a significant detriment to quality of life characterized by increased long-term dysfunction, disfigurement, and shoulder pain [50].

Taylor and colleagues [46] used the Neck Dissection Impairment Index (NDII) to show that the greatest factors affecting quality of life, in descending order of significance, were age and weight, radiation therapy, and the extent of neck dissection. Similarly, Rogers and colleagues [45], using the University of Washington Quality of Life (UW-QoL) scale coupled with the NDII and shoulder disability questionnaire (SDQ), found that patients treated with MRND or RND had the worst scores, whereas those who

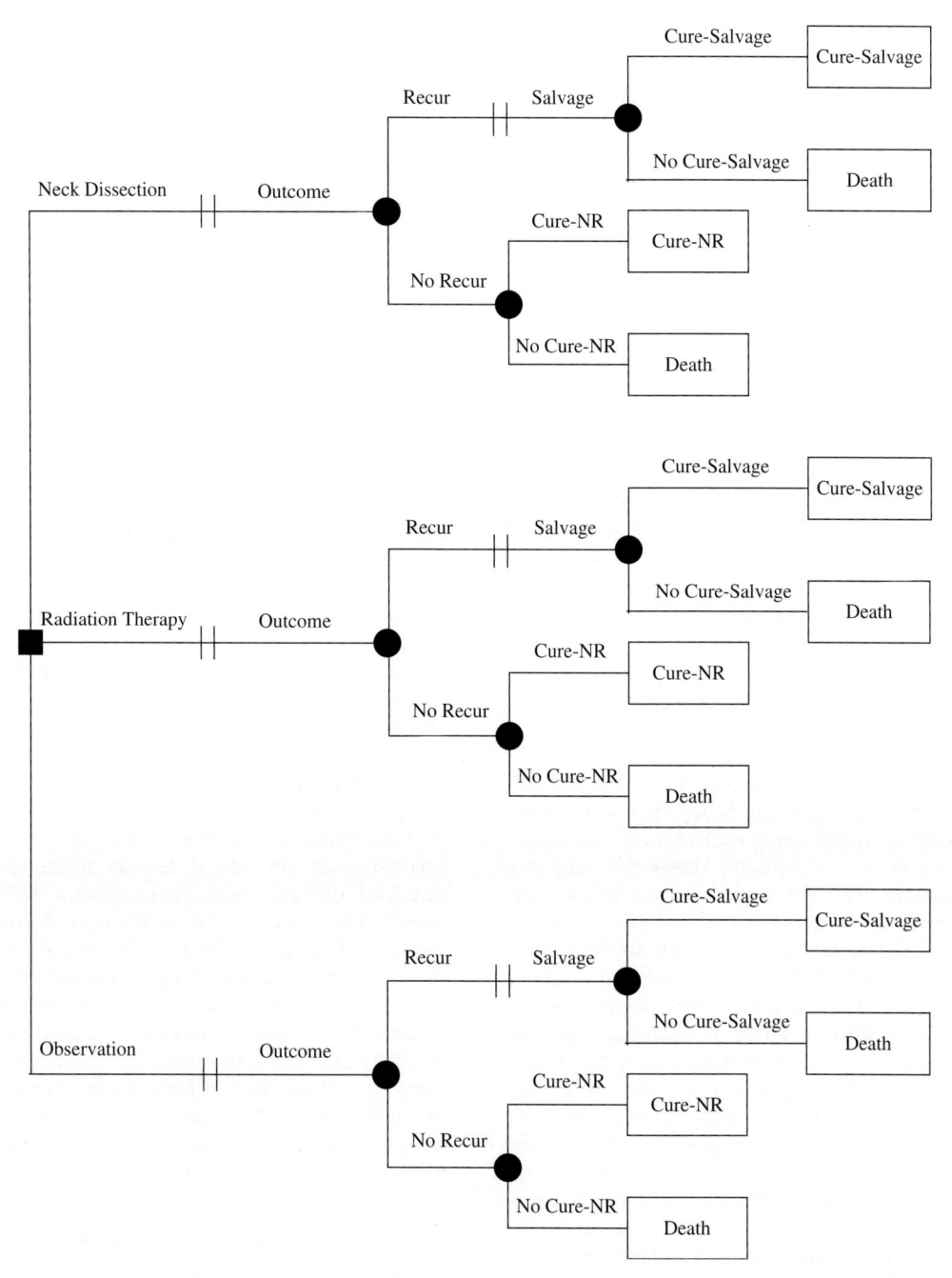

Fig. 1. Decision tree used by Weiss and colleagues [36] to perform a computer-assisted decision analysis. The figure depicts three alternative management strategies for the N0 neck. The filled box indicates the branching point between three different management strategies. Filled circles indicate branching points between two possible outcomes. Outcomes in boxes indicate the final outcome of that branch of the decision tree. Each of these outcomes was given a probability of occurrence and a desirability rating as quantified by the time tradeoff method. NR, no recurrence. (*Adapted from* Weiss MH, Harrison LB, Isaacs RS. Use of decision analysis in planning a management strategy for the stage N0 neck. Arch Otolaryngol Head Neck Surg 1994;120(7):699–702; with permission.)

had an SND of levels I through III had similar scores to those who underwent no neck dissection. Therefore, with the relatively low morbidity of SND compared with RND, the desirability values in the decision tree would certainly be different.

Quality of life must also be considered for patients followed up using the "wait and see" approach and later develop neck metastasis. Salvageable patients will be obligated to undergo a RND, possibly with chemoradiation therapy [20,51–53]. Given the findings of the studies mentioned earlier, the quality of life in these patients would be much lower even if a cure were obtained.

Thus, when the "wait and see" approach is used, failure results in decreased survival and quality of life. Of course, elective treatment is only advisable if it effectively prevents recurrences and decreases cancer-related mortality. Most studies on SND show that it prevents neck recurrence and controls occult neck metastasis [8,54]. Therefore, the negative impact on quality of life and survival using the "wait and see" approach must be considered.

Few prospective trials evaluating treatment algorithms

Weiss and colleagues' decision tree analysis is an important component in any algorithm used to decide on prescribing elective neck dissection. However, to the authors' knowledge, only one prospective series has attempted to evaluate the clinical usefulness of the 20% risk for occult metastasis as a threshold for elective treatment of the neck [26]. Most publications on elective treatment of the neck are retrospective and do not describe how the decision is reached regarding whether to operate and what diagnostic criteria exactly constitute a greater than 20% risk. Generally, the information on which the treatment decision is based is not provided and only the outcomes associated with each approach are reported. The original decisions in these retrospective studies were likely clinically based on the surgeon's experience and each patient's individual values. This approach does not allow an examination of the validity of the decision tree.

O'Brien and colleagues [26] reported on the application of the decision tree model, using clinical criteria, specifically tumor site, tumor stage, and the necessity of accessing the neck in resecting the primary tumor, in deciding when to electively treat the neck. In their series of 162 patients who had oral or oropharyngeal SCC and N0 necks, 58 patients underwent observation and 104 elective therapy in the form of an SND, radiation therapy, or these modalities combined. The decision to perform elective treatment of the neck was based on the clinical factors mentioned earlier, using 20% risk as the threshold for treatment.

Tumor stage was the strongest predictor in this study. In the elective treatment group, 30% of the neck dissection specimens had evidence of metastatic disease, and 4% of the patients, all of whom had positive nodes on initial neck dissection, developed unsalvageable neck recurrences. Among the observation group, 9% developed nodal metastasis, which were all N2 or greater, and the salvage rate was 80% at 3 years from primary surgery.

The disease-specific survival was 89% for the elective neck dissection group, 67% for the elective radiation therapy group, and 94% for the observation group. This result seems to indicate that using clinical criteria and a 20% risk threshold would have favorable results. That is, most patients who have occult metastasis would be treated electively, and the number of patients who develop neck recurrences while undergoing observation would be small and can be treated effectively with salvage therapy.

However, this study was purely a descriptive study, and did not include either a control group or randomization. Therefore, whether the high survival rates are related to use of the 20% threshold or some other factor unique to the investigators' practice, such as the clinical expertise of O'Brien and colleagues [26] in predicting risk for occult metastasis, is difficult to determine. Furthermore, an 80% salvage rate for neck recurrences is probably not transferable to most other oncology practices [23]. Even if the results are assumed to validate the decision tree analysis model, the surgeon and patient must still decide whether a 9% rate of neck recurrence and salvage surgery is an acceptable risk.

Elective neck dissection versus "wait and see"

Although the series by O'Brien and colleagues seems to be the only one that evaluated the decision tree, several studies advocate elective neck dissection over the "wait and see" approach, although very few were randomized and prospective. Only three prospective randomized trials seem to have compared the "wait and see" approach to the elective neck dissection, and only one evaluated the use of the SND (Table 1)

Table 1
Summary of data from randomized controlled trials on elective treatment of the N0 neck in patients who have oral SCC

Study	Elective therapy	Total patients	Occult metastasis on END[a]	Regional involvement on observation	Salvage[b]	Rate of DFS[c]
Vandenbrouck et al [21]	RND	75	49% (9%)	47%	Not reported	46% (58%) at 3 years
Fakih et al[d] [55]	RND	70	33% (14%)	57%	22% (30%)	64% (53%) at 12 months
Kligerman et al [54]	SND	67	33% (12%)	39%	25% (27%)	72% (49%) at 3 years

Abbreviations: DFS, disease-free survival; END, elective neck dissection; SCC, squamous cell carcinoma.
[a] Numbers in parentheses indicates neck recurrences after END.
[b] Salvage rates in neck recurrences only. Numbers in parentheses indicate salvage rates for neck recurrences in observation group. Minimum follow-up time shown.
[c] Numbers in parentheses indicate DFS in observation group.
[d] Study is specific to oral tongue SCC.

[21,54,55]. Vandenbrouck and colleagues [21] randomized 75 patients who had primary SCC of the oral cavity and no evidence of nodal metastasis to undergo either resection of the primary tumor without neck dissection or resection with a traditional RND. Patients in both groups remained on a monthly follow-up schedule for 3 years.

This series found that 49% of patients in the elective neck dissection group had occult metastasis and 47% in the "wait and see" group ultimately developed neck involvement and subsequently required salvage RND and radiation therapy. Moreover, a higher incidence of extracapsular spread was seen in the "wait and see" group. At 3 years, both groups had statistically equivalent survival patterns.

Despite being randomized, 21% of patients in the elective treatment group had T3 tumors compared with only 6% in the "wait and see" group. This difference in stage could be a potential confounder of the survival ratings. Furthermore, the reduced quality of life associated with RND and postoperative radiation therapy must be considered. Based on these results, Vandenbrouck and colleagues [21] recommended that elective neck dissection be offered to patients likely be lost to follow-up, but not necessarily to other patients. However, considering current risk assessment models, patients in the "wait and see" group who had larger nodes and higher incidence of extracapsular spread would be predicted to have a poorer prognosis and may have benefited from earlier treatment [24,53,56,57].

In 1989, Fakih and colleagues [55] published a study of 70 patients, with T1 and T2 oral tongue SCC and no evidence of neck involvement, who were randomized to either resection of the primary tumor without elective neck dissections or resection and an RND. They followed up their patients bimonthly for 1 year. This study found that 57% of patients in the "wait and see" group developed neck metastasis and 47% of the patients in the RND group had histologic evidence of occult metastasis.

At 1 year, the disease-free survival (DFS) of the "wait and see" group was 52% compared with 63% in the RND group, although this was not statistically significant. In the RND group, 4 of the 30 patients developed contralateral nodes, which were included in the count for occult metastasis, compared with none in the "wait and see" group.

Because all patients in the surgery group underwent ipsilateral neck dissections only, and without information on tumor location and whether the tumor violated the midline, some of those 4 patients may have been indicated for a contralateral SND, which might have affected the overall treatment outcome and the difference between the groups. In addition, the 1-year follow-up in this study is somewhat short, given that 95% of recurrences occur in the first 2 years [58]. This limited follow-up makes the effectiveness of salvage treatment in the "wait and see" group difficult to accurately evaluate.

Another criticism is that 28% of patients initially enrolled and who underwent initial therapy were lost to follow-up and removed from analysis. No data were provided as to which group these patients were lost, compromising the randomization and introducing a potential selection bias.

However, Fakih and colleagues did observe a significant difference in the presence of occult nodal metastasis among tumors with thickness greater than 4 mm (see later discussion).

Kligerman and colleagues [54] published the only prospective, randomized, controlled trial comparing elective SND of levels I through III with the "wait and see" approach for the N0 neck. This series randomly assigned 67 patients who had oral SCC and N0 necks to either resection alone of the primary tumor or in conjunction with a SND of levels I through III. These patients were followed up for at least 3 years postoperatively.

The investigators found a 21% rate of occult metastasis in the elective SND group and a 39% rate of recurrence in the neck in the "wait and see" group. Of significance, only 27% of patients who developed neck recurrences were salvageable. This finding is in sharp contrast to the 80% salvage rates reported by O'Brien and colleagues and is more consistent with other reported studies [23,26].

Kligerman and colleagues also reported that overall survival at 3 years was significantly improved in the elective neck dissection group. In contrast to the findings of Fakih and colleagues, no factors were found to be significantly associated with occult metastasis that could be used for prediction, including stage or depth of invasion.

Many retrospective, nonrandomized studies have also reported on the benefits of SND over the "wait and see" strategy in treating the neck [31,53,59–61]. These studies are summarized in Table 2. Keski-Santti and colleagues [60] found a significant improvement in survival despite more advanced primary tumors in the elective treatment groups, with 35% of patients in the observation group developing neck recurrences, and a 33% salvage rate.

Similarly, Capote and colleagues [31] found an 8% rate of neck recurrence in the elective neck dissection group versus a 26.8% rate in the observation group, with a 5-year survival rate of 91.7% and 77%, respectively. Again, success of salvage therapy was low at 32%.

In another nonrandomized retrospective review of 359 patients, Duvvuri and colleagues [59] found a 27% regional failure rate compared with 8% in the elective neck dissection group, although no difference in survival was seen at 5 years. Elective radiation therapy has also been shown to improve outcomes when used to manage the N0 neck [41].

A few studies have advised against elective treatment of the neck in favor of the "wait and see" approach [62–65]. In a retrospective analysis of 590 patients, Khafif and colleagues [65] found that patients who had occult metastasis who underwent an elective RND did not experience

Table 2
Summary of data from retrospective observational studies on elective treatment of the N0 neck

Study	Elective therapy	Total patients	Occult metastasis on END[a]	Regional involvement on observation	Salvage[b]	Rate of DFS[c]
Khafif et al[d] [65]	RND	590	42% (13%)	19%	49%	68% (88%) at 3 years
Nieuwenhuis et al[d] [63]	N/A	161	N/A	21%	(79%)	(79%) at 12 months
Duvvuri et al[d] [59]	SND	359	23% (8%)	27%	Not reported	66% (54%) at 3 years
Keski-Santti et al [60]	SND, RT or SND+RT	80	34% (13%)	24%	11% (47%)[e]	82% (81%) at 3 years
Capote et al [31]	END	154	Not reported (8%)	26.8%	32%[f]	92.5% (71.2%) at 5 years

Abbreviations: DFS, disease-free survival; END, elective neck dissection; RND, radical neck dissection; RT, radiation therapy; SCC, squamous cell carcinoma; SND, selective neck dissection.

[a] Numbers in parentheses indicates neck recurrences after END.
[b] Salvage rates are in neck recurrences only, unless otherwise noted. Numbers in parentheses indicate salvage rates for neck recurrences in observation group. Minimum follow-up time shown.
[c] Numbers in parentheses indicate DFS in observation group.
[d] Study not specific to oral cavity primaries; they may include oropharyngeal and laryngeal.
[e] Overall salvage rate for local and regional recurrences is shown.
[f] Overall neck salvage rate for both observation and END groups is shown.

a survival benefit compared with those who underwent observation and subsequently developed clinically apparent nodal involvement and required subsequent salvage RND.

However, these investigators assumed that pathologically N0 (pN0) necks did not have occult disease, although this assumption is not entirely accurate as evidenced by the 7% neck recurrence rate among patients who had pN0 necks in their study (see later discussion). When the elective RND group was analyzed, including patients who were pathologically positive and negative for nodal involvement, DFS was significantly improved over the salvage rate in the observation group (68% vs. 49%, respectively).

Khafif and colleagues [65] did not recommend elective treatment of the neck, based on the assumption that RND or radiation therapy would be used, which are both associated with significant morbidity. However, they supported using a more selective node sampling for staging purposes.

In a retrospective study of 891 patients who had oral SCC and N0/N+ necks, Layland and colleagues [62] showed that disease-specific survival was equivalent whether the neck was treated electively or after nodal disease became apparent. One criticism of this study is that the observation arm had a greater percentage of early T1 disease than T2 through T4 disease, a discrepancy that was not statistically addressed and could have confounded the outcome.

Assessing risk for occult metastasis

Elective treatment of the N0 neck is a complex decision because no accurate way exists to determine the risk for occult metastasis. The sensitivity of clinical examination to detect metastasis, even by expert surgeons, has been inadequate, with a sensitivity of 51% reported by one major head and neck surgery group [22]. Other groups have also reported on the low sensitivity of clinical examination, ranging from 60% to 70% [66–68].

Cancer is a heterogeneous disease, with significant biologic variability even among patients who have the same cancer. In this regard, SCC of the oral cavity is no different and is notorious for displaying a wide spectrum of clinical behavior. Much work has been devoted to dissecting these differences to create a risk assessment model for occult metastasis in oral SCC. However, no single parameter (or set) or adjunctive diagnostic technique has been sufficiently sensitive, and few have held up to further study.

Limitations of imaging

Imaging using CT, MRI, positron emission tomography (PET), ultrasound, and now PET/CT has been used to assess primary tumors. Unfortunately, despite improved resolution and software analysis, these techniques are still insufficiently sensitive for detecting occult neck metastases, with 20% to 45% of patients staged as N0 using these techniques having occult nodal involvement on pathologic evaluation of the neck [22,28,29].

For imaging techniques to be useful in treatment decisions, they must be able to detect metastatic nodes found in patients who have early-stage tumors, which are present only 20% to 45% of the time. These nodes are commonly small, with diameters as small as 3 to 10 mm. Also, the long axis of these nodes, which can be visualized accurately on pathology, is often not parallel to any of the planes used for anatomic imaging, causing even greater foreshortening [29,69].

The presence of structural changes, such as cystic changes or necrosis, aids detection, but these features are rarely present in occult disease [29]. In addition, these techniques must be not only sufficiently sensitive to detect microscopic disease but also specific enough such that frequent false-positive results do not cause universal prescription of elective neck treatment.

Anatomic imaging studies, such as MRI and CT, have been shown to have similar accuracies, with sensitivities ranging from 56% to 85% and specificities from 47% to 95% [70–73]. PET showed a sensitivity of 75% to 90% and specificity of 90% to 100%. Patients in these studies, however, did not have N0 necks exclusively. The sensitivity and specificity is expected to be much lower for detecting occult nodes in earlier-stage disease.

Multiple studies from one surgical oncology group have reported success using ultrasound-guided fine needle aspiration biopsy with a "wait and see" approach for patients who have N0 necks [63,66,74–76]. In one study using this strategy, Nieuwenhuis and colleagues [63] reported that 21% of their patients developed nodal disease during follow-up. These patients were then treated with a therapeutic neck dissection of levels I through V, with a salvage rate of 79% at 5 years. However, diagnosing occult metastasis with ultrasound seems to be highly technique-sensitive and user-specific, because other studies have been unable to replicate this success [22,77].

PET/CT is a recent imaging technology combining the improved sensitivity of PET for metastatic disease with the higher resolution and accuracy of CT. In a cohort of patients with N0 necks, Schoder and colleagues [69] found that PET/CT had a sensitivity and specificity of 67% and 85%, respectively. Using histopathology, they determined that nodes 3 mm or smaller could not be reliably detected with PET/CT. They therefore concluded that, despite overall high accuracy, PET/CT has limited clinical usefulness in this application because of the inadequate sensitivity for small nodes and high number of false-positives (13%). They also emphasize that the surgeons in their group had the PET/CT results before planning treatment, and that the information did not alter the decision to operate in any of the patients.

Nahmias and colleagues [78] also recently published a detailed study on the use of PET/CT in staging the neck. This study carefully mapped out each node from a neck dissection and then compared it with the corresponding node visualized on the preoperative PET/CT. Using this methodology, they examined the staging capacity of PET/CT on a node-by-node basis.

Their study included 70 patients who had oral cancer; 47 had N0 necks and 19 were clinically node-positive. The sensitivity and specificity of PET/CT for detecting metastatic nodal involvement in the 47 patients who had N0 necks patients were 79% and 82%, respectively, with positive (PPV) and negative predictive values (NPV) of 68% and 89%, respectively. Analysis on a node-by-node basis in patients who have N0 necks showed a sensitivity and specificity of 26% and 99%, respectively, with a PPV of 63% and NPV of 95%. The investigators concluded that, because of a NPV of 89% and a false-negative rate of 11%, PET/CT did not help rule out occult nodal metastasis to a degree that would affect a surgeon's decision to electively treat the neck.

Therefore, although it is a critical adjunct to treatment planning and diagnosing nodal metastasis, imaging is not sensitive enough to replace histopathologic staging using an elective neck dissection.

Tumor staging and risk of occult metastasis

Clinical factors, such as tumor staging and location, have long been associated with differential risk. Current convention is to use the American Joint Commission on Cancer (AJCC) TNM staging protocol [79]. Tumor staging is an important step in determining prognosis. Higher stages have been correlated with higher rates of positive margins on resection, higher rates of recurrence, and lower 5-year survival rates [1].

However, some debate exists on how accurate the current staging system is in prognosticating, especially regarding predicting nodal metastasis. More specifically, the AJCC system has been criticized for emphasizing certain features of the primary tumor, such as diameter, while excluding other factors that some studies suggest may play a larger role, such as perineural invasion, depth of tumor invasion, and the characteristics of the invasive front (discussed in more detail later).

Although advanced stage is used to predict risk for occult metastasis, multivariate analyses have shown that stage is not an independent risk factor for neck involvement when tumor thickness has been factored out [8,80]. Despite this fact, the simplicity of using the superficial diameter of a lesion as a prognostic tool, especially considering that it is likely to have some relationship to tumor thickness, still makes staging a frequently used measure that is recommended by most practices [22].

Significance of micrometastases

In addition, histopathologic review of nodes is not infallible. On more careful examination, several studies have found a high prevalence of micrometastases (ie, foci of tumor within lymph nodes smaller than 3 mm) when lymph nodes were serially sectioned, as opposed to the sampling technique of bisectioning lymph nodes that is used at most hospitals [81,82]. The rates of these micrometastases ranged from 16% to 25% in previously pathologically staged N0 necks. Although the prognostic significance of these micrometastases is still unclear, at least some of these tumor cells may be ultimately responsible for neck recurrences seen even in pathologically N0 necks.

The other implication is that previous studies on the prevalence of occult metastasis discovered through elective neck dissections may be grossly underestimating the actual prevalence of nodal involvement, and that many of these neck dissections are actually therapeutic. This possibility may explain the improved survival rates seen in elective treatment groups in several studies [54,60].

Role of tumor location in occult metastasis

The oral cavity has been divided into several subsites: lips, oral tongue, mandibular alveolar gingiva, maxillary alveolar gingiva, hard palate, floor of mouth, retromolar trigone, and buccal mucosa [79]. Much variability has been observed and described for tumors of different subsites regarding their effects on occult metastasis and survival.

SCC of the lip is generally considered to have a very favorable prognosis and low risk for regional metastasis if treated early. Tumors of the maxillary gingiva and hard palate have also been considered to have low incidence of regional metastasis. However, tumors of the oral tongue, floor of mouth, mandibular gingiva, and retromolar trigone are often reported to have high rates of occult metastasis [83]. Buccal mucosa tumors have also been shown to predict poor prognosis, with high rates of local and regional failure [84,85].

Several recent studies have challenged some of the aforementioned ideas, particularly the supposed indolent nature of maxillary SCC. In a series of 26 patients who had SCC of the maxilla, Simental and colleagues [86] found a 27% incidence of occult metastasis and a 34.6% rate for overall nodal metastasis. Similarly, Fernandes and colleagues [87] reported a 40% incidence of metastasis in a series of 15 patients. The senior author of this article also had this experience, with a 42.9% rate of cervical metastasis in 14 patients who had maxillary SCC [88].

Therefore, all intraoral tumors seem to possess some risk for regional metastasis, and therefore a worse prognosis, despite conventional thinking. Using the purported characteristics of different subsites within the oral cavity as a reason not to address the neck is not currently justified. However, SCC of the lip is still unlikely to have the same risk, and elective neck treatment can be deferred unless the tumor is advanced in stage or adjacent subsites are involved, or if nodal involvement is clinically detectable.

Limitations of histopathologic grading

Histologic grading has been used for some time to predict the behavior of benign and malignant tumors. However, although useful in some tumors, its prognostic value in SCC is controversial. Broders' [89,90] classification of the degree of malignancy has been used for many decades and was the first attempt to develop a grading system for head and neck SCC. It classifies tumors as well differentiated, moderately well differentiated, poorly differentiated, or undifferentiated based on the proportion of well-differentiated cells within the tumor. Broders showed that degree of differentiation was able to predict rates of metastasis in lip carcinomas [91].

Byers and colleagues [22] also found the Broders system of tumor differentiation correlated with nodal metastasis in a mixed group of patients who had N0 and N+ necks, although whether it would be as useful in evaluating the N0 neck independently was unclear. Unfortunately, it has not correlated well with patient prognosis or risk for regional involvement when studied by other groups, probably because of the ambiguity of the definitions used in the Broders system and its oversimplicity [92,93]. To improve the predictive value of grading, several groups have tried to create multifactorial malignancy grading systems that include several histopathologic criteria [92–100]. The large number of these systems is a reflection of the complexity of quantifying malignancy in oral SCC.

Modified versions of the grading system published by Anneroth and colleagues [92,93,101] are probably the most widely used today. They include several factors, such as degree of keratinization, nuclear polymorphism, number of mitoses per high power field, pattern of invasion, and lymphoplasmacytic infiltration. Other factors that have been studied include tumor shape (reductive or expansive), growth pattern (endophytic or exophytic), perineural invasion, vascular invasion, muscular invasion, and depth of invasion. Using the Anneroth malignancy grading system with modifications by Woolgar and colleagues, Kademani and colleagues [102], found it to be predictive of DFS and neck metastasis in a series of 215 patients who had oral SCC.

In an exhaustive study of 71 patients with SCC of the oral tongue, Po Wing Yuen and colleagues [80] evaluated the Anneroth, Bryne, and Martinez-Gimeno grading systems, and stage, perineural invasion, vascular invasion, lymphovascular invasion, shape, stage, growth pattern, and thickness. After careful analysis, only tumor thickness was an independent risk factor for nodal metastasis. In a similarly thorough study of 29 patients, which also included immunohistochemical analysis of tumors for vascular endothelial growth factors (VEGF) and health-related behaviors, Warburton and colleagues [103] also found tumor thickness to be the only independent predictor of nodal metastasis. Clark and colleagues [8] also reached the same conclusion in 164 patients.

used cost-minimization and -effectiveness analyses. Unfortunately, a dearth of research exists on the economic ramifications of elective treatment of the neck in oral SCC [124].

In an extensive study published in 2006 by Speight and colleagues [125] on data from two hospitals in the United Kingdom, patients who had oral SCC of earlier stage had shorter hospital stays and a smaller mean per-patient cost. Initial diagnosis and treatment costs were $3443 for precancer patients compared with $24,890 in patients who had stage IV cancer. The report concluded that prevention and early intervention would be the most cost-effective way to address the substantial costs of oral cancer. Similarly, in 2004 Lang and colleagues [126] used Surveillance, Epidemiology, and End Result–Medicare data to show that patients who had regional and distant metastasis had twice the hospital stay and related costs compared with patients who had localized cancer.

Although these studies do not directly address the question of elective treatment of the N0 neck, it can be hypothesized that patients who have early cancer and undergo elective neck dissections would probably generate lower costs, because they are clinically staged as I or II, than patients who develop clinically apparent metastases after treatment with the "wait and see" approach. The latter would be stage IV and would require RND, longer intensive care unit admissions, and exceedingly expensive chemoradiation therapy [127]. Considering that neck failure occurs 20% to 45% of the time in the "wait and see" approach, one might expect the overall economic burden to be larger in this group. Further investigation is needed to clarify this issue.

Summary

In light of recent quality of life studies, SND is much less morbid than RND. In long-term studies, quality of life in patients who undergo SND is equivalent to that of patients who did not undergo neck dissection. Therefore, the decision tree analysis which analyzed the threshold for elective RND use, should be revisited to set a new and likely lower threshold for elective treatment with SND. In addition, given the inability to accurately assess risk for neck metastasis using clinical, histopathologic, radiologic, or molecular techniques; the added morbidity of the "wait and see" approach; and the effectiveness of SND in preventing neck failure in a randomized clinical trial, the authors believe that elective neck dissection should be offered to all patients who have oral SCC at any intraoral site.

How to treat

Surgery is not the only treatment option available for elective treatment of the neck. Radiation therapy is also efficacious in managing the N0 neck and is often used in head and neck cancer for this application [41]. However, surgery remains the preferred modality in elective treatment of the N0 neck in oral SCC, for various reasons.

It is preferable to select the same treatment modality for the neck that is being used to treat the primary tumor, if possible. Although radiation therapy has been shown to be effective in treating oropharyngeal, nasopharyngeal, hypopharyngeal, and laryngeal SCC, it has compared unfavorably with surgery as a primary therapy for oral SCC because of its considerable morbidity and poor cancer control rates [128,129].

Toxicities include mucositis, xerostomia and its dental sequelae, erythematous skin changes, subcutaneous fibrosis, carotid artery stenosis, and osteoradionecrosis [130]. Furthermore, speech and ability to swallow are often more severely affected with radiation therapy. These adverse reactions lead to a protracted recovery that likely contributes to the lower quality of life scores that are correlated with radiation therapy [46,131,132]. Because surgery is the preferred treatment for primary oral SCC tumors, and SND is better tolerated by patients than radiation therapy, it is sensible to prescribe SND rather than radiation therapy for the N0 neck in oral SCC.

Despite treatment with curative intent, oral SCC has a relatively high recurrence rate [133]. The use of radiation therapy as a primary therapy precludes its future use as adjunctive or salvage therapy. Surgery in an irradiated field is a considerable challenge, making the salvage surgery more difficult and complicated. Reserving radiation therapy to the neck for oral SCC for adjunctive or second-line therapy makes sense.

Probably the most important reason to choose surgery over radiation therapy to treat the N0 neck is the staging information that histopathologic review of the neck specimen provides [134,135]. Although the accuracy of lymph node staging has limitations, the histopathologic review of the neck is still invaluable. The presence of extracapsular spread and multiple occult nodes can significantly alter prognosis and signals the need for additional treatment [24,56].

Extent of neck dissection

Since Crile's [136] description of the RND in 1905 and 1906, treatment of the neck has become less radical and more conservative, such as sparing nonlymphatic structures (spinal accessory nerve, sternocleidomastoid muscle, and internal jugular vein) and decreasing the number of levels of neck lymphatics removed [18,38]. The clinical significance is a marked reduction in postoperative morbidity, particularly with avoiding sacrifice of the spinal accessory nerve and preventing trauma to this nerve by foregoing dissection of the posterior triangle [48]. Currently, SND of levels I through III is the most frequently used surgical option to treat the N0 neck in patients who have oral SCC [19]. Fig. 2 illustrates the levels of neck as classified in 2002 by Robbins and colleagues [137].

This selectivity is based on the observation that oral SCC follows predictable patterns of lymphatic metastasis [8,19,138–141]. Lindberg's [140] classic study in 1972 showed that in primary SCC tumors of the oral cavity, neck metastases could be found in the submandibular triangle, submental triangle, upper jugular chain, and midjugular chain of lymph nodes. Lindberg also described the prevalence of "skip metastases," wherein metastatic tumors could "skip" the upper echelon of nodes (ie, the jugulodigastric or submandibular nodes) and be found in the midjugular chain. These skip metastases were not found in the lower jugular chain (level IV) or in the posterior triangle of the neck (level V).

Several subsequent studies have confirmed Lindberg's observations. In a series of 1119 RNDs for primary oral SCC tumors, Shah and colleagues [19] found that level V nodes were never involved when levels I through IV were negative. Similarly, in a cohort of 1123 patients who had head and neck SCC, Davidson and colleagues [138] reported that only 1% of patients staged clinically as N0 had metastasis to level V. In 2004, Dias and colleagues [139] published a series of 339 patients in which only 1.5% who had N0 necks had skip metastasis to level IV, and none had skip metastases to level V.

In addition to these findings on the patterns of cervical metastasis, several groups have shown the efficacy of SND in treating the N0 neck [8,54,59]. This efficacy has been shown to be comparable to RND [30,33,142,143].

Level IIB

In an effort to further delineate the selectivity of elective neck dissection, the inclusion of sublevels of the neck has been debated. In 2002, a reclassification of the neck dissection was published that divided level II into IIA and IIB using the spinal accessory nerve as the dividing line, and level V into VA and VB using a horizontal plane that crosses the inferior border of the anterior cricoid arch as a dividing line (see Fig. 2) [137].

The purpose of this reclassification was to distinguish sublevels IIB and VA for potential preservation, based on the premise that IIB nodes (also known as the *supraretrospinal triangle*, *supraspinal accessory lymph node pad*, or *submuscular recess*) were rarely involved in occult metastasis and that dissection of those nodes may lead to traction of the spinal accessory nerve and subsequent shoulder dysfunction [50].

Several studies have confirmed that occult metastases to level IIB are rare. Silverman and colleagues [144] only found 1.6% of 74 patients who had IIB metastasis. Elsheikh and colleagues [145] found no positive IIB nodes using reverse transcriptase polymerase chain reaction molecular techniques, except in SCC of the oral tongue. In this subsite, they found that

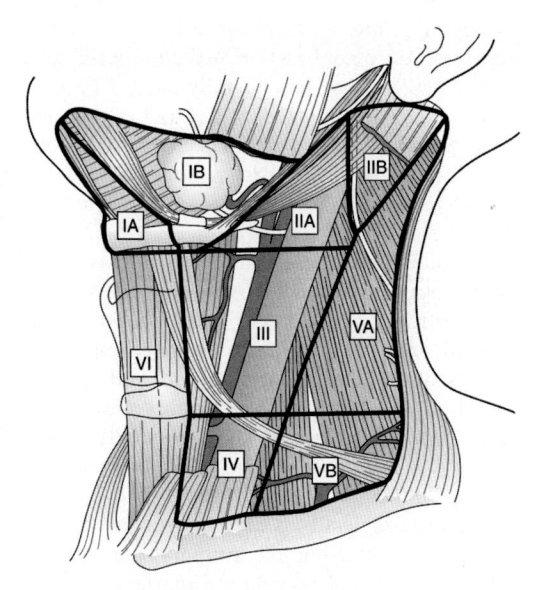

Fig. 2. Illustration of the levels and sublevels of the neck. Notice that level II is divided into IIA and IIB by the spinal accessory nerve and level V is divided by a horizontal plane from the inferior border of the cricoid arch into VA and VB.

10% of patients had molecular evidence of tumor cells in IIB nodes. Lim and colleagues [146] also only found 5% of metastasis to this level in 74 patients.

Contemporary practice at the University of California, San Francisco (UCSF) is still to includes level IIB in the neck specimen. The clinical reasoning behind this approach is that no significant amount of shoulder dysfunction has been seen from including this level, nor have any quality of life studies evaluated the benefits of preservation of level IIB. However, dissection of level IIB in the setting of recurrence will certainly be much more difficult than addressing this area at initial surgery. Therefore, the authors recommend that IIB nodes be included in SND.

Level IV

Some controversy also surrounds the inclusion of level IV nodes in the SND. Although several groups have shown that level IV nodes are rarely involved in skip metastases [8,139], others have found the opposite [147]. Byers and colleagues [147] found that skip metastases to level IV occurred at the alarming rate of 15.8%. Some of these differences may be caused by the anatomic variability of the omohyoid muscle position, which is commonly used to determine the inferior border of level III and superior border of level IV [148].

The current practice within the Department of Oral and Maxillofacial Surgery at UCSF is to not include level IV in SND. However, level IV is examined clinically in situ during surgery. If physical findings suggesting metastasis are noted, such as nodal induration or enlargement, level IV is included with the specimen. The rationale behind this approach is twofold. First, in this department's experience, skip metastasis to level IV has not been observed and dissection of these nodes is of low yield. Second, dissection of level IV may damage the phrenic nerve and, when operating on the left, the thoracic duct.

Bilateral neck dissection

Contralateral occult metastasis is also observed, particularly in tumors that encroach on the midline [140]. Prescribing a bilateral SND is recommended for patients who have oral SCC that violates the midline [137], including any SCC tumor requiring a wide resection that crosses the midline to achieve a 1-cm margin.

Sentinel node biopsy

Perhaps the best example of the shift toward ultra-selectivity in managing the N0 neck is the advent of the sentinel node biopsy. This technique involves injection of radiolabeled tracer around the periphery of the tumor, allowing the tracer to drain through the lymphatic system to the first echelon of nodes. The sentinel nodes are delineated with a gamma probe, followed by their surgical removal in a manner that preserves oncologic safety. After excision, the nodes are examined initially with frozen section. If micrometastases are identified, patients undergo SND.

Postoperatively, the nodes from the permanent specimen are examined thoroughly with serial sectioning, as opposed to bisectioning, which is the technique typically used to sample lymph nodes for histopathologic review. If micrometastases are located in the permanent serial sections, patients return to the operating room for a conventional SND, if not already performed [149].

This technique, which has been used effectively to treat melanoma and breast cancer, shows great promise for treating the neck in oral SCC [150,151]. Preliminary results from a multicenter trial in 2004 were favorable [152]. In addition, a recent clinical trial published by Stoeckli and colleagues [149] showed that the use of sentinel node biopsy had very high sensitivity and specificity for detecting occult metastases, with a false-negative rate of only 6%. Furthermore, in nine patients (13%) who had laterally located floor of mouth and oral tongue SCC, use of sentinel node biopsy identified drainage to contralateral nodes and level IV nodes, regions that would not have been addressed with a conventional SND.

Despite this promise, some concerns have been raised regarding the use of sentinel node biopsy. One criticism is that the radiolabeled tracer injected into an oral SCC tumor, especially tumors of the floor of mouth and oral tongue, would obscure gamma probe readings in the first echelon nodes because of their proximity to the primary tumor, negating any benefit from the exercise. Stoeckli and colleagues [149] circumvented this problem by going against conventional practice and excising the primary tumor first, before the sentinel nodes were marked out and addressed.

Another criticism is that if micrometastasis is detected later, only after serial sectioning of the permanent specimen, patients would be subjected to a second surgery. Knowing the high rates of occult metastasis, this would likely result in 20% to 45% of patients requiring second surgeries. Studies evaluating this technique are generally small; more are needed before the efficacy of sentinel node biopsy can be adequately compared with conventional SND, with its attendant low morbidity.

It seems unlikely that removing level I and II nodes would be significantly less morbid than removing levels I through III, in contrast with performing two separate operations instead of one. Although sentinel node biopsy is certainly very promising and warrants further investigation, it is still too early to recommend it as a treatment for the N0 neck except in select cases.

Summary

The, surgical management of the N0 neck is ideally performed through SND of levels I through III. Level IIB should be included in this dissection, because it does not add significant morbidity to the surgery. Level IV should be spared because removing this level is of low yield and may damage the phrenic nerve and possibly the thoracic duct if operating on the left neck.

Conclusion

The management of the N0 neck, particularly the timing of elective treatment, is highly controversial, with no single standard of care agreed on by all practitioners. However, because current methods to assess the risk for occult metastasis are insufficiently accurate and prone to underestimation of actual risk; the limited number of studies available favor elective treatment of the N0 neck; and SND has a minimal long-term detriment to quality of life, the authors believe that all patients who have oral SCC, excluding lip SCC, should undergo elective treatment of the neck lymphatics. Because of the morbidity of radiation therapy and because the treatment of the primary tumor is surgical, elective neck dissection is the preferred treatment. In deciding the extent of the neck dissection, several retrospective studies and one randomized clinical trial have shown SND of levels I through III to be highly efficacious.

References

[1] Sutton DN, Brown JS, Rogers SN, et al. The prognostic implications of the surgical margin in oral squamous cell carcinoma. Int J Oral Maxillofac Surg 2003;32(1):30–4.

[2] Shah JP, Johnson NW, Batsakis JG. Oral cancer. London New York: Martin Dunitz; Distributed in the United States by Thieme New York; 2003.

[3] Parkin DM, Pisani P, Ferlay J. Global cancer statistics. CA Cancer J Clin 1999;49(1):33–64 31.

[4] Fielding LP, Fenoglio-Preiser CM, Freedman LS. The future of prognostic factors in outcome prediction for patients with cancer. Cancer 1992; 70(9):2367–77.

[5] Kowalski LP, Magrin J, Waksman G, et al. Supraomohyoid neck dissection in the treatment of head and neck tumors. Survival results in 212 cases. Arch Otolaryngol Head Neck Surg 1993;119(9):958–63.

[6] Leemans CR, Tiwari R, Nauta JJ, et al. Regional lymph node involvement and its significance in the development of distant metastases in head and neck carcinoma. Cancer 1993;71(2):452–6.

[7] Shah JP, Andersen PE. Evolving role of modifications in neck dissection for oral squamous carcinoma. Br J Oral Maxillofac Surg 1995;33(1): 3–8.

[8] Clark JR, Naranjo N, Franklin JH, et al. Established prognostic variables in N0 oral carcinoma. Otolaryngol Head Neck Surg 2006;135(5):748–53.

[9] Lavertu P, Adelstein DJ, Saxton JP, et al. Management of the neck in a randomized trial comparing concurrent chemotherapy and radiotherapy with radiotherapy alone in resectable stage III and IV squamous cell head and neck cancer. Head Neck 1997;19(7):559–66.

[10] Looser KG, Shah JP, Strong EW. The significance of "positive" margins in surgically resected epidermoid carcinomas. Head Neck Surg 1978; 1(2):107–11.

[11] Loree TR, Strong EW. Significance of positive margins in oral cavity squamous carcinoma. Am J Surg 1990;160(4):410–4.

[12] Partridge M, Brakenhoff R, Phillips E, et al. Detection of rare disseminated tumor cells identifies head and neck cancer patients at risk of treatment failure. Clin Cancer Res 2003;9(14):5287–94.

[13] Partridge M, Li SR, Pateromichelakis S, et al. Detection of minimal residual cancer to investigate why oral tumors recur despite seemingly adequate treatment. Clin Cancer Res 2000;6(7): 2718–25.

[14] Slootweg PJ, Hordijk GJ, Schade Y, et al. Treatment failure and margin status in head and neck cancer. A critical view on the potential value of molecular pathology. Oral Oncol 2002;38(5):500–3.

[15] Vikram B, Strong EW, Shah JP, et al. Failure at the primary site following multimodality treatment in advanced head and neck cancer. Head Neck Surg 1984;6(3):720–3.

[16] van Es RJ, van Nieuw Amerongen N, Slootweg PJ, et al. Resection margin as a predictor of recurrence at the primary site for T1 and T2 oral cancers.

[17] Byers RM. Modified neck dissection. A study of 967 cases from 1970 to 1980. Am J Surg 1985;150(4):414–21.
[18] Byers RM. Neck dissection: concepts, controversies, and technique. Semin Surg Oncol 1991;7(1):9–13.
[19] Shah JP. Patterns of cervical lymph node metastasis from squamous carcinomas of the upper aerodigestive tract. Am J Surg 1990;160(4):405–9.
[20] Snow GB, Annyas AA, van Slooten EA, et al. Prognostic factors of neck node metastasis. Clin Otolaryngol Allied Sci 1982;7(3):185–92.
[21] Vandenbrouck C, Sancho-Garnier H, Chassagne D, et al. Elective versus therapeutic radical neck dissection in epidermoid carcinoma of the oral cavity: results of a randomized clinical trial. Cancer 1980;46(2):386–90.
[22] Byers RM, El-Naggar AK, Lee YY, et al. Can we detect or predict the presence of occult nodal metastases in patients with squamous carcinoma of the oral tongue? Head Neck 1998;20(2):138–44.
[23] Ord RA, Kolokythas A, Reynolds MA. Surgical salvage for local and regional recurrence in oral cancer. J Oral Maxillofac Surg 2006;64(9):1409–14.
[24] Woolgar JA, Rogers SN, Lowe D, et al. Cervical lymph node metastasis in oral cancer: the importance of even microscopic extracapsular spread. Oral Oncol 2003;39(2):130–7.
[25] Zbaren P, Nuyens M, Caversaccio M, et al. Elective neck dissection for carcinomas of the oral cavity: occult metastases, neck recurrences, and adjuvant treatment of pathologically positive necks. Am J Surg 2006;191(6):756–60.
[26] O'Brien CJ, Traynor SJ, McNeil E, et al. The use of clinical criteria alone in the management of the clinically negative neck among patients with squamous cell carcinoma of the oral cavity and oropharynx. Arch Otolaryngol Head Neck Surg 2000;126(3):360–5.
[27] Okada Y, Mataga I, Katagiri M, et al. An analysis of cervical lymph nodes metastasis in oral squamous cell carcinoma. Relationship between grade of histopathological malignancy and lymph nodes metastasis. Int J Oral Maxillofac Surg 2003;32(3):284–8.
[28] Spiro JD, Spiro RH, Shah JP, et al. Critical assessment of supraomohyoid neck dissection. Am J Surg 1988;156(4):286–9.
[29] Woolgar JA. Pathology of the N0 neck. Br J Oral Maxillofac Surg 1999;37(3):205–9.
[30] Yu S, Li J, Li Z, et al. Efficacy of supraomohyoid neck dissection in patients with oral squamous cell carcinoma and negative neck. Am J Surg 2006;191(1):94–9.
[31] Capote A, Escorial V, Munoz-Guerra MF, et al. Elective neck dissection in early-stage oral squamous cell carcinoma–does it influence recurrence and survival? Head Neck 2007;29(1):3–11.
[32] Ferlito A, Rinaldo A, Silver CE, et al. Elective and therapeutic selective neck dissection. Oral Oncol 2006;42(1):14–25.
[33] Hosal AS, Carrau RL, Johnson JT, et al. Selective neck dissection in the management of the clinically node-negative neck. Laryngoscope 2000;110(12):2037–40.
[34] Nahum AM, Mullally W, Marmor L. A syndrome resulting from radical neck dissection. Arch Otolaryngol 1961;74:424–8.
[35] Byers RM, Wolf PF, Ballantyne AJ. Rationale for elective modified neck dissection. Head Neck Surg 1988;10(3):160–7.
[36] Weiss MH, Harrison LB, Isaacs RS. Use of decision analysis in planning a management strategy for the stage N0 neck. Arch Otolaryngol Head Neck Surg 1994;120(7):699–702.
[37] Barkley HT Jr, Fletcher GH, Jesse RH, et al. Management of cervical lymph node metastases in squamous cell carcinoma of the tonsillar fossa, base of tongue, supraglottic larynx, and hypopharynx. Am J Surg 1972;124(4):462–7.
[38] Bocca E, Pignataro O, Oldini C, et al. Functional neck dissection: an evaluation and review of 843 cases. Laryngoscope 1984;94(7):942–5.
[39] Lee DJ, Koch WM, Yoo G, et al. Impact of chromosome 14q loss on survival in primary head and neck squamous cell carcinoma. Clin Cancer Res 1997;3(4):501–5.
[40] Levendag P, Vikram B. The problem of neck relapse in early stage supraglottic cancer–results of different treatment modalities for the clinically negative neck. Int J Radiat Oncol Biol Phys 1987;13(11):1621–4.
[41] Mendenhall WM, Million RR, Cassisi NJ. Elective neck irradiation in squamous-cell carcinoma of the head and neck. Head Neck Surg 1980;3(1):15–20.
[42] Ogura JH, Biller HF, Wette R. Elective neck dissection for pharyngeal and laryngeal cancers. An evaluation. Ann Otol Rhinol Laryngol 1971;80(5):646–50.
[43] Simes RJ, Coates AS. Patient preferences for adjuvant chemotherapy of early breast cancer: how much benefit is needed? J Natl Cancer Inst Monogr 2001;(30):146–52.
[44] Sweeney KJ, Ryan E, Canney M, et al. Justifying adjuvant chemotherapy in breast cancer: a survey of women and healthcare professionals. Eur J Surg Oncol 2007;33(7):838–42.
[45] Rogers SN, Scott B, Lowe D. An evaluation of the shoulder domain of the University of Washington quality of life scale. Br J Oral Maxillofac Surg 2007;45(1):5–10.
[46] Taylor RJ, Chepeha JC, Teknos TN, et al. Development and validation of the neck dissection impairment index: a quality of life measure. Arch Otolaryngol Head Neck Surg 2002;128(1):44–9.

[47] Terrell JE, Ronis DL, Fowler KE, et al. Clinical predictors of quality of life in patients with head and neck cancer. Arch Otolaryngol Head Neck Surg 2004;130(4):401–8.

[48] Terrell JE, Welsh DE, Bradford CR, et al. Pain, quality of life, and spinal accessory nerve status after neck dissection. Laryngoscope 2000;110(4): 620–6.

[49] Laverick S, Lowe D, Brown JS, et al. The impact of neck dissection on health-related quality of life. Arch Otolaryngol Head Neck Surg 2004;130(2): 149–54.

[50] Cheng PT, Hao SP, Lin YH, et al. Objective comparison of shoulder dysfunction after three neck dissection techniques. Ann Otol Rhinol Laryngol 2000;109(8 Pt 1):761–6.

[51] Bernier J, Domenge C, Ozsahin M, et al. Postoperative irradiation with or without concomitant chemotherapy for locally advanced head and neck cancer. N Engl J Med 2004;350(19):1945–52.

[52] Cooper JS, Pajak TF, Forastiere AA, et al. Postoperative concurrent radiotherapy and chemotherapy for high-risk squamous-cell carcinoma of the head and neck. N Engl J Med 2004;350(19): 1937–44.

[53] Andersen PE, Cambronero E, Shaha AR, et al. The extent of neck disease after regional failure during observation of the N0 neck. Am J Surg 1996; 172(6):689–91.

[54] Kligerman J, Lima RA, Soares JR, et al. Supraomohyoid neck dissection in the treatment of T1/T2 squamous cell carcinoma of oral cavity. Am J Surg 1994;168(5):391–4.

[55] Fakih AR, Rao RS, Borges AM, et al. Elective versus therapeutic neck dissection in early carcinoma of the oral tongue. Am J Surg 1989;158(4): 309–13.

[56] Woolgar JA, Rogers S, West CR, et al. Survival and patterns of recurrence in 200 oral cancer patients treated by radical surgery and neck dissection. Oral Oncol 1999;35(3):257–65.

[57] Greenberg JS, Fowler R, Gomez J, et al. Extent of extracapsular spread: a critical prognosticator in oral tongue cancer. Cancer 2003;97(6):1464–70.

[58] Kissun D, Magennis P, Lowe D, et al. Timing and presentation of recurrent oral and oropharyngeal squamous cell carcinoma and awareness in the outpatient clinic. Br J Oral Maxillofac Surg 2006; 44(5):371–6.

[59] Duvvuri U, Simental AA Jr, D'Angelo G, et al. Elective neck dissection and survival in patients with squamous cell carcinoma of the oral cavity and oropharynx. Laryngoscope 2004;114(12): 2228–34.

[60] Keski-Santti H, Atula T, Tornwall J, et al. Elective neck treatment versus observation in patients with T1/T2 N0 squamous cell carcinoma of oral tongue. Oral Oncol 2006;42(1):96–101.

[61] Lee JG, Krause CJ. Radical neck dissection: elective, therapeutic, and secondary. Arch Otolaryngol 1975;101(11):656–9.

[62] Layland MK, Sessions DG, Lenox J. The influence of lymph node metastasis in the treatment of squamous cell carcinoma of the oral cavity, oropharynx, larynx, and hypopharynx: N0 versus N+. Laryngoscope 2005;115(4):629–39.

[63] Nieuwenhuis EJ, Castelijns JA, Pijpers R, et al. Wait-and-see policy for the N0 neck in early-stage oral and oropharyngeal squamous cell carcinoma using ultrasonography-guided cytology: is there a role for identification of the sentinel node? Head Neck 2002;24(3):282–9.

[64] Umeda M, Yokoo S, Take Y, et al. Lymph node metastasis in squamous cell carcinoma of the oral cavity: correlation between histologic features and the prevalence of metastasis. Head Neck 1992; 14(4):263–72.

[65] Khafif RA, Gelbfish GA, Tepper P, et al. Elective radical neck dissection in epidermoid cancer of the head and neck. A retrospective analysis of 853 cases of mouth, pharynx, and larynx cancer. Cancer 1991;67(1):67–71.

[66] Castelijns JA, van den Brekel MW. Imaging of lymphadenopathy in the neck. Eur Radiol 2002; 12(4):727–38.

[67] van den Brekel MW, Castelijns JA. What the clinician wants to know: surgical perspective and ultrasound for lymph node imaging of the neck. Cancer Imaging 2005;5(Spec No A):S41–9.

[68] Woolgar JA, Vaughan ED, Scott J, et al. Pathological findings in clinically false-negative and false-positive neck dissections for oral carcinoma. Ann R Coll Surg Engl 1994;76(4):237–44.

[69] Schoder H, Carlson DL, Kraus DH, et al. 18F-FDG PET/CT for detecting nodal metastases in patients with oral cancer staged N0 by clinical examination and CT/MRI. J Nucl Med 2006; 47(5):755–62.

[70] Adams S, Baum RP, Stuckensen T, et al. Prospective comparison of 18F-FDG PET with conventional imaging modalities (CT, MRI, US) in lymph node staging of head and neck cancer. Eur J Nucl Med 1998;25(9):1255–60.

[71] Di Martino E, Nowak B, Hassan HA, et al. Diagnosis and staging of head and neck cancer: a comparison of modern imaging modalities (positron emission tomography, computed tomography, color-coded duplex sonography) with panendoscopic and histopathologic findings. Arch Otolaryngol Head Neck Surg 2000;126(12):1457–61.

[72] Hannah A, Scott AM, Tochon-Danguy H, et al. Evaluation of 18 F-fluorodeoxyglucose positron emission tomography and computed tomography with histopathologic correlation in the initial staging of head and neck cancer. Ann Surg 2002; 236(2):208–17.

[73] Ng SH, Yen TC, Liao CT, et al. 18F-FDG PET and CT/MRI in oral cavity squamous cell carcinoma: a prospective study of 124 patients with histologic correlation. J Nucl Med 2005;46(7):1136–43.

[74] van den Brekel MW, Castelijns JA, Reitsma LC, et al. Outcome of observing the N0 neck using ultrasonographic-guided cytology for follow-up. Arch Otolaryngol Head Neck Surg 1999;125(2): 153–6.

[75] van den Brekel MW, Castelijns JA, Stel HV, et al. Occult metastatic neck disease: detection with US and US-guided fine-needle aspiration cytology. Radiology 1991;180(2):457–61.

[76] van den Brekel MW, Stel HV, Castelijns JA, et al. Lymph node staging in patients with clinically negative neck examinations by ultrasound and ultrasound-guided aspiration cytology. Am J Surg 1991;162(4):362–6.

[77] Takes RP, Knegt P, Manni JJ, et al. Regional metastasis in head and neck squamous cell carcinoma: revised value of US with US-guided FNAB. Radiology 1996;198(3):819–23.

[78] Nahmias C, Carlson ER, Duncan LD, et al. Positron emission tomography/computerized tomography (PET/CT) scanning for preoperative staging of patients with oral/head and neck cancer. J Oral Maxillofac Surg 2007;65(12):2524–35.

[79] Greene FL, Page DL, Fleming ID, editors. AJCC cancer staging manual. 6th edition. New York: Springer-Verlag; 2002.

[80] Po Wing Yuen A, Lam KY, Lam LK, et al. Prognostic factors of clinically stage I and II oral tongue carcinoma—a comparative study of stage, thickness, shape, growth pattern, invasive front malignancy grading, Martinez-Gimeno score, and pathologic features. Head Neck 2002;24(6):513–20.

[81] van den Brekel MW, van der Waal I, Meijer CJ, et al. The incidence of micrometastases in neck dissection specimens obtained from elective neck dissections. Laryngoscope 1996;106(8):987–91.

[82] Woolgar JA. Micrometastasis in oral/oropharyngeal squamous cell carcinoma: incidence, histopathological features and clinical implications. Br J Oral Maxillofac Surg 1999;37(3):181–6.

[83] Shah JP, Patel SG, Shah JPH. Chapter 6: Oral and Oropharynx, Chapter 9: Cervical Lymph Nodes. In: Shah JP, Patel SG, editors. Head and neck surgery and oncology. 3rd edition. Edinburgh (UK): Mosby; 2003. p. 179, 356.

[84] Diaz EM Jr, Holsinger FC, Zuniga ER, et al. Squamous cell carcinoma of the buccal mucosa: one institution's experience with 119 previously untreated patients. Head Neck 2003;25(4):267–73.

[85] Sieczka E, Datta R, Singh A, et al. Cancer of the buccal mucosa: are margins and T-stage accurate predictors of local control? Am J Otolaryngol 2001;22(6):395–9.

[86] Simental AA Jr, Johnson JT, Myers EN. Cervical metastasis from squamous cell carcinoma of the maxillary alveolus and hard palate. Laryngoscope 2006;116(9):1682–4.

[87] Fernandes R, Lee J, Goldman N, et al. Cervical metastasis from maxillary alveolar squamous cell carcinoma. Oral Oncology Supplement 2007;2(1):130.

[88] Montes DM, Schmidt BL. Oral maxillary squamous carcinoma: management of the clinically negative neck. J Oral Maxillofac Surg 2008;66(4): 762–6.

[89] Broders AC. Carcinoma of the mouth: types and degrees of malignancy. American Journal of Roentgenology and Radium Therapy 1927;17:90–3.

[90] Broders AC. The microscopic grading of cancer. Surg Clin North Am 1941;21:947–62.

[91] Broders AC. Squamous cell epithelioma of the lip; a study of five hundred and thirty-seven cases. JAMA 1920;74:656–64.

[92] Anneroth G, Batsakis J, Luna M. Review of the literature and a recommended system of malignancy grading in oral squamous cell carcinomas. Scand J Dent Res 1987;95(3):229–49.

[93] Bryne M, Koppang HS, Lilleng R, et al. Malignancy grading of the deep invasive margins of oral squamous cell carcinomas has high prognostic value. J Pathol 1992;166(4):375–81.

[94] Bryne M, Koppang HS, Lilleng R, et al. New malignancy grading is a better prognostic indicator than Broders' grading in oral squamous cell carcinomas. J Oral Pathol Med 1989;18(8):432–7.

[95] Jakobsson PA, Eneroth CM, Killander D, et al. Histologic classification and grading of malignancy in carcinoma of the larynx. Acta Radiol Ther Phys Biol 1973;12(1):1–8.

[96] Martinez-Gimeno C, Rodriguez EM, Vila CN, et al. Squamous cell carcinoma of the oral cavity: a clinicopathologic scoring system for evaluating risk of cervical lymph node metastasis. Laryngoscope 1995;105(7 Pt 1):728–33.

[97] Odell EW, Jani P, Sherriff M, et al. The prognostic value of individual histologic grading parameters in small lingual squamous cell carcinomas. The importance of the pattern of invasion. Cancer 1994;74(3):789–94.

[98] Shintani S, Matsuura H, Hasegawa Y, et al. The relationship of shape of tumor invasion to depth of invasion and cervical lymph node metastasis in squamous cell carcinoma of the tongue. Oncology 1997;54(6):463–7.

[99] Woolgar JA, Scott J. Prediction of cervical lymph node metastasis in squamous cell carcinoma of the tongue/floor of mouth. Head Neck 1995; 17(6):463–72.

[100] Yuen AP, Lam KY, Wei WI, et al. A comparison of the prognostic significance of tumor diameter, length, width, thickness, area, volume, and clinicopathological features of oral tongue carcinoma. Am J Surg 2000;180(2):139–43.

[101] Woolgar JA, Beirne JC, Vaughan ED, et al. Correlation of histopathologic findings with clinical and

radiologic assessments of cervical lymph-node metastases in oral cancer. Int J Oral Maxillofac Surg 1995;24(1 Pt 1):30–7.
[102] Kademani D, Bell RB, Bagheri S, et al. Prognostic factors in intraoral squamous cell carcinoma: the influence of histologic grade. J Oral Maxillofac Surg 2005;63(11):1599–605.
[103] Warburton G, Nikitakis NG, Roberson P, et al. Histopathological and lymphangiogenic parameters in relation to lymph node metastasis in early stage oral squamous cell carcinoma. J Oral Maxillofac Surg 2007;65(3):475–84.
[104] Jones KR, Lodge-Rigal RD, Reddick RL, et al. Prognostic factors in the recurrence of stage I and II squamous cell cancer of the oral cavity. Arch Otolaryngol Head Neck Surg 1992;118(5):483–5.
[105] O'Brien CJ, Lauer CS, Fredricks S, et al. Tumor thickness influences prognosis of T1 and T2 oral cavity cancer—but what thickness? Head Neck 2003;25(11):937–45.
[106] Sheahan P, Colreavy M, Toner M, et al. Facial node involvement in head and neck cancer. Head Neck 2004;26(6):531–6.
[107] Spiro RH, Huvos AG, Wong GY, et al. Predictive value of tumor thickness in squamous carcinoma confined to the tongue and floor of the mouth. Am J Surg 1986;152(4):345–50.
[108] Mohit-Tabatabai MA, Sobel HJ, Rush BF, et al. Relation of thickness of floor of mouth stage I and II cancers to regional metastasis. Am J Surg 1986;152(4):351–3.
[109] Califano J, van der Riet P, Westra W, et al. Genetic progression model for head and neck cancer: implications for field cancerization. Cancer Res 1996;56(11):2488–92.
[110] Bova RJ, Quinn DI, Nankervis JS, et al. Cyclin D1 and p16INK4A expression predict reduced survival in carcinoma of the anterior tongue. Clin Cancer Res 1999;5(10):2810–9.
[111] Kastan MB, Onyekwere O, Sidransky D, et al. Participation of p53 protein in the cellular response to DNA damage. Cancer Res 1991;51(23 Pt 1):6304–11.
[112] Kawano K, Yanagisawa S. Predictive value of laminin-5 and membrane type 1-matrix metalloproteinase expression for cervical lymph node metastasis in T1 and T2 squamous cell carcinomas of the tongue and floor of the mouth. Head Neck 2006;28(6):525–33.
[113] Keum KC, Chung EJ, Koom WS, et al. Predictive value of p53 and PCNA expression for occult neck metastases in patients with clinically node-negative oral tongue cancer. Otolaryngol Head Neck Surg 2006;135(6):858–64.
[114] Mineta H, Miura K, Takebayashi S, et al. Cyclin D1 overexpression correlates with poor prognosis in patients with tongue squamous cell carcinoma. Oral Oncol 2000;36(2):194–8.

[115] Nakayama S, Sasaki A, Mese H, et al. Establishment of high and low metastasis cell lines derived from a human tongue squamous cell carcinoma. Invasion Metastasis 1998;18(5–6):219–28.
[116] Rubin Grandis J, Melhem MF, Barnes EL, et al. Quantitative immunohistochemical analysis of transforming growth factor-alpha and epidermal growth factor receptor in patients with squamous cell carcinoma of the head and neck. Cancer 1996;78(6):1284–92.
[117] Rubin Grandis J, Melhem MF, Gooding WE, et al. Levels of TGF-alpha and EGFR protein in head and neck squamous cell carcinoma and patient survival. J Natl Cancer Inst 1998;90(11):824–32.
[118] Schipper JH, Unger A, Jahnke K. E-cadherin as a functional marker of the differentiation and invasiveness of squamous cell carcinoma of the head and neck. Clin Otolaryngol Allied Sci 1994;19(5):381–4.
[119] Tanaka N, Odajima T, Ogi K, et al. Expression of E-cadherin, alpha-catenin, and beta-catenin in the process of lymph node metastasis in oral squamous cell carcinoma. Br J Cancer 2003;89(3):557–63.
[120] Yin Y, Tainsky MA, Bischoff FZ, et al. Wild-type p53 restores cell cycle control and inhibits gene amplification in cells with mutant p53 alleles. Cell 1992;70(6):937–48.
[121] Chung CH, Parker JS, Karaca G, et al. Molecular classification of head and neck squamous cell carcinomas using patterns of gene expression. Cancer Cell 2004;5(5):489–500.
[122] Pinkel D, Albertson DG. Array comparative genomic hybridization and its applications in cancer. Nat Genet 2005;37(Suppl):S11–7.
[123] Snijders AM, Schmidt BL, Fridlyand J, et al. Rare amplicons implicate frequent deregulation of cell fate specification pathways in oral squamous cell carcinoma. Oncogene 2005;24(26):4232–42.
[124] Menzin J, Lines LM, Manning LN. The economics of squamous cell carcinoma of the head and neck. Curr Opin Otolaryngol Head Neck Surg 2007;15(2):68–73.
[125] Speight PM, Palmer S, Moles DR, et al. The cost-effectiveness of screening for oral cancer in primary care. Health Technol Assess 2006;10(14):1–144, iii–iv.
[126] Lang K, Menzin J, Earle CC, et al. The economic cost of squamous cell cancer of the head and neck: findings from linked SEER-Medicare data. Arch Otolaryngol Head Neck Surg 2004;130(11):1269–75.
[127] Braaksma M, van Agthoven M, Nijdam W, et al. Costs of treatment intensification for head and neck cancer: concomitant chemoradiation randomised for radioprotection with amifostine. Eur J Cancer 2005;41(14):2102–11.
[128] Wolfensberger M, Zbaeren P, Dulguerov P, et al. Surgical treatment of early oral carcinoma-results

[129] Robertson AG, Soutar DS, Paul J, et al. Early closure of a randomized trial: surgery and postoperative radiotherapy versus radiotherapy in the management of intra-oral tumours. Clin Oncol (R Coll Radiol) 1998;10(3):155–60.

[130] Rowell NP. Radiotherapy in the management of orofacial cancer. In: Ward Booth P, Schendel SA, Hausamen J-E, editors. . 2nd editionMaxillofacial surgery, vol 1St. Louis (MO): Churchill Livingstone; 2007. p. 331–51.

[131] Denham JW, Peters LJ, Johansen J, et al. Do acute mucosal reactions lead to consequential late reactions in patients with head and neck cancer? Radiother Oncol 1999;52(2):157–64.

[132] Pauloski BR, Rademaker AW, Logemann JA, et al. Speech and swallowing in irradiated and nonirradiated postsurgical oral cancer patients. Otolaryngol Head Neck Surg 1998;118(5):616–24.

[133] Leon X, Quer M, Diez S, et al. Second neoplasm in patients with head and neck cancer. Head Neck 1999;21(3):204–10.

[134] Greenberg JS, El Naggar AK, Mo V, et al. Disparity in pathologic and clinical lymph node staging in oral tongue carcinoma. Implication for therapeutic decision making. Cancer 2003;98(3):508–15.

[135] Henick DH, Silver CE, Heller KS, et al. Supraomohyoid neck dissection as a staging procedure for squamous cell carcinomas of the oral cavity and oropharynx. Head Neck 1995;17(2):119–23.

[136] Crile G III. On the technique of operations upon the head and neck. Ann Surg 1906;44(6):842–50.

[137] Robbins KT, Clayman G, Levine PA, et al. Neck dissection classification update: revisions proposed by the American Head and Neck Society and the American Academy of Otolaryngology-Head and Neck Surgery. Arch Otolaryngol Head Neck Surg 2002;128(7):751–8.

[138] Davidson BJ, Kulkarny V, Delacure MD, et al. Posterior triangle metastases of squamous cell carcinoma of the upper aerodigestive tract. Am J Surg 1993;166(4):395–8.

[139] Dias FL, Lima RA, Kligerman J, et al. Relevance of skip metastases for squamous cell carcinoma of the oral tongue and the floor of the mouth. Otolaryngol Head Neck Surg 2006;134(3):460–5.

[140] Lindberg R. Distribution of cervical lymph node metastases from squamous cell carcinoma of the upper respiratory and digestive tracts. Cancer 1972;29(6):1446–9.

[141] Skolnik EM, Yee KF, Friedman M, et al. The posterior triangle in radical neck surgery. Arch Otolaryngol 1976;102(1):1–4.

[142] Mira E, Benazzo M, Rossi V, et al. Efficacy of selective lymph node dissection in clinically negative neck. Otolaryngol Head Neck Surg 2002;127(4):279–83.

[143] Results of a prospective trial on elective modified radical classical versus supraomohyoid neck dissection in the management of oral squamous carcinoma. Brazilian Head and Neck Cancer Study Group. Am J Surg 1998;176(5):422–7.

[144] Silverman DA, El-Hajj M, Strome S, et al. Prevalence of nodal metastases in the submuscular recess (level IIb) during selective neck dissection. Arch Otolaryngol Head Neck Surg 2003;129(7):724–8.

[145] Elsheikh MN, Mahfouz ME, Elsheikh E. Level IIb lymph nodes metastasis in elective supraomohyoid neck dissection for oral cavity squamous cell carcinoma: a molecular-based study. Laryngoscope 2005;115(9):1636–40.

[146] Lim YC, Song MH, Kim SC, et al. Preserving level IIb lymph nodes in elective supraomohyoid neck dissection for oral cavity squamous cell carcinoma. Arch Otolaryngol Head Neck Surg 2004;130(9):1088–91.

[147] Byers RM, Weber RS, Andrews T, et al. Frequency and therapeutic implications of "skip metastases" in the neck from squamous carcinoma of the oral tongue. Head Neck 1997;19(1):14–9.

[148] Mizen KD, Mitchell DA. Anatomical variability of omohyoid and its relevance in oropharyngeal cancer. Br J Oral Maxillofac Surg 2005;43(4):285–8.

[149] Stoeckli SJ. Sentinel node biopsy for oral and oropharyngeal squamous cell carcinoma of the head and neck. Laryngoscope 2007; Publish Ahead of Print.

[150] Krag DN, Weaver DL, Alex JC, et al. Surgical resection and radiolocalization of the sentinel lymph node in breast cancer using a gamma probe. Surg Oncol 1993;2(6):335–9 [discussion: 340].

[151] Morton DL, Wen DR, Wong JH, et al. Technical details of intraoperative lymphatic mapping for early stage melanoma. Arch Surg 1992;127(4):392–9.

[152] Ross GL, Soutar DS, Gordon MacDonald D, et al. Sentinel node biopsy in head and neck cancer: preliminary results of a multicenter trial. Ann Surg Oncol 2004;11(7):690–6.

[153] Shahnavaz SA, Regezi JA, Bradley G, et al. p53 gene mutations in sequential oral epithelial dysplasias and squamous cell carcinomas. J Pathol 2000;190(4):417–22.

[154] Saunders ME, MacKenzie R, Shipman R, et al. Patterns of p53 gene mutations in head and neck cancer: full-length gene sequencing and results of primary radiotherapy. Clin Cancer Res 1999;5(9):2455–63.

[155] Juarez J, Clayman G, Nakajima M, et al. Role and regulation of expression of 92-kDa type-IV collagenase (MMP-9) in 2 invasive squamous-cell-carcinoma cell lines of the oral cavity. Int J Cancer 1993;55(1):10–8.

[156] Riedel F, Gotte K, Schwalb J, et al. Expression of 92-kDa type IV collagenase correlates with angiogenic markers and poor survival in head and neck squamous cell carcinoma. Int J Oncol 2000;17(6): 1099–105.

[157] Impola U, Uitto VJ, Hietanen J, et al. Differential expression of matrilysin-1 (MMP-7), 92 kD gelatinase (MMP-9), and metalloelastase (MMP-12) in oral verrucous and squamous cell cancer. J Pathol 2004;202(1):14–22.

[158] Nozaki S, Endo Y, Kawashiri S, et al. Immunohistochemical localization of a urokinase-type plasminogen activator system in squamous cell carcinoma of the oral cavity: association with mode of invasion and lymph node metastasis. Oral Oncol 1998;34(1):58–62.

[159] Clayman G, Wang SW, Nicolson GL, et al. Regulation of urokinase-type plasminogen activator expression in squamous-cell carcinoma of the oral cavity. Int J Cancer 1993;54(1):73–80.

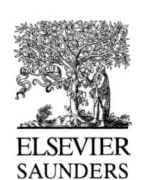

Management of the Node-Positive Neck in Oral Cancer

Dimitrios Nikolarakos, BDSc, MBBS, FRACDS(OMS)[a],
R. Bryan Bell, DDS, MD, FACS[a,b,*]

[a]*Oral and Maxillofacial Surgery Service, Legacy Emanuel Hospital and Health Center, 2801 N. Gantenbein Avenue, Portland, OR 97227, USA*
[b]*Department of Oral and Maxillofacial Surgery, Oregon Health & Science University, 611 S.W. Campus Drive, Portland, OR 97201, USA*

It has long been established that cancer of the upper aerodigestive tract metastasizes to the regional lymphatics of the neck. The presence of such lymphatic metastasis is one of the most important negative prognostic indicators, conferring approximately a 50% reduction in cure rates compared with those obtainable if such metastases are not present [1–5]. The treatment of patients with clinical or radiographic evidence of cervical metastasis has traditionally been surgical. More recently, this has been extended to include roles for adjuvant radiotherapy and chemoradiotherapy. In the treatment of some oropharyngeal tumors, chemoradiotherapy is used primarily with surgery reserved for salvage of regional failure.

Surgical therapy

Neck dissection classification

Robbins and colleagues [6] outlined the conceptual guidelines for neck dissection classification:

- The radical neck dissection (RND) is the standard procedure for the comprehensive removal of at-risk lymph node groups (levels I–V) and all other procedures represent alterations to this procedure.
- When the alteration involves preservation of one or more nonlymphatic structures routinely removed in the RND, the procedure is termed modified RND (MRND). This remains a comprehensive form of neck dissection.
- When the alteration involves preservation of one or more lymph node levels routinely removed in the RND, the procedure is termed selective neck dissection (SND). This is therefore a less than comprehensive form of neck dissection.
- When the alteration involves removal of additional lymph node groups or nonlymphatic structures relative to the RND, the procedure is termed extended neck dissection.

Comprehensive neck dissections

If modern oncologic principles are to be followed, the safest surgical procedure for management of cervical lymph node metastasis from oral cancer is the removal of the diseased nodal group and the comprehensive clearance of all remaining lymphatics on the affected side of the neck (ie, levels I through V).

Radical neck dissection

The first cervical lymphadinectomy procedure was described in Europe as early as 1888 [7]. The procedure was popularized by Crile [8] in a 1906 publication, when it was first termed the RND. The RND involves the *en bloc* removal of all five lateral lymph node levels along with the removal of the sternocleidomastoid muscle (SCM), the internal jugular vein (IJV), and the spinal accessory nerve (SAN). Bears and Martin helped to further establish the procedure and widen its use in the 1950s. The RND became the most extensively used surgical procedure through the

---

Received from: Oral and Maxillofacial Surgery Service, Legacy Emanuel Hospital and Health Center, Portland, Oregon.

* Corresponding author. 1849 NW Kearney, Suite 300, Portland, OR 97209
 E-mail address: bellb@hsna1.com (R.B. Bell).

1950s and into the 1960s for cervical metastases, and was shown to confer a survival benefit. It is still considered the gold standard by which all other interventions are measured.

Modified radical neck dissection

The cosmetic deformity and significant shoulder disability associated with the removal of the SCM, IJV, and SAN [9] prompted Suárez [10,11], Bocca and Pignataro [12] to introduce modifications to the RND. The rationale for these modifications is that the fibrofatty lymph node–containing tissues lie within fascial layers that invest these structures. The dissection can be maintained within these planes, essentially skeletonizing the SCM, IJV, and SAN, thus not violating the oncologic principal of comprehensive *en bloc* lymphadenectomy. Each of these structures can be preserved if they are not directly involved by tumor.

The work of Bocca and colleagues [13] and Byers [14] established that the MRND is as effective as the RND in the treatment of cervical metastasis and this has become the accepted standard for the treatment of all but the bulkiest neck disease that directly involves the SCM, IJV, and SAN [15].

There are many classifications of modified neck dissection. Each of the three simplest preserves one, two, or all three nonlymphatic structures. Type I MRND preserves the SAN; type II MRND preserves the SAN and IJ; and type III MRND preserves the SAN, IJV, and SCM.

Selective neck dissection (less than comprehensive)

To further ameliorate the morbidity of therapeutic neck dissection, surgeons have introduced an even more conservative approach, which is aimed at removing only the affected lymph nodes along with the nodal groups at most risk of also containing micrometastsis. SND was discussed as early as the 1960s [15]. It has been extensively investigated for the management of the clinically negative neck (N0) in oral cancer and has become the standard of care in this setting. The application of this therapy in the management of clinically evident cervical metastasis (node-positive or N+ neck) is far more controversial. The SND contravenes the oncologic principal of *en bloc* lymphadenectomy with the division of lymphatic channels and the retention of nodal groups that are potentially diseased by tumor cells.

The current understanding of the embolic nature of tumor metastasis, along with the extensive studies of the lymphatic drainage pathways and patterns of cervical metastatic spread, has given theoretic merit to the concept of a more selective neck dissection, even in the presence of clinically evident neck disease [2,4,16–18]. It is now well appreciated that oral cancer has a predilection for spread to levels I through III and rarely to level IV and V, in the absence of concurrent involvement of levels I through III [19–21]. Furthermore, in the presence of metastasis in levels I through III, the risk of disease in level IV increases from 3% to 17%, but the risk of level V involvement remains less than 3% [19]. It is logical, therefore, to conclude that it is safe to dissect only levels I through III in oral cancer with clinically N0 necks and levels I through IV if there is clinically evident nodal disease in levels I through II.

No prospective randomized controlled studies have been performed to test the efficacy of the SND compared with comprehensive types of neck dissection in the clinically N+ neck. All studies currently available are small retrospective case series with the expected lack of statistical power and potential for selection bias. They are further confounded by the range of protocols that exist for nodal levels to be dissected and administration of adjuvant radiotherapy. It is unlikely that an appropriately prospective randomized study will ever be undertaken given the large number of patients that would be required to provide statistical significance.

In 1985, Byers [14] reviewed 967 cases that underwent modified neck dissection (including supraomohyoid neck dissection). When radiation therapy was administered to patients with a pathologically positive node larger than 3 cm, extracapsular disease or multiple involved nodes, the overall recurrence rate for the modified procedures were similar to that previously reported for RND. He concluded that supraomohyoid neck dissection (SOHND levels I–III) is adequate for early stage disease if postoperative radiotherapy is administered for ECS or if multiple levels are involved. Kowalski and Carvalho [22] analyzed 164 oral cavity cancer patients with clinically N1 and N2 necks who were submitted to therapeutic RND. The investigators found that 42.1% of these necks turned out to be pathologically N0. Of those clinically N1, 57.4% were actually pathologically N0. Only 1 patient with multiple positive nodes had a metastatic node in level IV while none had positive nodes in level V. These patients would therefore have been candidates for SOHND.

A 1989 series by Medina and Byers [23] included 114 patients who were clinically N+. Most were N1. Of these, only 79.8% actually had pathologic evidence of metastasis. SND alone had a neck recurrence rate of 10% in the pathologically N1 necks without ECS and 24% if multiple nodes or ECS was present. Postoperative radiotherapy reduced this to 15%.

Chepeha and colleagues [24] analyzed a group of 52 patients undergoing 58 SNDs. Twenty-six were clinically N0 and 26 were clinically N+. Postoperative radiation was administered if more than two nodes were found involved on pathologic examination, if ECS was present, or if the primary was staged as T3/4. The neck recurrence rate was 6% and was considered comparable to the recurrence rate reported in the literature for MRND with similar indications for radiotherapy. Two of the 6 patients with neck recurrences had those recurrences outside the dissected field. In a similar study, Traynor and colleagues [25] reviewed 29 patients who had 36 SNDs for clinically and pathologically N+ (N1 to N2c). Twenty patients underwent postoperative radiotherapy for similar indications. The 4-year regional failure rate was 4%. No recurrences occurred outside the dissected field.

In a 1996 study, Ambrosch and colleagues [26] reported on 167 patients who underwent SND. They found a neck recurrence rate of 6.6% for patients with pathologically N+ necks. More recently, the same group reported on SND for clinically N0 and pathologically N+ in 503 patients. The 3-year neck recurrence rates were 4.7% pathologically N0, 4.9% for pathologically N1, and 12.1% for pathologically N2. Postoperative radiotherapy trended to improve the recurrence rate in N1 and definitely improved the recurrence rate in patients with multiple positive nodes or those with ECS [27].

Pelliteri and colleagues [28] reported on a review of 82 patients undergoing 94 SNDs for clinically N0 to N3 disease using similar indications for postoperative radiotherapy. The recurrence rate for pathologically N2 and above was 11.5% despite the presence of ECS. In addition, this recurrence rate was not statistically different to that found in the N1 cohort (12.5%).

In a 2002 multi-institution study, Anderson and colleagues [29] reviewed 129 patients with both clinically and pathologically positive necks (N1 to N2c). All underwent SND and postoperative radiotherapy was administered for histologic evidence of multiple levels of nodal involvement or the presence of ECS. ECS was found in 34% of patients and was correlated with recurrence in the neck (2.4% if no evidence of ECS versus 21.9% if ECS was present) and 5-year disease-specific survival (75.3% versus 55.8% respectively). The overall regional control rate was 94.3%. All ipsilateral recurrences occurred within the field of dissection (none outside the expected drainage pathway and none in level V). The investigators recommended that SND was appropriate in selected patients with N1 and N2 disease. They recommended comprehensive neck dissection in the presence of massive adenopathy, evidence of nodal fixation, or obvious ECS, a history of neck surgery, and radiotherapy. In addition, the surgeon should be prepared to alter the plan for unexpected findings, such as involvement of IJV, SCM, and SAN, and if suspicious nodes are encountered in lower levels.

Controversy also exists over the appropriate extent of SND. Byers and colleagues [30] found that 15% of patients with oral tongue cancer presented with only level III or IV disease. This was confirmed by Woolgar [31], who found the incidence of skip metastasis to level IV to be 10%. Shah [1] found a 15% incidence of positive nodes in level IV in clinically positive necks treated with MRND. As SND limited to levels I through III may not remove these nodes, leading to inadequate staging and perhaps undertreatment if the indications for radiotherapy are based on the number of nodes found to be diseased. Based on this data, dissection of levels I to IV would be most appropriate for management of the N+ neck in oral cancer.

Furthermore the role of postoperative radiotherapy, especially when only one pathologic node is detected (N1), is unclear. There is no consistent interinstitutional protocol for the use of radiotherapy in the pathologically N1 neck.

Byers and colleagues [32] analyzed 363 patients who underwent SND for necks that were clinically N0, N1, N2a, or N2b. The recurrence rate reported was 35.7% in the N1 necks not treated with postoperative radiotherapy. This was reduced to 5.6% when radiotherapy was undertaken. The recurrence rate for N2b necks dropped from 14% to 8.3% with radiotherapy. They concluded than the SOHND in conjunction with postoperative radiotherapy is highly effective in controlling neck metastasis in patients with limited disease in the neck.

In a retrospective study of 176 patients, Muzaffar [33] found no statistical difference in the incidence of recurrence and disease-free survival between matched cohorts with pathologically N+ necks treated with SND, MRND, and RND. All patients had postoperative radiotherapy. Spiro and colleagues [34] reported on 296 SOHNDs performed for clinically N0 and N1 disease. All underwent postoperative radiotherapy. Of the pathologically N0 necks, 5% failed in the neck. Six percent of pathologically N+ necks failed. Only 1 recurrence occurred outside the dissected field. They also concluded that the SOHND in conjunction with postoperative radiotherapy was highly effective in controlling neck metastasis in patients with limited disease in the neck.

In a 2005 study, Schiff and colleagues [35] investigated the effectiveness of SND versus MRND in 220 patients with squamous cell carcinoma of the oral tongue. They found no significant difference in the neck recurrence rate between the two procedures. There was, however, selection bias in that there was a much larger tumor burden in the final pathology of those patients selected for MRND (78.9% pathologically N2b or greater) compared with those selected for SND (40% N2b or greater). Of the cohort with N2 or greater disease, 4 of 16 SND had regional failure while none of 14 MRND had recurrence. They were otherwise matched for ECS and radiotherapy. The investigators suggest that while SND may be effective treatment for many N+ necks, more aggressive surgery and adjunctive therapies may be required for significant tumor burden. In addition to this, they found that, of the N1 cohort (50 patients), 2 of 25 that did not have radiotherapy had regional failure while none of the 25 that did have radiotherapy failed. They concluded that all N+ necks should receive radiotherapy.

ECS is a significant negative prognostic indicator associated with increased local recurrence rate and decreased disease-free survival. The incidence of ECS increases to 75% in positive nodes larger than 3 cm [36–38]. With the paucity of data available regarding the use of SND in nodes larger than 3 cm in mind, most investigators continue to support the role of MRND over SND in the treatment of bulky nodal disease.

Recent quality-of-life studies have confirmed the improvement in shoulder function and postoperative pain with the more conservative types of neck dissection, which is ultimately the motivation for the drive toward the use of SND over the comprehensive forms of neck dissection. While MRND is definitely an improvement over RND, patients undergoing MRND have been shown to have significantly worse shoulder function than those undergoing SND [39–41].

The body of evidence now available supports the use of SND for the management of N1 and N2 neck disease from oral squamous cell carcinoma and limited to one or two levels. Disease control is comparable to that achieved with comprehensive neck dissections with significantly reduced morbidity. The dissection should include levels I to IV to remove the most at-risk nodes. It is unnecessary to extend the dissection to level V because of the very low risk of metastasis to these nodes. Postoperative radiotherapy is strongly recommended for disease N2 and above if multiple levels are involved or if there is evidence of ECS. There is some evidence to support the use of adjuvant radiotherapy for isolated N1 disease, although more research is required to clarify this further.

SND is not recommended in the presence of massive adenopathy. Relative contraindications include nodal fixation, gross ECS, and a history of neck surgery and radiotherapy. The surgeon should be prepared to extend the neck dissection to include resection of nonlymphatic structures found to be invaded by tumor intraoperatively. This would include tumor adhesion to the IJV, SCM, or SAN.

Postoperative chemoradiotherapy for advanced-stage squamous cell carcinoma

Until recently, primary surgery of locally advanced head and neck squamous cell carcinoma was traditionally followed by postoperative radiotherapy alone. Despite such relatively aggressive bimodality treatment, this approach yielded loco-regional recurrence of 30%, distant metastasis of 25%, and 5-year survival rates of 40%. In 2004, the European Organization for Research and Treatment of Cancer (EORTC) and Radiation Therapy Oncology Group (RTOG) published the results of two randomized trials (EORTC trial #22,931 and RTOG trial #9501) that evaluated the role of concomitant chemotherapy-enhanced radiation therapy (CERT) in the postoperative setting for this group of patients [42,43]. Level I evidence was reached with the publication of the results of these two studies, which, except for the primary endpoints chosen and definition of high risk, had been designed similarly. Both trials demonstrated that, compared with postoperative radiation alone, adjuvant CERT was more efficacious in terms of loco-regional control and disease-free survival. However, there is some discordance between the trials in terms of overall survival in that the EORTC study revealed a highly significant difference in overall survival, whereas the RTOG trial showed only a marginal improvement. Both studies compared the addition of concomitant relatively high doses of cisplatin (100 mg/m^2 administered intravenously on days 1, 22, and 43) to radiotherapy versus radiotherapy alone given after surgery in patients with high-risk cancers of the oral cavity, oropharynx, larynx, or hypopharynx.

To clarify the differences between the RTOG and EORTC trials, a comparative analysis of the selection criteria, clinical and pathologic risk factors, and treatment outcomes was performed using data pooled from both studies [44]. Extracapsular extension (ECE) and/or microscopically involved surgical margins were the only risk factors for which the impact of CERT was significant in both trials. There was also a trend in favor of CERT in the group of patients who had stage III or IV disease, perineural infiltration, vascular embolisms, or clinically enlarged level IV or V lymph nodes secondary to tumors arising in the oral cavity or oropharynx. Patients who had two or more histopathologically involved lymph nodes without ECE as their only risk factor did not seem to benefit from the addition of chemotherapy in this analysis. Subject to the usual caveats of retrospective subgroup analysis, the data suggested that in locally advanced head and neck cancer, microscopically involved resection margins and ECS of tumor from neck nodes are the most significant prognostic factors for poor outcome. The addition of concomitant cisplatin to postoperative radiotherapy otherwise improved outcome in patients with one or both of these risk factors who were medically fit to receive chemotherapy.

It is clear that the addition of chemotherapy to radiotherapy exacts a cost of increased toxicity and potential long-term effects that may make this approach unfeasible for many patients. As toxic deaths can occur, patients must be properly selected for combined-modality treatment, be monitored closely, receive appropriate drug-dose reductions, and be provided with optimal supportive care. An additional meta-analysis published in 2007 pooled the evidence from four existing randomized trials [42,43,45,46] studying nearly 1000 patients. This meta-analysis also supported the addition of concomitant chemotherapy to postoperative radiotherapy for patients with resectable head and neck cancer considered at high risk for cancer recurrence [47]. Sizeable differences in acute severe adverse events with chemoradiotherapy compared with radiotherapy alone were observed in some studies (77% versus 34%, $P = .0001$). The most common grade-adverse events were mucositis or dysphagia, followed by various hematologic events and nausea and vomiting. Treatment-related deaths occurred in 1% to 2% of the patients.

With regards to the neck, the data support the use of postoperative chemoradiotherapy for the purpose of achieving better local-regional control and improving survival when compared with adjuvant radiotherapy alone. However, the data also suggest that patients with two or more positive lymph nodes as a solitary risk factor might benefit less from chemoradiotherapy, with the corollary that nodal burden as assessed by tumor-node-metastasis (TNM) stage might better identify patients benefiting from combined-modality therapy. Therefore, patients with solitary nodal disease (N1) may not benefit from the addition of chemotherapy, given the associated toxicity, if no additional adverse histopathologic features are present (ECE, positive resection margins, or perineural invasion).

Fig. 1 provides a treatment algorithm for the management of cervical metastasis from oral squamous cell carcinoma.

Management of the node-positive neck in organ preservation treatment regimens

To preserve organ function (eg, base of tongue, oropharynx, and larynx), concurrent chemoradiation has become routine as the primary treatment of some advanced-stage head and neck cancers. When chemotherapy is combined with radiotherapy to avoid surgery, it achieves comparable local control and overall survival compared with radical resection and postoperative radiotherapy without the considerable loss of quality of life, diminished oral function, and changes in facial appearance associated with this type of surgery [48–51].

Additional surgical management of the positive neck when chemoradiotherapy is used as the primary treatment modality is controversial. Experience with conventional single-modality radiotherapy yielded lower regional control rates of N2 and N3 neck disease than those for combined surgery and radiotherapy. Surgical salvage of recurrence was very difficult and rarely achieved.

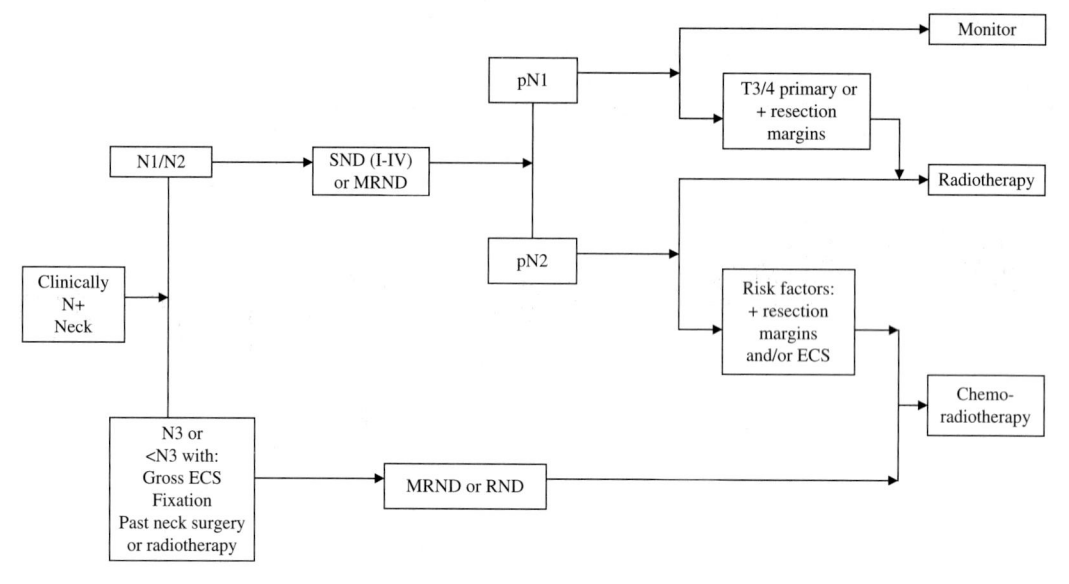

Fig. 1. Management of the clinically positive neck. pN, pathologic N stage.

These results were influential when guidelines were being developed for the management of advanced nodal disease when organ preservation protocols were introduced.

Generally, patients with initial N1 necks do not require neck dissection unless there is evidence of persistent disease after the chemoradiotherapy. Similarly, it is agreed that partial responders to the initial therapy based on clinical and radiological evidence of residual disease should proceed to neck dissection.

The options for N2 and N3 neck disease that has had a complete response to chemoradiotherapy are planned neck dissection (either pre- or postchemoradiotherapy) or a watch-and-wait policy with surgery reserved for salvage of recurrent neck disease.

Many cancer centers recommended neck dissection for all N2 and N3 disease post–organ-sparing therapy regardless of response. This was in part due to the fear of higher recurrence rates, borne out of the data on the use of radiotherapy alone for neck disease mentioned previously. Additionally, studies emerged that demonstrated a high rate of identifiable tumor cells in the lymph nodes removed during planned neck dissection in patients who had a complete clinical and radiological response to the initial therapy. No clinical parameters were identified that could reliably predict which of the complete clinical responders would have pathologically evident residual disease [7–13]. Furthermore, there is a small, but not an insignificant, rate of regional recurrence following apparent complete clinical response to chemoradiotherapy. Up to 65% of these patients are subsequently deemed not to be candidates for salvage surgery because of comorbidities or the presence of unresectable disease. Salvage surgery is also more difficult to perform because of extensive radiation-induced soft tissue changes and generally has a very poor prognosis [52–58].

The many interinstitutional variations in treatment protocols and limited numbers of patients treated in individual centers have resulted in a paucity of studies of sufficient quality and power to define the role of neck dissection in patients with bulky neck disease who have had a complete clinical response to chemoradiotherapy. There appears, however, to be a trend in the available research supporting a more conservative approach to this conundrum.

Whether neck dissection postchemoradiotherapy provides better regional control compared to chemoradiotherapy alone is debatable. Overall survival in these patients with N2 or N3 disease is similar regardless of the addition of neck dissection and reflects the high incidence of distant metastasis associated with such advanced disease [59,60].

Some patients who have undergone neck dissection following complete clinical response have been found to have residual nodal disease, but it is questionable whether the tumor detected is viable [58]. Despite this, the regional control rates for chemoradiotherapy alone seem comparable to those achieved with the addition of surgery.

Armstrong and colleagues [61] reported on a series of 54 patients with N+ cancer treated with induction chemotherapy followed by radiotherapy. Seventeen of 44 patients with complete clinical response did not proceed to planned neck dissection. Only 1 patient had a neck recurrence and the neck control rate in this cohort was 94%. Garden and colleagues [62] reported no neck recurrences in 27 patients who completely responded to chemoradiotherapy. Similarly, Robbins and colleagues [63] reported that 33 of 56 (59%) necks had complete response to chemoradiotherapy. There were no recurrences in the 17 of these that did not proceed to neck dissection. Interestingly, of the 16 complete responders who had neck dissections, none had residual disease, and, of the 18 partial responders, only 14 (78%) had pathologically positive nodal disease [63]. Corry and colleagues [64] reported on 25 complete responders who did not undergo neck dissection. None of these responders developed recurrence, supporting the watch-and-wait approach in these patients.

Stenson and colleagues [58] reported on 69 patients who had neck dissections after chemoradiotherapy. Thirty-five percent had pathologically residual disease that did not correlate with the clinical or radiographic response. Clayman and colleagues [65] found that 36% of 66 patients had complete response to chemoradiotherapy. These patients had better regional control than did partial responders. Of the partial responders, those who proceeded to neck dissection had improved regional control and overall survival than those who did not.

In 2004, Argiris and colleagues [59] reported on 131 patients with N2 or N3 neck disease treated with chemoradiotherapy. Ninety-two (70%) had a clinically complete response and 62 of these received a neck dissection. There was no significant difference in the regional recurrence rate between those complete responders who had a neck dissection and with those who did not. In the N3 group, regardless of response, there was a trend toward improved survival with neck dissection. The investigators concluded that there was benefit in neck dissection for patients with N3 disease but that planned neck dissection for patients achieving complete response to chemoradiotherapy conferred no additional benefit.

Brizel and colleagues [52] evaluated 108 patients with N2 or N3 disease and found a 4-year disease-free survival benefit ($P = .08$) for complete responders who underwent neck dissection. These investigators recommended routine planned neck dissection for all patients undergoing primary chemoradiotherapy.

The reported complication rates from a neck dissection after concurrent chemoradiotherapy ranged from 26% to 61%. The rate is highest in the first year postoperatively (77% compared with 20% after the first year) [66]. Mostly this reflects poor wound healing [53,66,67]. Such serious surgical morbidity is difficult to justify given the unproven benefits of neck dissection in patients who have had a complete response to chemoradiation.

The current standard of care is to recommend neck dissection for patients with N1 or N2 neck disease with only partial or no response following chemoradiotherapy. The literature presented above supports a watch-and-wait approach for those patients determined to have had a complete clinical response. Patients with N3 disease may have a survival benefit from planned neck dissection regardless of complete response to chemoradiotherapy.

Methods available to assess response include physical examination and diagnostic imaging. Physical evaluation is often inaccurate because of the presence of soft tissue fibrosis and scarring of the neck mass posttreatment. As discussed, neck dissections in patients with clinically complete response have detected residual tumor. Conversely, 55% of partial clinical responders have had negative necks pathologically [68].

CT, MRI, and ultrasound imaging modalities also have significant error rates [68]. False-positive rates for CT evaluation of nodal status have been reported in up to 57% of cases. MRI does not seem to add further diagnostic accuracy in predicting the presence of residual tumor [68–79]. Physiologic posttreatment imaging with positron emission tomography may become the most useful modality to detect the presence of viable residual disease. Sensitivity in detecting recurrent disease of 96% and negative predictive values of 83% to 91% have been reported [71–74]. The optimal standardized uptake value threshold has not been established to take into account the inflammatory changes caused by the chemoradiation. Similarly, the optimal timing of such a scan to ensure resolution of the inflammation and still allow for early detection of residual disease is yet to be determined. Currently, to assist in deciding whether to recommend a follow-up neck dissection, it is reasonable is to require a positron emission tomography scan for patients who have had a clinically complete response to chemoradiotherapy at 12 weeks posttreatment [75].

Fig. 2 provides a treatment algorithm for the management of cervical metastasis when organ preservation treatment is undertaken.

Carotid artery involvement

Involvement of the carotid artery by cervical metastasis from head and neck cancer imparts an extremely poor prognosis. Without treatment, the tumor invades the arterial wall, which can result in carotid rupture and fatal exsanguination. The patients often suffer from fistula formation and erosion into the pharynx or skin, all of which greatly impact on dignity and quality of life. Total removal of the tumor, including the involved carotid artery is likely to improve loco-regional control. Unfortunately, advanced tumors are associated with a higher incidence of distant metastasis, therefore limiting the impact of such aggressive treatment on disease-free survival.

Imaging criteria for carotid artery invasion have been defined as greater than 25% effacement of the circumference of the artery on CT or the loss of the fascial plane around the artery on T2-weighted MRI [76]. The cancer rarely invades the lumen of the artery. Scaring surrounding the artery from previous surgical or radiation therapy occasionally hinders the identification of tumor invasion radiographically.

Untreated carcinoma with cervical metastasis and direct carotid involvement should be treated with full-course radiation and chemotherapy. Often, the response is sufficient to eliminate the need to sacrifice the carotid artery and the vagus, hypoglossal, and sympathetic nerves [77].

The treatment options available for the management of persistent or recurrent neck disease with direct involvement of the carotid artery include supportive/palliative care, surgery, and chemotherapy. The surgical options are resection of the carotid artery with or without reconstruction or a surgical peel. The decision to proceed with carotid artery resection should be made during the treatment-planning phase to allow for appropriate informed consent and coordination of the surgical team.

Some investigators have argued that peeling cancer off the carotid violates oncologic principles because it leaves microscopic tumor adherent to the artery with 42% of resected arteries showing invasion of the arterial wall [78]. It provides only a very narrow margin of resection and is thought to weaken the arterial wall, predisposing to postoperative rupture [79]. It may, however, be necessary in the setting of unexpected involvement without preoperative workup, inability to reconstruct the artery due to deficient collateral cerebral

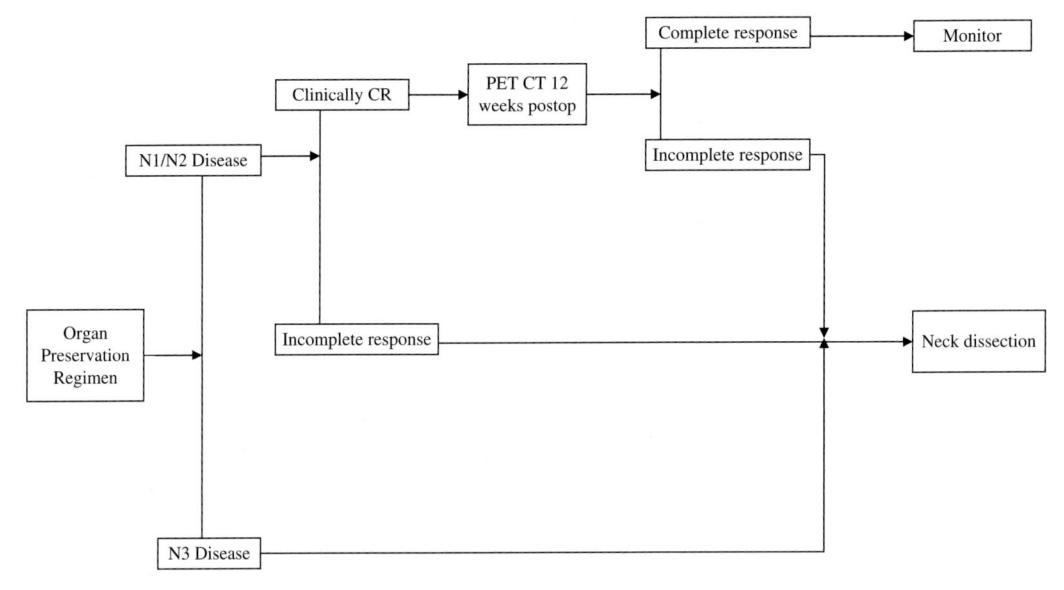

Fig. 2. Management of neck metastasis during organ preservation regimens. CR, complete response; PET, positron emission tomography.

circulation, and management of unresectable disease. The weakened artery should be covered with well-vascularized, nonirradiated tissue to prevent carotid blowout.

Carotid resection remains a controversial treatment option because of the risk of neurologic complications. Reports of the results of carotid resection were disappointing, with rates of neurologic complications (permanent hemiplegia, coma, and death) of about 30% [80,81]. Advances in cerebral perfusion studies and surgical techniques have resulted in a significant decrease in morbidity and mortality associated with the procedure. The preoperative assessment is aimed at predicting the patient's tolerance of interruption of carotid arterial flow.

Intraoperative measurement of the internal carotid artery stump pressure following temporary occlusion of the vessel provides the most accurate information on collateral cerebral blood flow. This can be combined with intraoperative measurement of somatosensory evoked potentials to detect alteration in brain function during the occlusion. Patients with stump systolic pressures below 50 mm Hg are at high risk of neurologic injury if the carotid artery is ligated and carotid reconstruction is indicated [82]. Pressures over 70 mm Hg are sufficient to allow safe ligation of the artery without adjunctive measures. Patients with pressures ranging from 50 to 70 mm Hg who undergo ligation benefit from postoperative heparinization [83].

Carotid backpressure can now be measured preoperatively, at the time of angiography, by using a balloon catheter to temporarily occlude the artery. This has been supplemented with cold xenon CT techniques, single photon emission CT (SPECT) studies, and positron emission tomographic studies conducted during the balloon occlusion test as quantitative measures of cerebral ischemia. deVries and colleagues [82] reported on 136 patients who underwent this evaluation, of which 22 had a favorable study and went on to have ligation of the carotid artery without complication.

Chazono and colleagues [84] reported on the occurrence of intraoperative cerebral infarctions in 2 of 12 patients despite favorable preoperative studies. This has led some investigators to recommend carotid artery reconstruction whenever possible, regardless of balloon occlusion test results. When reconstruction is not possible, preoperative permanent occlusion of the carotid artery while the patient is hemodynamically stable may be safer than intraoperative ligation. The internal carotid artery is occluded with radiologically guided placement of coils proximal to the ophthalmic branch 2 weeks before surgery, allowing for full heparinization, tight blood-pressure control, and fixation of the coils to the artery wall. If there is inadequate collateral cerebral circulation on preoperative assessment and reconstruction is technically not possible, then nonsurgical means of palliation should be chosen [72].

Carotid artery reconstruction with vein grafts following tumor resection was first reported by Conley [85] in 1953. Stoney and Wylie [86] reported on the use of arterial grafts for reconstruction in 1970. Lore and Boulos [87] described the currently used two-step procedure with bypass of the affected segment of carotid to allow tumor extirpation and limit the disruption to cerebral flow, followed by immediate reconstruction of the artery. When carcinoma involves the skull base, extracranial-intracranial carotid bypass surgery can be undertaken. This can be staged over two separate procedures to minimize the risk of ischemia caused by the temporary occlusion of the middle cerebral artery [88].

In a meta-analysis of the literature reporting outcomes of carotid reconstruction, Katsuno and colleagues [89] found that the rate of major neuromorbidity was 4.7% and of mortality was 6.8%. The combined major morbidity and mortality rate was 10.1%. The overall complication rate is 50% [77]. This, they felt, balanced favorably with the oncologic effectiveness of the procedure, with 2-year survival rates reported up to 35% [89]. Whether this translates to a long-term survival benefit is unclear, but advocates of this approach report that carotid resection provides improved regional control [81,90].

Carotid artery involvement by advanced cervical metastasis is associated with a very poor prognosis. In select cases, resection of the tumor along with the carotid artery is possible and may provide improvements in local control rates and quality of life but has not been shown to impart a survival benefit. The surgeon and patient must choose a treatment plan that best balances the significant and potentially devastating complications associated with carotid resection surgery against the natural progression of the disease if left untreated. When resection of the carotid artery is planned, interpositional grafting should be undertaken whenever possible to minimize neuromorbidity.

Summary

With more than 100 years of clinical experience, surgery continues to play a prominent role in the management of patients with loco-regionally advanced squamous cell carcinoma of the upper aerodigestive tract. The preponderance of evidence supports the use of comprehensive neck dissection for N+ disease. The literature also supports the use of modified radical neck dissection for all but the most bulky adenopathy (N3 disease) or in the radiated or operated neck. While there may never be level 1 data specifically comparing comprehensive versus selective neck dissection in the face of cervical metastasis, there is evolving evidence that SND clearing levels I through IV results in similar failure rates to those of modified RND in patients with N1 or N2 disease. The evidence for performing a less than comprehensive neck dissection in N3 patients is less compelling.

There is also reasonable evidence to suggest that planned neck dissection following definitive radiation therapy and chemoradiation therapy is unnecessary in the great majority of patients with N1 or N2 neck disease who exhibit a complete response. Once again, however, the evidence for less aggressive therapy (ie, observation following organ-preservation therapy) is much less compelling in patients with bulky adenopathy and many centers continue to advocate mandatory neck dissection following radiation or chemoradiation for N3 necks. The extent of the neck dissection in this setting remains controversial and, while the evidence certainly supports comprehensive neck dissection, there is growing enthusiasm for selective or even super-selective neck dissection for surgical salvage.

Finally, when cervical disease is so advanced as to involve the carotid artery, the current body of evidence continues to portend a dismal prognosis, regardless of the extent of neck dissection. Resection of carotid artery rarely impacts survival but may improve loco-regional control. The decision to resect the carotid artery as part of an extended radical neck dissection should be made judiciously.

References

[1] Shah JP. Patterns of cervical lymph node metastasis from squamous cell carcinomas of the upper aerodigestive tract. Am J Surg 1990;160(4):405–9.
[2] Shah JP, Medina JE, Shaha AR, et al. Cervical lymph node metastasis. Curr Probl Surg 1993; 30(3):1–335.
[3] Kowalski LP, Medina JP. Nodal metastases: predictive factors. Otolaryngol Clin North Am 1998;31(4): 621–37.
[4] Woolgar JA, Scott J, Vaughan ED, et al. Survival, metastasis, and recurrence of oral cancer in relation to pathological features. Ann R Coll Surg Engl 1995; 77(5):325–31.
[5] Layland MK, Sessions DG, Lenox J. The influence of lymph node metastasis in the treatment of squamous cell carcinoma of the oral cavity, oropharynx, larynx, and hypopharynx: N0 versus N+. Laryngoscope 2005;115(4):629–39.
[6] Robbins KT, Clayman G, Levine PA, et al. American Head and Neck Society; American Academy of Otolaryngology—Head and Neck Surgery. Neck dissection classification update: revisions proposed by the American Head and Neck Society and the American Academy of Otolaryngology—Head and Neck Surgery. Arch Otolaryngol Head Neck Surg 2002;128(7):751–8.
[7] Ferlito A, Johnson JT, Rinaldo A, et al. European surgeons were the first to perform neck dissection. Laryngoscope 2007;117(5):797–802.
[8] Crile G. Excision of cancer of the head and neck—with special reference to the plan of dissection based on one hundred and thirty-two operations. JAMA 1906;47:1780–6.
[9] Short SO, Kaplan JN, Laramore GE, et al. Shoulder pain and function after neck dissection with or without preservation of the spinal accessory nerve. Am J Surg 1984;148(4):478–82.
[10] Suárez O. El problema de las metastasis linfáticas y alejadas del cáncer de laringe e hipofaringe. Rev Otorrinolaringol 1963;23:83–99.
[11] Ferlito A, Rinaldo A. Osvaldo Suárez: often-forgotten father of functional neck dissection (in the non–Spanish-speaking literature). Laryngoscope 2004; 114(7):1177–8.
[12] Bocca E, Pignataro O. A conservative technique in radical neck dissection. Ann Otol Rhinol Laryngol 1967;76(5):975–87.
[13] Bocca E, Pignataro O, Oldini C, et al. Functional neck dissection: an evaluation and review of 843 cases. Laryngoscope 1984;94(7):942–5.
[14] Byers RM. Modified neck dissection. A study of 967 cases from 1970 to 1980. Am J Surg 1985;150(4): 414–21.
[15] Jesse RH, Ballantyne AJ, Larson D. Radical or modified neck dissection: a therapeutic dilemma. Am J Surg 1978;136(4):516–9.
[16] Rouvie're H. Lymphatic system of the head and neck. In: Tobias MJ, editor. Anatomy of the human lymphatic system. Ann Arbor (MI): Edwards Brothers; 1938. p. 5–28.
[17] Fisch UP, Sigel ME. Cervical lymphatic system as visualized by lymphography. Ann Otol Rhinol Laryngol 1964;73:870–82.
[18] Werner JA, Dünne AA, Myers JN. Functional anatomy of the lymphatic drainage system of the upper

aerodigestive tract and its role in metastasis of squamous cell carcinoma. Head Neck 2003;25(4): 322–32.
[19] Shah JP, Candela FC, Poddar AK. The patterns of cervical lymph node metastases from squamous carcinoma of the oral cavity. Cancer 1990;66(1):109–13.
[20] Davidson BJ, Kulkarny V, Delacure MD, et al. Posterior triangle metastases of squamous cell carcinoma of the upper aerodigestive tract. Am J Surg 1993;166(4):395–8.
[21] Lindberg R. Distribution of cervical lymph node metastases from squamous cell carcinoma of the upper respiratory and digestive tracts. Cancer 1972;29(6):1446–9.
[22] Kowalski LP, Carvalho AL. Feasibility of supraomohyoid neck dissection in N1 and N2a oral cancer patients. Head Neck 2002;24(10):921–4.
[23] Medina JE, Byers RM. Supraomohyoid neck dissection: rationale, indications and surgical technique. Head Neck Surg 1989;11(2):111–22.
[24] Chepeha DB, Hoff PT, Taylor RJ, et al. Selective neck dissection for the treatment of neck metastasis from squamous carcinoma of the head and neck. Laryngoscope 2002;112(3):434–8.
[25] Traynor SJ, Cohen JI, Gray J, et al. Selective neck dissection and the management of the node-positive neck. Am J Surg 1996;172(6):654–7.
[26] Ambrosch P, Freudenberg L, Kron M, et al. Selective neck dissection in the management of squamous cell carcinoma of the upper digestive tract. Eur Arch Otorhinolaryngol 1996;253(6):329–35.
[27] Ambrosch P, Kron M, Pradier O, et al. Efficacy of selective neck dissection: a review of 503 cases of elective and therapeutic treatment of the neck in squamous cell carcinoma of the upper aerodigestive tract. Otolaryngol Head Neck Surg 2001;124(2): 180–7.
[28] Pellitteri PK, Robbins KT, Neuman T. Expanded application of selective neck dissection with regard to nodal status. Head Neck 1997;19(4):260–5.
[29] Andersen PE, Warren F, Spiro J, et al. Results of selective neck dissection in the management of the node-positive neck. Arch Otolaryngol Head Neck Surg 2002;128(10):1180–4.
[30] Byers RM, Weber RS, Andrews T, et al. Frequency and therapeutic implications of "skip metastasis" in the neck from squamous cell carcinoma of the oral tongue. Head Neck 1997;19(1):14–9.
[31] Woolgar JA. The topography of cervical lymph node metastases revisited: the histological findings in 526 sides of neck dissection from 439 previously untreated patients. Int J Oral Maxillofac Surg 2007;36(3):219–25.
[32] Byers RM, Clayman GL, McGill D, et al. Selective neck dissections for squamous carcinoma of the upper aerodigestive tract: patterns of regional failure. Head Neck 1999;21(6):499–505.
[33] Muzaffar K. Therapeutic selective neck dissection: a 25-year review. Laryngoscope 2003;113(9):1460–5.

[34] Spiro RH, Morgan GJ, Strong EW, et al. Supraomohyoid neck dissection. Am J Surg 1996;172(6): 650–3.
[35] Schiff BA, Roberts DB, El-Naggar A, et al. Selective vs modified radical neck dissection and postoperative radiotherapy vs observation in the treatment of squamous cell carcinoma of the oral tongue. Arch Otolaryngol Head Neck Surg 2005;131(10): 874–8.
[36] Alvi A, Johnson JT. Extracapsular spread in the clinically negative neck (N0): implications and outcome. Otolaryngol Head Neck Surg 1996;114(1): 65–70.
[37] Hosal AS, Carrau RL, Johnson JT, et al. Selective neck dissection in the management of the clinically node-negative neck. Laryngoscope 2000;110(12): 2037–40.
[38] Johnson JT, Barnes EL, Myers EN, et al. The extracapsular spread of tumors in cervical node metastsis. Arch Otolaryngol 1981;107(12):725–9.
[39] Taylor RJ, Chepeha JC, Teknos TN, et al. Development and validation of the neck dissection impairment index: a quality of life measure. Arch Otolaryngol Head Neck Surg 2002;128(1):44–9.
[40] Terrell JE, Welsh DE, Bradford CR, et al. Pain, quality of life, and spinal accessory nerve status after neck dissection. Laryngoscope 2000;110(4):620–6.
[41] Chepeha DB, Taylor RJ, Chepeha JC, et al. Functional assessment using Constant's shoulder scale after modified radical and selective neck dissection. Head Neck 2002;24(5):432–6.
[42] Bernier J, Domenge C, Ozsahin M, et al. European Organization for Research and Treatment of Cancer trial 22931. Postoperatve irradiation with or without concomitant chemotherapy for locally advanced head and neck cancer. N Engl J Med 2004;350(19): 1945–52.
[43] Cooper JS, Pajak TF, Forastiere AA, et al. Radiation therapy oncology group 9501/intergroup. Postoperative concurrent radiotherapy and chemotherapy for high-risk squamous-cell carcinoma of the head and neck. N Engl J Med 2004;350(19): 1937–44.
[44] Bernier J, Cooper JS, Pajak RF, et al. Defining risk levels in locally advanced head and neck cancers: a comparative analysis of concurrent postoperative radiation plus chemotherapy trials of the EORTC (#22931) and RTOG (#9501). Head Neck 2005; 27(10):843–50.
[45] Bachaud JM, Cohen-Jonathan E, Alzieu C, et al. Combined postoperative radiotherapy and weekly cisplatin infusion for locally advanced head and neck carcinoma: final report of a randomized trial. Int J Radiat Oncol Biol Phys 1996;36(5):999–1004.
[46] Smid L, Budihna M, Zakotnik B, et al. Postoperative concomitant irradiation and chemotherapy with mitomycin C and bleomycin for advanced head and neck carcinoma. Int J Radiat Oncol Biol Phys 2003;56(4):1055–62.

[47] Winquist E, Oliver T, Gilbert R. Postoperative chemoradiotherpy for advanced squamous cell carcinoma of the head and neck: a systematic review with meta-analysis. Head Neck 2007;29(1):38–46.

[48] Pignon JP, Bourhis J, Domenge C, et al. Chemotherapy added to locoregional treatment for head and neck squamous-cell carcinoma: three meta-analyses of updated individual data. MACH-NC collaborative group. Meta-analysis of chemotherapy on head and neck cancer. Lancet 2000;355(9208): 949–55.

[49] Munro AJ. An overview of randomised controlled trials of adjuvant chemotherapy in head and neck cancer. Br J Cancer 1995;71(1):83–91.

[50] Forastiere AA, Goepfert H, Maor M, et al. Concurrent chemotherapy and radiotherapy for organ preservation in advanced laryngeal cancer. N Engl J Med 2003;349(22):2091–8.

[51] Denis F, Garaud P, Bardet E, et al. Final results of the 94-01 French head and neck oncology and radiotherapy group randomized trial comparing radiotherapy alone with concomitant radiochemotherapy in advanced-stage oropharynx carcinoma. J Clin Oncol 2004;22(1):69–76.

[52] Brizel DM, Prosnitz RG, Hunter S, et al. Necessity for adjuvant neck dissection in setting of concurrent chemoradiation for advanced head-and-neck cancer. Int J Radiat Oncol Biol Phys 2004;58(5): 1418–23.

[53] Lavertu P, Adelstein DJ, Saxton JP, et al. Management of the neck in a randomized trial comparing concurrent chemotherapy and radiotherapy with radiotherapy alone in resectable stage III and IV squamous cell head and neck cancer. Head Neck 1997;19(7):559–66.

[54] Lee HJ, Zelefsky MJ, Kraus DH, et al. Long-term regional control after radiation therapy and neck dissection for base of tongue carcinoma. Int J Radiat Oncol Biol Phys 1997;38(5):995–1000.

[55] McHam SA, Adelstein DJ, Rybicki LA, et al. Who merits a neck dissection after definitive chemoradiotherapy for N2–N3 squamous cell head and neck cancer? Head Neck 2003;25(10):791–8.

[56] Mendenhall WM, Villaret DB, Amdur RJ, et al. Planned neck dissection after definitive radiotherapy for squamous cell carcinoma of the head and neck. Head Neck 2002;24(11):1012–8.

[57] Roy S, Tibesar RJ, Daly K, et al. Role of planned neck dissection for advanced metastatic disease in tongue base or tonsil squamous cell carcinoma treated with radiotherapy. Head Neck 2002;24(5): 474–81.

[58] Stenson KM, Haraf DJ, Pelzer H, et al. The role of cervical lymphadenectomy after aggressive concomitant chemoradiotherapy: the feasibility of selective neck dissection. Arch Otolaryngol Head Neck Surg 2000;126(8):950–6.

[59] Argiris A, Stenson KM, Brockstein BE, et al. Neck dissection in the combined-modality therapy of patients with locoregionally advanced head and neck cancer. Head Neck 2004;26(5):447–55.

[60] Homma A, Furuta Y, Oridate N, et al. "Watch-and-see" policy for the clinically positive neck in head and neck cancer treated with chemoradiotherapy. Int J Clin Oncol 2006;11(6):441–8.

[61] Armstrong J, Pfister D, Strong E, et al. The management of the clinically positive neck as part of a larynx preservation approach. Int J Radiat Oncol Biol Phys 1993;26(5):759–65.

[62] Garden AS, Glisson BS, Ang KK, et al. Phase I/II trial of radiation with chemotherapy "boost" for advanced squamous cell carcinomas of the head and neck: toxicities and responses. J Clin Oncol 1999;17(8):2390–5.

[63] Robbins KT, Wong FS, Kumar P, et al. Efficacy of targeted chemoradiation and planned selective neck dissection to control bulky nodal disease in advanced head and neck cancer. Arch Otolaryngol Head Neck Surg 1999;125(6):670–5.

[64] Corry J, Rischin D, Smith J, et al. Radiation with concurrent late chemotherapy intensification ('chemo-boost') for locally advanced head and neck cancer. Radiother Oncol 2000;54(2):123–7.

[65] Clayman GL, Johnson CJ II, Morrison W, et al. The role of neck dissection after chemoradiotherapy for oropharyngeal cancer with advanced nodal disease. Arch Otolaryngol Head Neck Surg 2001;127(2): 135–9.

[66] Sassler AM, Esclamado RM, Wolf GT. Surgery after organ preservation therapy. Analysis of wound complications. Arch Otolaryngol Head Neck Surg 1995;121(2):162–5.

[67] Newman JP, Terris DJ, Pinto HA, et al. Surgical morbidity of neck dissection after chemoradiotherapy in advanced head and neck cancer. Ann Otol Rhinol Laryngol 1997;106(2):117–22.

[68] Velázquez RA, McGuff HS, Sycamore D, et al. The role of computed tomographic scans in the management of the N-positive neck in head and neck squamous cell carcinoma after chemoradiotherapy. Arch Otolaryngol Head Neck Surg 2004;130(1):74–7.

[69] Ojiri H, Mendenhall WM, Stringer SP, et al. Post-RT CT results as a predictive model for the necessity of planned post-RT neck dissection in patients with cervical metastatic disease from squamous cell carcinoma. Int J Radiat Oncol Biol Phys 2002;52(2): 420–8.

[70] Anzai Y, Brunberg JA, Lufkin RB. Imaging of nodal metastasis in the head and neck. J Magn Reson Imaging 1997;7(5):774–83.

[71] Adams S, Baum RP, Stuckensen T, et al. Prospective comparison of 18F-FDG PET with conventional imaging modalities (CT, MRI, US) in lymph node staging of the head and neck cancer. Eur J Nucl Med 1998;25(9):1255–60.

[72] Wong RJ, Lin DT, Schöder H, et al. Diagnostic and prognostic value of [(18)F]fluorodeoxyglucose positron emission tomography for recurrent head and

neck squamous cell carcinoma. J Clin Oncol 2002; 20(20):4199–208.
[73] Ware RE, Matthews JP, Hicks RJ, et al. Usefulness of fluorine-18 fluorodeoxyglucose positron emission tomography in patients with residual structural abnormality following definitive treatment for squamous cell carcinoma of the head and neck. Head Neck 2004;26(12):1008–17.
[74] Kubota K, Yokoyama J, Yamaguchi K, et al. FDG-PET delayed imaging for the detection of head and neck cancer recurrence after radio-chemotherapy: comparison with MRI/CT. Eur J Nucl Med Mol Imaging 2004;31(4):590–5.
[75] Pellitteri PK, Ferlito A, Rinaldo A, et al. Planned neck dissection following chemoradiotherapy for advanced head and neck cancer: Is it necessary for all? Head Neck 2006;28(2):166–75.
[76] Brennan JA, Jafek BW. Elective carotid artery resection for advanced squamous cell carcinoma of the neck. Laryngoscope 1994;104(3 Pt 1): 259–63.
[77] Freeman SB, Hamaker RC, Borrowdale RB, et al. Management of neck metastasis with carotid artery involvement. Laryngoscope 2004;114(1):20–4.
[78] Huvos AG, Leaming RH, Moore OS. Clinicopathologic study of the resected carotid artery. Am J Surg 1973;126(4):570–4.
[79] Kennedy JT, Krause CJ, Loevy S. The importance of tumor attachment to the carotid artery. Arch Otolaryngol Head Neck Surg 1977;103(2):70–3.
[80] Konno A, Togawa K, Iizuka K. Analyis of factors affecting complications of carotid ligation. Ann Otol Rhinol Laryngol 1981;90(3 Pt 1):222–6.
[81] Snyderman CH, D'Amico F. Outcome of carotid resection for neoplastic disease: a meta-analysis. Am J Otolaryngol 1992;13(6):373–80.
[82] deVries EJ, Sekhar LN, Horton JA, et al. A new method to predict safe resection of the internal carotid artery. Laryngoscope 1990;100(1):85–8.
[83] Ehrnefeld WK, Stoney RJ, Wylie EJ. Relation of carotid stump pressure to safety of carotid artery ligation. Surgery 1983;93(2):299–305.
[84] Chazono H, Okamoto Y, Matsuzaki Z, et al. Carotid artery resection: preoperative temporary occlusion is not always an accurate predictor of collateral blood flow. Acta Otolaryngol 2005;125(2):196–200.
[85] Conley JJ. Free autogenous vein graft to the internal and common carotid arteries in the treatment of tumors of the neck. Ann Surg 1953;137(2):205–14.
[86] Stoney RJ, Wylie EJ. Arterial autografts. Surgery 1970;67(1):18–25.
[87] Loré JM, Boulos EJ. Resection and reconstruction of the carotid artery in metastatic squamous cell carcinoma. Am J Surg 1981;142(4):437–42.
[88] Chazono H, Okamoto Y, Matsuzaki Z, et al. Extracranial-intracranial bypass for reconstruction of internal carotid artery in the management of head and neck cancer. Ann Vasc Surg 2003;17(3):260–5.
[89] Katsuno S, Takemae T, Ishiyama T, et al. Is carotid reconstruction for advanced cancer in the neck a safe procedure? Otolaryngol Head Neck Surg 2001; 124(2):222–4.
[90] Németh Z, Dömötör Gy, Tálos M, et al. Resection and replacement of the carotid artery in metastatic head and neck cancer: literature review and case report. Int J Oral Maxillofac Surg 2003;32(6):645–50.

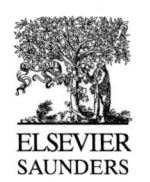

Tracheotomy: Elective and Emergent
Eric J. Dierks, DMD, MD, FACS[a,b],*

[a]Department of Oral and Maxillofacial Surgery, Oregon Health & Science University,
611 S.W. Campus Drive, Portland, OR 97239, USA
[b]Legacy Emanuel Hospital, 2801 N. Gantenbein Avenue, Portland, OR 97227, USA

History

Tracheotomy has been practiced since ancient times [1]. As early as 3600 BC, the procedure was depicted on Egyptian engravings from the Abydos and Sakkara regions of Egypt. Tracheotomy and cricothyroidotomy passed through an era of great controversy and Hippocrates condemned the operation due to the risk of carotid damage. This period was followed by general acceptance of the procedure' life-saving potential. The name of Chevalier Jackson [2] will always be associated with tracheotomy. In 1921, he described the indications and techniques for tracheostomy and also condemned what he referred to as "high tracheostomy," or cricothyroidotomy.

Indications

The indications for tracheotomy fall into four general categories:

1. To protect the larynx and trachea from the damage produced by prolonged translaryngeal intubation in patients who require prolonged ventilatory support.
2. To remove the airway from a surgical field in the maxillofacial region, pharynx, or larynx.
3. To bypass upper airway obstruction, not manageable by simpler means.
4. To facilitate pulmonary toilet by the use of a tube within the trachea that is shorter than an endotracheal tube.

Contraindications

There are no absolute contraindications to tracheotomy. The rarely encountered anatomic variant of a high position of the innominate artery that crosses the trachea above the sternal notch would preclude standard tracheotomy technique.

Elective adult tracheotomy: anatomy and technique

Elective tracheotomy can be performed under either local or general anesthesia, although general anesthesia is preferred. The head and neck are tilted backward, either with the aid of a shoulder roll or by placing the head on a suitably positioned Mayfield horseshoe headholder. The purpose of this position is to distract the larynx and trachea, increasing the distance from the cricoid cartilage to the sternal notch.

Following administration of local anesthesia with epinephrine, a transverse incision is made between the medial borders of the sternocleidomastoids, at a level approximately half the distance between the cricoid and the sternal notch. The subcutaneous fat is bluntly separated with a gauze sponge to avoid damage to the anterior jugular veins, which can often be identified, but not injured, by this maneuver. The median raphe between the paired, paramedian sternohyoid and sternothyroid muscles is identified and entered with a Crile hemostat, thereby passing through the superficial layer of the deep cervical fascia. The strap muscles are retracted laterally with an Army-Navy retractor as the operation proceeds in the midline toward the trachea.

The trachea is mobile in the transverse plane and periodic reassessment of the midline is necessary.

---

* Head & Neck Surgical Associates, 1849 NW Kearney #300, Portland, OR 97209
  E-mail address: dierksej@hnsa1.com

The thyroid isthmus is identified and is usually retracted superiorly. If the isthmus is enlarged, or if it lies directly in the path of the planned tracheotomy, it can be dissected off the trachea and divided between suture-ligatures or with electrocautery. The pretracheal fascia is swept off the trachea with a gauze sponge and the tracheal rings are identified.

Once the trachea has been visualized, the surgeon will request the appropriate sized tracheotomy (or "trach") tube, usually a #8 for a man and a #6 for a woman. The scrub nurse will inflate and deflate the tube' cuff to test for leaks and will lubricate the tube and cuff with water-soluble lubricant to help avoid cuff tears upon insertion. The scrub nurse will also place the stylet within the trach tube lumen. The cricoid is palpated through the wound and is hooked from beneath its inferior border with a cricoid hook to allow the assistant to provide anterior-superior traction. This serves to both elevate and transfix the trachea within what would otherwise seem to be a deep hole. If the location of the thyroid isthmus interferes with hooking the cricoid ring, the first tracheal ring can be hooked. If desired, "stay sutures" can be placed through the tracheal ring cartilage on either side of the planned tracheal opening.

After alerting the anesthesiologist, a scalpel is used to make the tracheal incision of choice, usually a midline vertical incision between rings two, three and often four. T-shaped or transverse incisions between the tracheal rings can also be used, but care is taken to avoid laceration of the membranous posterior tracheal wall. Calcified rings may need to be cut with a heavy scissor such as a curved Mayo. The Army-Navy retractors are removed, but the cricoid hook is left in place until successful positioning of the trach tube has been confirmed.

A Trousseau or other tracheal dilator is placed and deployed to aid passage of the tube into the trachea. The trach tube is then inserted with a curving motion. The stylet is removed and, if a dual lumen trach tube is used, the inner cannula is placed and connected to the ventilator tubing. Once end-tidal CO_2 is confirmed and/or chest auscultation performed, the cricoid hook is removed and the flange of the trach tube is sutured to skin in four quadrants. A circumferential tie is then placed around the neck. A portable chest radiograph is obtained in the recovery room to confirm proper positioning of the tube and to assess for pneumothorax.

Complications and misadventures in elective tracheotomy

Intraoperative

Paratracheal or pretracheal placement of the trach tube is occasionally encountered following what seemed to be accurate passage of the tube into the trachea. This problem is usually rapidly identified by the lack of end-tidal CO_2 registration on the capnograph monitor or by the lack of appropriate breath sounds upon chest auscultation. If there is doubt, a tracheal suction catheter can be quickly passed and the tube' malposition can be determined by the lack of a cough response in a lightly anesthetized patient or by the lack of normal aspiration of sputum or bloody tracheal secretions.

Pneumothorax can occur following routine tracheotomy but it would logically be more likely following a difficult trach or one with excessive lateral dissection. A portable chest radiograph has traditionally been used to identify this potential complication.

Bleeding during or following tracheotomy is probably the most frequent complication of tracheotomy. Bleeding identified shortly after the skin incision is most likely due to laceration of an anterior jugular vein. Bleeding deeper within the wound more likely arises from the highly vascular thyroid gland. If division of the thyroid isthmus is needed, the isthmus should be carefully and completely elevated from the trachea with a right-angle dissector such as a Mixter or Dietrich, and the stumps suture-ligated. Alternatively, thorough electrocautery can be used to divide the isthmus. Deeper bleeding arising lateral to the trachea can occur from vessels of the lateral vascular arcade that nourish the trachea. Bipolar cautery is useful in this area due to the proximity of the underlying recurrent laryngeal nerve which courses near the tracheo-esophageal groove.

Postoperative

The appearance of buds of granulation tissue around the trach tube is common and is occasionally problematic due to bleeding. Silver nitrate application can be helpful.

Peri-tracheostomal wound infection can occur following tracheotomy and generally responds to wound hygiene and wet-to-dry packing around the trach tube. Such infections can produce necrosis of the adjacent tissues, however, healing around the trach tube by granulation is to be expected (Figs. 1 and 2).

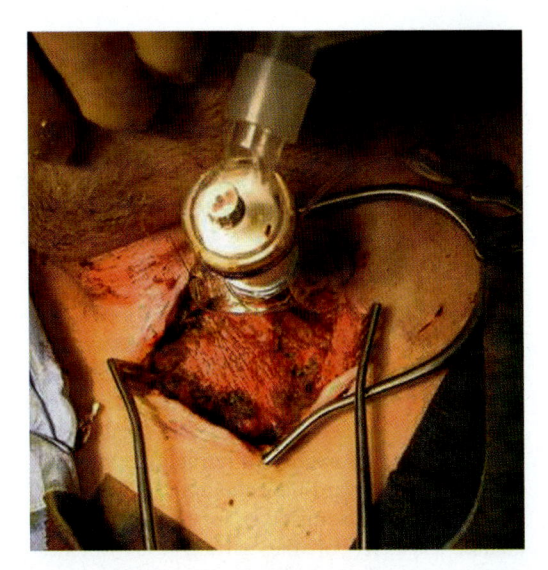

Fig. 1. Necrotizing peri-tracheal wound after cleaning with serial wet-to-dry dressings.

Tracheocutaneous fistula is much more common following tracheotomy in children than adults, where it is generally a function of the duration of the trach tube. Electrocautery of the fistula walls may be all that is required to produce fistula closure in children, whereas formal excision of the fistula with layered wound closure, including interposition of the adjacent strap muscles, is often needed among adults.

Tracheo-innominate fistula (TIF) can develop months after tracheotomy and is usually due to erosion of the anterior tracheal wall by the tube tip. This erosion extends anteriorly to involve the posterior wall of the innominate artery as it crosses the trachea in the upper mediastinum. Standard tracheal incisions in the second and third tracheal ring will invariably place a part of the trach tube tip near the aspect of the trachea

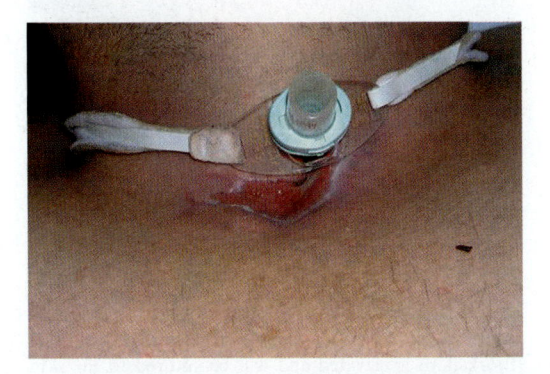

Fig. 2. Peritracheal wound healed by granulation.

where the innominate artery crosses [3]. TIF usually presents as an initial sentinel or herald bleed that is followed hours to weeks later by a fatal, ex-sanguinating hemorrhage. TIF is initially managed by attempting to inflate the cuff of the trach tube or an endotracheal tube at the site of the fistula. If this fails, the Utley maneuver involves opening the inferior aspect of the tracheotomy site to allow blunt finger dissection into the anterior mediastinum [4]. Anterior compression of the innominate artery against the manubrium will diminish the hemorrhage until an emergency thoracotomy can be performed.

Tracheal stenosis is often cited as a complication of tracheotomy but it may often be caused by prolonged translaryngeal intubation before tracheotomy. In a series of 1130 tracheotomies of Goldenberg and colleagues [5] identified 21 cases of tracheal stenosis, all of which occurred in patients who had been intubated for at least 12 days before tracheotomy.

Slow displacement of the trach tube out of the trachea into the peri-tracheal soft tissues can occur in two forms, one of which can be life-threatening.

Type I slow displacement results from a progressive increase in the distance from the anterior tracheal wall to the neck skin, usually due to postoperative edema occurring within the first few postoperative days. It occurs primarily among patients with thick or obese necks. As the trach tube approaches complete distraction out of the trachea, the edges of the adjacent tracheal rings will provide mechanical interference with a suction catheter as it is passed though the end of the trach tube. Difficulty passing a suction catheter into the trachea is a danger sign. Visual inspection of the trach site is unremarkable as the trach flange lies in normal contact with the skin, flange sutures are intact, and air is passing through the trach tube. A portable lateral chest radiograph may help confirm type I slow displacement phenomenon, but consideration should be given to immediate placement of a longer trach tube under controlled conditions. When the tip of the trach tube slips completely out of the trachea into the neck soft tissues, immediate and catastrophic airway obstruction can occur (Fig. 3).

Type II slow displacement occurs in the absence of an increased distance from the anterior tracheal wall to the neck skin. It is seen in patients with normal neck size and occurs later than type I displacement, often in patients ready for decannulation. Like type I displacement, the hallmark is

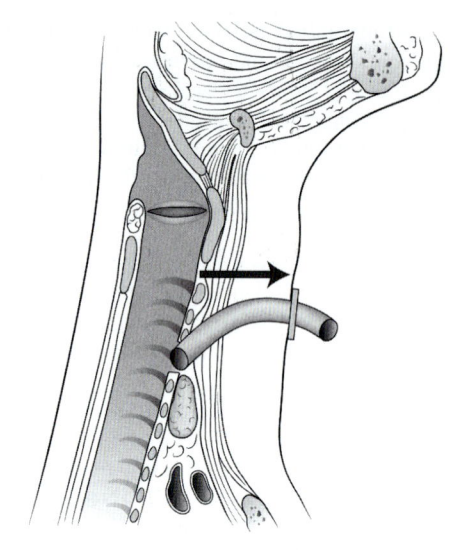

Fig. 3. Type I displacement. Tip of trach tube has been drawn out of trachea into peritracheal tissue due to increase in distance from the skin to tracheal anterior wall.

the report by the bedside nurse that passage of the suction catheter is difficult. In type II displacement, it may be impossible to pass the catheter as the trach tube may already be completely out of the trachea. Visual inspection of the trach site slows elevation the trach tube flange off the skin by 1 cm or more (Fig. 4). The patient is often breathing without difficulty and is able to phonate. In this scenario, the trach tube has migrated out of the trachea due to loose trach ties or the absence of sutures in the trach tube flange, in a patient whose airway is otherwise intact and is ready to decannulate. The trach tube is then simply removed, if no longer needed for other purposes.

Special considerations

Pediatric tracheotomy

The technique of pediatric tracheotomy differs somewhat from that of adult tracheotomy. The mobility of the trachea within the neck is more pronounced than that of adults and distances between anatomic landmarks are smaller. As a result, modestly exuberant retraction can direct the dissection toward the common carotid artery, which can easily be mistaken for the trachea. The greater elasticity of the cartilaginous tracheal rings allows effective placement and subsequent use of stay sutures to open the trachea. Children that require long-term tracheostomy may benefit from construction of a tracheal stoma with an inferiorly-based flap of the anterior tracheal wall sutured to the inferior skin of the trach stoma (Bjork flap) (Fig. 5). The size of the trach tube must be accurately matched to the trachea as standard pediatric trach tubes are cuffless, relying on close fit of the tube to the tracheal lumen for seal. Following placement of the trach tube, an intraoperative chest radiograph is usually obtained to check position of the tube to avoid right mainstem bronchus intubation.

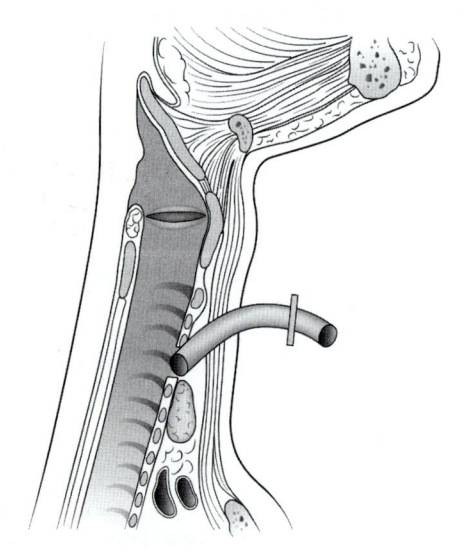

Fig. 4. Type II displacement with characteristic elevation of trach flange off the underlying skin surface.

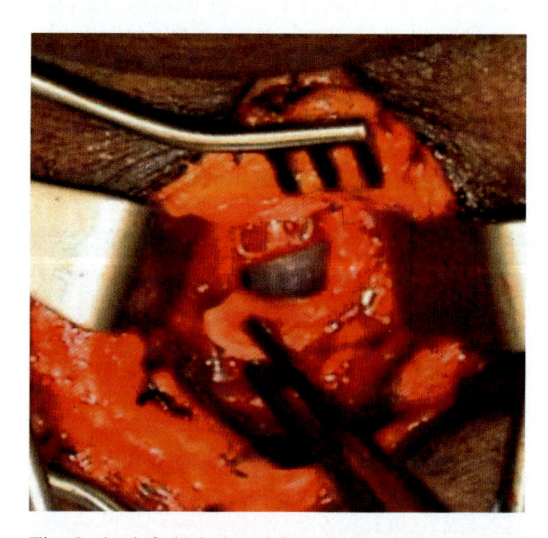

Fig. 5. An inferiorly-based flap of the anterior tracheal (Bjork flap) is elevated and will be sutured to the skin at the inferior border of the tracheal stoma.

Pediatric tracheotomy is associated with a higher incidence of complications. Carr and colleagues [6] noted a 43% incidence of serious loss of airway due to accidental decannulation, tube occlusion, or requirement of a separate surgical procedure. These authors also noted a 0.7% mortality due to tracheotomy-related complications. Following tracheal decannulation, the incidence of tracheocutaneous fistula is much higher among children than adults.

Tracheotomy in the obese patient

The obese neck presents several problems when the obese patient requires tracheotomy. Critical assessment of the obese patient' neck may reveal that although the patient may be obese, the low, anterior neck may not be obese and a standard tracheotomy may be appropriate. The obese patient with an obese neck is more the norm; the increased distance from the skin of the anterior neck to the anterior tracheal wall must be managed to avoid complications and potential catastrophe. The excision of fat from the area of the tracheotomy is usually helpful; the construction of a tracheal stoma via an inferiorly based Bjork flap to form the inferior wall of the stoma, combined with a superiorly based skin flap to form the superior wall, will result in a tracheostomy that stands open upon removal (or dislodgement) of the trach tube (Fig. 6). A 43% overall complication rate was encountered in a series of defatting tracheotomies among obese patients [7]. Specialized trach tubes with an increased length of the proximal part of the trach tube are very helpful in the obese neck (Fig. 7). If such a tube is not available, a standard endotracheal tube can be split and tailored to create an extended-length trach tube [8].

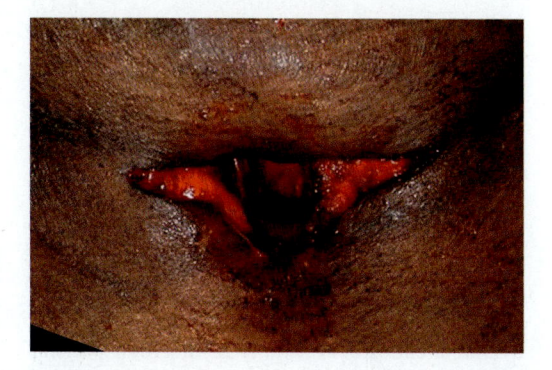

Fig. 6. Tracheal stoma for an obese patient constructed with a Bjork flap inferiorly and a skin flap sutured to the superior aspect of the tracheal opening.

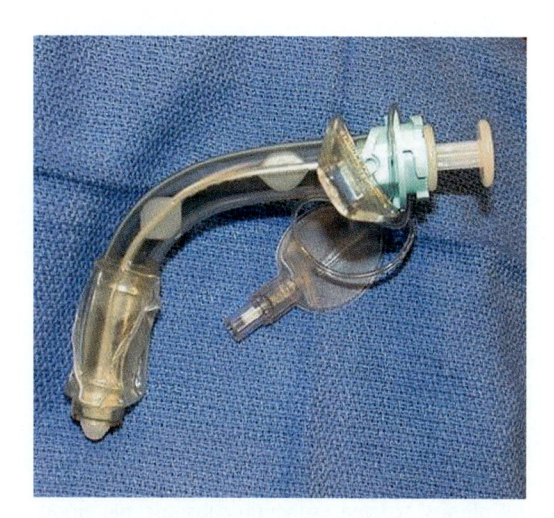

Fig. 7. Shiley XLT tracheotomy tube with proximal extension is very useful for obese patients.

Percutaneous dilational tracheotomy

Percutaneous dilational tracheotomy (PDT) is a bedside technique based upon the Seldinger dilational process that creates a track for trach tube placement via serial dilation of the orifice over a guide wire placed by percutaneous puncture. Ciaglia and colleagues [9] introduced this as a dilational technique in 1985 and it has been widely used since. This technique is primarily applied to the intubated patient who requires conversion to tracheotomy for prolonged ventilatory support.

The advantages of PDT include the cost savings and scheduling convenience of the procedure when performed at bedside in the ICU as compared with open tracheotomy in the operating room. Although originally developed as a technique to be done blindly, many pulmonologists, intensivists and others who use PDT do so with bronchoscopic guidance. The guidance confirms intra-tracheal placement of the guide wire and tube, but diminishes some of the potential cost savings. Specific training is the technique is required. Kost [10] noted a 9.2% overall complication rate with complications increasing to 15% when the BMI exceeded 30.

Emergency surgical airway: cricothyroidotomy and emergency tracheotomy

Emergency cricothyroidotomy or "crike"

Cricothyroidotomy has also been termed "coniotomy" as it involves entry through the conus elasticus, a fibro-elastic membrane extending from the cricoid cartilage superiorly and medially to the inferior edge of the anterior aspect of the thyroid cartilage. The median cricothyroid ligament is a readily discernible anteromedial condensation of the conus elasticus. Cricothyroidotomy or "crike" has gained popularity as an emergency airway access technique due to its straightforward nature and the fact that it does not require formal surgical training to either learn or perform. It is less dependent on optimal patient positioning and can be performed with alacrity in most patients.

Patients requiring emergency cricothyroidotomy fall into one of two general morphologic categories: those whose cricothyroid membranes can be readily palpated and those who by virtue of obesity, edema, subcutaneous air or blood, cannot. In the former category, cricothyroidotomy can be readily executed by stabilizing the cricoid with the non-dominant hand while creating a transverse skin incision over the cricothyroid membrane. The surgeon will repalpate the cricothyroid membrane through the skin incision, followed by a second transverse incision through the membrane that enters the airway. Thin patients may undergo this procedure with one incision through skin and membrane, often necessitating a sawing motion. Finger dilation or dilation produced by twisting the scalpel handle in the membrane opening is followed swiftly by placement of a small endotracheal or tracheotomy tube.

The latter category of patients poses a challenge as the location of the cricothyroid membrane via external palpation is obscured. The surgeon may wisely opt for a large vertical incision that allows a wider range of palpation to identify the location of the cricothyroid membrane. The membrane is then entered via transverse incision and the tube of choice placed.

Bennett and colleagues [11] measured the cricothyroid membrane in a series of fresh adult cadavers and found a vertical midline measurement mean of 13.69 mm (range from 8–19 mm) and width between the cricothyroid muscles mean of 12.39 (range of 9–19 mm). These authors point out that the diameter of an endotracheal or tracheotomy tube placed through a cricothyroidotomy should not exceed 8.5 mm in external diameter, which corresponds to the external diameter of a size #4 Shiley tracheostomy tube. In the heat of an emergency airway obstruction, it is obvious that any tube that can be passed will suffice.

Once the emergency cricothyroidotomy patient has been stabilized, consideration should be given to converting the cricothyroidotomy to a formal tracheotomy. This potentially minimizes the trauma to the cricothyroid muscle and the articulation of the cricoid and thyroid cartilages. In some situations, the tracheotomy can be performed through the crike incision. If the crike incision is too high to allow this, it can be loosely closed following conversion.

"Slash" tracheotomy

The sailors' adage "any port in a storm" applies to the rapid placement of a deep vertical neck incision down to trachea without regard for hemostasis, in a desperate attempt to secure a surgical airway. Although cricothyroidotomy is clearly preferable, "slash" trachs are occasionally appropriate and necessary. One such scenario is that of the elective tracheotomy "gone bad" with loss of control of the airway during an elective procedure in which the endotracheal tube has become dislodged and the patient falls into the "cannot intubate/cannot ventilate" predicament. Here, a "reverse slash" can be performed by placing the scalpel deep within the wound and incising outward and upward in a vertical fashion, cutting through everything overlying the trachea and larynx including skin. This inverted T-shaped wound allows much wider access for palpation of the cricoid and trachea, allowing entry into the airway. The blood-filled wound may not allow visual inspection and the surgeon must proceed via palpation alone. Any emergency surgical airway procedure that results in a living patient is a success, regardless of collateral damage to the cricoid, trachea, thyroid cartilage, lung, or other adjacent structures.

Emergent re-opening of a trach site

Following decannulation, airway obstruction can recur, necessitating re-establishment of the tracheotomy. Should this scenario present as an airway emergency, the tracheotomy tract can be quickly reopened by forcing a Crile or other hemostat through the healing wound and into the trachea, followed by opening the hemostat, which will allow the insertion a trach tube or other available endotracheal tube. In the adult patient, this maneuver can be performed though a healed incision at the prior tracheotomy site up to several months after decannulation.

Controversies

Elective cricothyroidotomy

In 1976, two cardiothoracic surgeons published a provocative paper regarding their experience with 655 elective cricothyroidotomies among a population of elective thoracic surgery patients [12]. Their retrospective study cited the advantages of cricothyroidotomy as simplicity, absence of cross-contamination among median sternotomy patients, and safety, with a 6.1% complication rate. Their paper was widely referenced and also widely criticized. A wave of enthusiasm for elective cricothyroidotomy followed, but a subsequent prospective study identified five cases of subglottic stenosis in a series of 76 elective cricothyroidotomies [13].

Skin incision

The transverse incision has been generally accepted as the incision of choice for elective tracheotomy, due to its ease of execution and cosmetics. The vertical incision is associated with wider access as well as decreased bleeding; the vertical incision is reserved for emergency applications and possibly for those situations in which hemostasis considerations are paramount.

Tracheal incision

The type of incision into the trachea probably has less to do with subsequent tracheal stenosis than it does with the duration of intubation preceding the tracheotomy and other factors. A dog study comparing vertical, horizontal, and window excision tracheal entry failed to show a significant difference in reduction of tracheal lumen diameter, with all three techniques resulting in an average of about 25% reduction [14].

Timing of elective tracheotomy

Optimal timing of elective tracheotomy in the ventilator-dependent patient has been the subject of a controversy that is summarized well by McWhorter [15]. An initial Glasgow Coma Score of seven or less has been identified as an indicator for early tracheotomy among trauma patients [16]. A survey of critical care nurses noted that 92% would personally prefer a tracheotomy to prolonged intubation if they personally required intubation for greater than 10 days [17].

Tracheal stay sutures

Stay sutures entail the placement of suture through the tracheal rings on either side of the tracheal opening, draping these sutures through the wound and taping them to the chest wall. In the event of tube dislodgement, traction can be applied to these sutures to spread the tracheal opening, facilitating tube re-placement. Stay sutures work well in the pediatric patient as the cartilaginous nature of the tracheal rings allows reasonably secure suture placement as well as the flexibility to open upon traction of the sutures. Stay sutures are significantly less effective in the adult patient. The progressive ossification of the tracheal rings allows the ring to crack and split upon suture placement. Suture traction on a calcified tracheal ring does not allow the wide dilation seen in the pediatric patient and, in an emergency, the stay sutures in an adult can interfere with of tube replacement. This author has abandoned their use in the adult patient.

The establishment of a surgical airway via tracheotomy or cricothyroidotomy represents a skill set shared by multiple surgical disciplines. Although the risk-to-benefit ratio of this group of procedures is generally highly favorable, it behooves surgeons to periodically revisit this interdisciplinary topic to provide the highest level of care to their patients.

References

[1] Frost EA. Tracing the tracheostomy. Ann Otol Rhinol Laryngol 1976;85:618–24.
[2] Jackson C. High tracheotomy and other errors. The chief causes of chronic laryngeal stenosis. Surg Gynecol Obstet 1921;32:392–8.
[3] Oshinsky AE, Rubin JS, Gwozdz CS. The anatomical basis for post-tracheotomy innominate artery rupture. Laryngoscope 1988;98:1061–4.
[4] Utley JR, Singer MM, Roe BB. Definitive management of innominate artery hemorrhage complicating tracheostomy. JAMA 1972;4:577–9.
[5] Goldenberg D, Ari EG, Golz A, et al. Tracheotomy complications: a retrospective study of 1130 cases. Otolaryngol Head Neck Surg 2000;123:495–500.
[6] Carr MM, Poje CP, Kingston L, et al. Complications in pediatric tracheostomies. Laryngoscope 2001;111:1925–8.
[7] Gross ND, Cohen JI, Andersen PE, et al. "Defatting" tracheotomy in morbidly obese patients. Laryngoscope 2002;112:1940–4.
[8] Bettez M, Maves MD. The endotracheal tube as a tracheotomy tube. Otolaryngol Head Neck Surg 1991;105:480–2.
[9] Ciaglia P, Firsching R, Syniec C. Elective percutaneous dilational tracheostomy, a new simple

bedside procedure, preliminary report. Chest 1985; 87:715–9.

[10] Kost KM. Endoscopic percutaneous dilatational tracheotomy: a prospective evaluation of 500 consecutive cases. Laryngoscope 2005;115:1–30.

[11] Bennett JDC, Guha SC, Sankar AB. Cricothyroidotomy: the anatomical basis. J R Coll Surg Edinb 1996;41:57–60.

[12] Brantigan CO, Grow JB. Cricothyroidotomy: elective use in respiratory problems requiring tracheostomy. J Thorac Cardiovasc Surg 1976;71:72–81.

[13] Sise MJ, Shacksord SR, Cruickshank JC, et al. Cricothyroidotomy for long term tracheal access. Ann Surg 1984;200:13–7.

[14] Bryant LR, Mujia D, Greenberg S, et al. Evaluation of tracheal incisions for tracheostomy. Am J Surg 1978;135:675–9.

[15] McWhorter AJ. Tracheotomy: timing and techniques. Curr Opin Otolaryngol Head Neck Surg 2003;11:473–9.

[16] Lanza DC, Koltai PJ, Parnes SM, et al. Predictive value of the Glasgow coma scale for tracheotomy in head-injured patients. Ann Otol Rhinol Laryngol 1990;99:38–41.

[17] Astrachan DI, Kirchner JC, Goodwin WJ. Prolonged intubation vs. tracheotomy: complications, practical and psychosocial considerations. Laryngoscope 1988;98:1165–9.

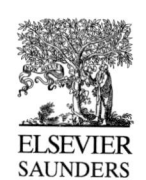

Preparation of the Neck for Microvascular Reconstruction of the Head and Neck

Jason K. Potter, MD, DDS[a,b,*], Timothy M. Osborn, DDS, MD[c]

[a]Plastic and Maxillofacial Surgery, Dallas, TX, USA
[b]Department of Oral and Maxillofacial Surgery, Baylor College of Dentistry, Dallas, TX, USA
[c]Department of Oral and Maxillofacial Surgery, Oregon Health & Science University, Portland, OR, USA

Reconstruction of congenital, developmental, or acquired head and neck defects remains a significant challenge for the oral and maxillofacial surgeon. Arguably, in no other anatomic location is the quality of both form and function of the reconstructed part more critically appraised by the patient, surgeon, and society.

Reconstruction of head and neck defects was previously limited by the paucity of local tissues available to reconstruct complex wounds. The development of pedicled flaps during the 1970s and 1980s (deltopectoral, pectoralis major, latissimus dorsi) revolutionized head and neck surgery and quickly became the workhorse procedures of the reconstructive surgeon. Critical review of these techniques, however, has illuminated the shortcomings of pedicled flaps for routine use in the reconstruction of composite head and neck defects: (1) the pedicled transfer of bone-containing soft tissue flaps is unpredictable and limited because of extreme arcs of rotation; (2) large, axial pattern rotational flaps, such as the pectoralis major myocutaneous flap, commonly result in unsightly contours and an unfavorable donor site defect; and (3) the use in midface and upper facial reconstruction is limited. Pedicled flaps and nonvascularized bone grafting techniques continue to play an important role in reconstructive oral and maxillofacial surgery. It has become clear, however, that microvascular free tissue transfer has several advantages over nonvascularized bone grafts and pedicled soft tissue flaps that currently make it the modality of choice for the reconstruction of extirpative defects of the head and neck. The advantages of microvascular free flaps include (1) predictable composite tissue transfer from a variety of donor sites at a single stage (immediate reconstruction); (2) radiation tolerance; and (3) minimal donor site morbidity. Although there is little argument that microvascular surgery increases the complexity of the reconstructive procedure, it has been shown to carry success rates of greater than 90% in experienced hands [1–8].

Quality microvascular reconstruction begins, as with any surgical procedure, with sound preoperative planning. Preoperative planning focuses on the characteristics of the missing or anticipated missing tissues, but no matter how aesthetic the final result looks on the table it is as successful as the microsurgical portion of the procedure. What separates a consistently successful microvascular surgeon is the attention to details in the setup of the microsurgery that facilitates a smooth and timely procedure without unanticipated difficulties. The preoperative planning must also include detailed attention to the technical aspects of the microvascular procedure. This includes a thorough understanding of the vascular anatomy of the patient's neck, vascular anatomy of the various flaps including pedicle lengths, anticipation of the needed pedicle length given defect location and probable inflow-outflow vessels, and knowledge of how to facilitate microvascular surgery in the neck and to manage complicating factors in the difficult neck.

* Corresponding author.
E-mail address: potterplasticsurgery@comcast.net (J.K. Potter).

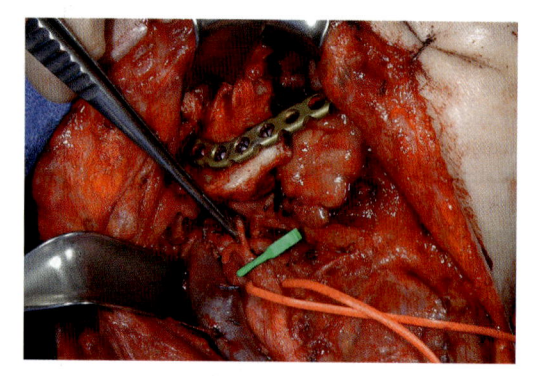

Fig. 2. View of vascular structures of the right neck following removal of posterior digastric and stylohyoid muscles. Note improved visualization of and access to branches of external carotid artery.

The internal jugular vein is the authors' preferred choice for venous outflow. It is prepared by dissecting 360 degrees for several centimeters to free it from the surrounding structures (Fig. 5). This allows for unhindered manipulation of the vessel and placement of vascular clamps proximally and distally that does not interfere with the microsurgical field. Care must be taken to protect the vagus nerve during these maneuvers. Frequently, the stump of the common facial vein may be preserved by the ablative surgeon. When it provides an excellent size match to the flap vein it may be used for venous outflow. The

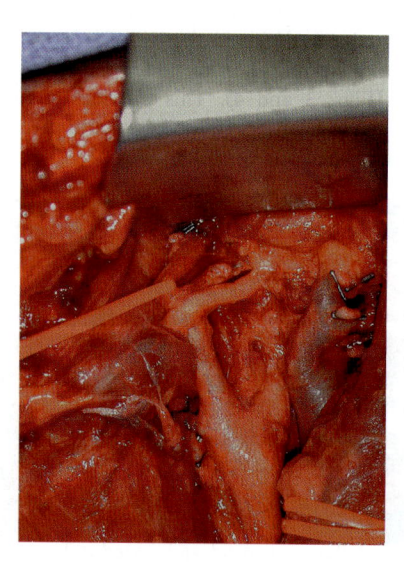

Fig. 3. Note position of distal external carotid artery (left neck) in relation to hypoglossal nerve and inferior border of mandible (behind retractor). Significant tension on vessel loop is needed to visualize adequate length of vessel.

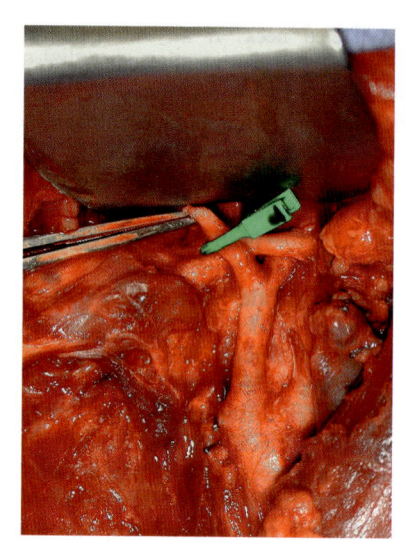

Fig. 4. Significantly improved access and length of vessel is provided by dividing vessel, dissecting it free, and flipping it from under to hypoglossal nerve. The vessel now lies superficial to hyoglossal and is unimpeded for microsurgery.

surgeon should be cautioned to avoid using it in situations where size match is not ideal. An end-to-side anastomosis into the internal jugular is technically more feasible and likely more reliable in this situation. Occasionally, the internal jugular vein may be resected, fibrotic, or otherwise unsuitable. In these situations the external jugular may be used. This vessel may be divided and transposed for end-to-end anastomosis or used in an end-to-side fashion.

Once vessels are selected and prepared, the head is positioned to the contralateral side and dura hooks or lone star hooks are used to provide

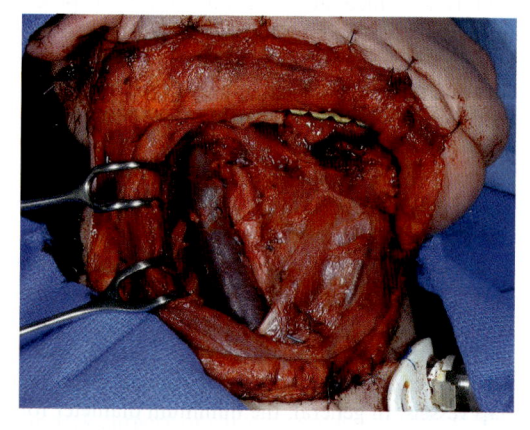

Fig. 5. Internal jugular vein access following careful and meticulous dissection is now ready for microsurgery.

wide exposure while using the surgical microscope. This is best accomplished with retraction of the sternocleidomastoid muscle posterolaterally and the mandible superiorly (Fig. 6).

Proper vessel care is essential throughout preparation of the neck and during time under the microscope. Desiccation caused by inattention can lead to sloughing of vessel endothelium and vessel thrombosis. During flap elevation and before flap division, 4% lidocaine or papaverine is applied on moistened cottonoids as a topical vasodilator. This technique also serves to protect vessels from desiccation.

Microvascular anastomosis

The microvascular anastomosis is arguably the most important component of microvascular tissue transfer and beyond the scope of this article. The vessels must be prepared appropriately to facilitate appropriate coaptation of the vessels and inset in such a way so that there is no tension on the vessels. The sequence of anastomosis (ie, artery first, vein first, and so forth) is dictated by the relation of vessels to each other so that the first anastomosis does not sit on top of the next vessel to be sutured. The arterial and venous anastomosis is performed using 8–0 or 9–0 suture under the microscope. If available, the authors use a dual venous outflow of the flap. After the anastomosis is completed, the clamps are released and the patency and seal of the site is verified.

The vessel-depleted neck

In situations in which the primary recipient vessels are no longer available because of previous ablation, prior free tissue transfer, or poor quality or caliber, selection of alternative vasculature is necessary. Alternative vessels are often at a greater distance from the recipient site, which makes pedicle length a limiting factor. The ideal flap for the reconstruction may not have sufficient pedicle length and the pedicle must be lengthened. Options to increase pedicle length include interposition vein grafts, cephalic transposition, creation of an arteriovenous loop, or selection of an alternative flap with a long pedicle.

The decision to use an interposition vein graft was based on the distance between flap and recipient vessels. When the gap is less than 10 cm, a reversed interposition vein graft is used; however, when the gap is greater than 10 cm, an arteriovenous loop is created. The saphenous vein is the most convenient conduit for vein graft or arteriovenous loop creation. The arteriovenous loop can be used as a one-stage or two-stage reconstruction, with the second stage division and anastomosis of the arteriovenous loop and flap occurring approximately 1 week later. Another technique that can be used is cephalic transposition where the cephalic vein is divided distally and transposed to the neck.

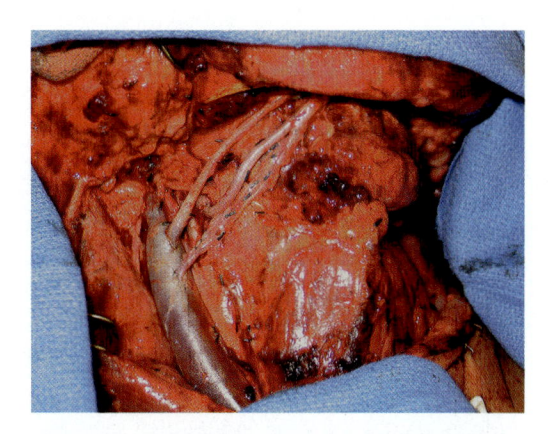

Fig. 6. Retraction hooks placed into the sternocleidomastoid muscle and at inferior border of mandible provide a stable, wide surgical field for successful microsurgery.

In previously operated necks, it may also be necessary to use vasculature outside of the carotid system. The transverse cervical vessels have been shown to be suitable as recipient vessels in more than 90% of cases and should be used in difficult head and neck reconstruction [24]. Patients who have had previous neck dissection should not be excluded from having microvascular free flap reconstruction. Free flaps in these patients have been shown to be highly effective despite a paucity of potential cervical vessels with reliance on flaps with long vascular pedicles [25]. Patients who have failed free flaps should not be excluded from another free flap reconstruction because they often are able to have a second free flap reconstruction [26].

Survival of free flaps depends on an adequate venous drainage system. In free flap reconstruction of head and neck defects, the ablative procedure or prior surgery may precipitate internal jugular vein thrombosis. Studies in which the internal jugular vein was preserved with neck dissection demonstrated a 14% to 33% thrombosis rate [27,28]. Prevention of internal jugular vein thrombosis is partially under the control of the surgeon and risk can be minimized by atraumatic manipulation of the vein, avoiding desiccation, maintaining optimal flow characteristics by ligation of jugular side branches far enough away to prevent constriction, but close enough to prevent blind jugular side pouches, which may contribute to retrograde thrombosis [27]. Although there is a high incidence of internal jugular vein thrombosis, free flap success is still 90% to 95% and there does not seem to be an effect on ultimate free flap survival rates [29].

References

[1] Blackwell KE. Unsurpassed reliability of free flaps for head and neck reconstruction. Arch Otolaryngol Head Neck Surg 1999;125:295.

[2] Pryor SG, Moore EJ, Kasperbauer JL. Implantable Doppler flow system: experience with 24 microvascular free flap operations. Otolaryngol Head Neck Surg 2006;135:714.

[3] Heden PG, Hamilton R, Arnander C, et al. Laser Doppler surveillance of the circulation of free flaps and replanted digits. Microsurgery 1985;6:11.

[4] Payette JR, Kohlenberg E, Leonardi L, et al. Assessment of skin flaps using optically based methods for measuring blood flow and oxygenation. Plast Reconstr Surg 2005;115:539.

[5] Velanovich V, Smith DJ Jr, Robson MC, et al. The effect of hemoglobin and hematocrit levels on free flap survival. Am Surg 1988;54:659.

[6] Qiao Q, Zhou G, Chen GY, et al. Application of hemodilution in microsurgical free flap transplantation. Microsurgery 1996;17:487.

[7] Chung TL, Pumplin DW, Hotlon LH, et al. Prevention of microsurgical anastomotic thrombosis using aspirin, heparin, and the glycoprotein IIb/IIIa inhibitor Tirofiban. Plast Reconstr Surg 2007;120:1281.

[8] Chien W, Varvares MA, Hadlock T, et al. Effects of aspirin and low-dose heparin in head and neck reconstruction using microvascular free flaps. Laryngoscope 2005;115:973.

[9] Nahabedian MY, Singh N, Deune EG, et al. Recipient vessel analysis for microvascular reconstruction of the head and neck. Ann Plast Surg 2004;52:148.

[10] Serletti JM, Higgins JP, Moran S, et al. Factors affecting outcome in free tissue transfer in the elderly. Plast Reconstr Surg 2000;106:66.

[11] Ueda K, Harii K, Nakasuka T, et al. Comparison of end-to-end and end-to-side venous anastomosis in free tissue transfer following resection of head and neck tumors. Microsurgery 1996;17:146.

[12] Beckman JA, Thakore A, Kalinowski BH, et al. Radiation therapy impairs endothelium-dependent vasodilation in humans. J Am Coll Cardiol 2001; 37:761.

[13] Drake DB, Oishi SN. Wound healing considerations in chemotherapy and radiation therapy. Clin Plast Surg 1995;22:31.

[14] Cooley BC, Hanel DP, Anderson RB, et al. The influence of diabetes on free flap transfer: I. Flap survival and microascular healing. Ann Plast Surg 1992; 99:156.

[15] Cooley BC, Hanel DP, Lan M, et al. The influence of diabetes on free flap transfer: II. The effect of ischemia on flap survival. Ann Plast Surg 1992;29:58.

[16] Tapp RJ, Balkau B, Shaw JE, et al, The DESIR Study Group. Association of glucose metabolism, smoking and cardiovascular risk factors with incident peripheral arterial disease: the DESIR study. Atherosclerosis 2007;190:84.

[17] Schusterman MA, Miller MJ, Reece GP, et al. A single center's experience with 308 free flaps for repair of head and neck cancer defects. Plast Reconstr Surg 1994;93:472–80.

[18] Krueger JK, Rohrich RJ. Clearing the smoke: the scientific rationale for tobacco abstention with plastic surgery. Plast Reconstr Surg 2001;108(4):1063.

[19] German G, Steinau HU. The clinical reliability of vein grafts in free flap transfer. J Reconstr Microsurg 1996;9:245.

[20] Miller MJ, Schusterman MA, Reece GP, et al. Interposition vein grafting in head and neck reconstructive microsurgery. J Reconstr Microsurg 1993;125: 869.

[21] Rand RP, Gruss JB. The saphenous arteriovenous fistula in microsurgical head and neck reconstruction. Am J Otolaryngol 1994;15:215.

[22] Kroll SS, Miller MJ, Reece GP, et al. Anticoagulants and hematomas in free flap surgery. Plast Reconstr Surg 1995;96:643.

[23] Webb RM, Baker NJ. Division of digastric tendon improves access for microvascular anastomosis in the neck. J Oral Maxillofac Surg 2008;66(2):408–9.

[24] Yu P. The transverse cervical vessels as recipient vessels for previously treated head and neck cancer patients. Plast Reconstr Surg 2005;115:1253.

[25] Head C, Sercarz JA, Abemayor E, et al. Microvascular reconstruction after previous neck dissection. Arch Otolaryngol Head Neck Surg 2002;128:328.

[26] Urken ML, Weinberg H, Buchbinder ML, et al. Microvascular free flaps in head and neck reconstruction. Arch Otolaryngol Head Neck Surg 1994;120: 633.

[27] Brown DH, Mulholland S, Yoo JHJ, et al. Internal jugular vein thrombosis following modified neck dissection: implications for head and neck flap reconstruction. Head Neck 1998;20:169.

[28] Leotonsins TG, Currie AR, Mannell A. Internal jugular vein thrombosis. Laryngoscope 1995;95:169.

[29] Wax MK, Quraishi H, Rodman S, et al. Internal jugular vein patency in patients undergoing microvascular reconstruction. Laryngoscope 1997;107:1245.

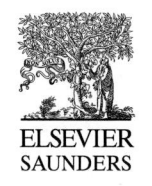

Index

Note: Page numbers of article titles are in **boldface** type.

A

Adenoma, pleomorphic, 449–450
    metastasizing, 449–450

Aerodigestive tract, upper, cancer of, neck masses in, 330–331

Anastomosis, microvascular, in head and neck reconstructive surgery, 525

Anatomy, neck, cervical spine, 381–383
    atlas (C1), 381–382
    axis (C2), 382
    occipital condyles, 381
    occiput-C1-C2 relationship, 382
    spinal cord, 383
    subaxial spine (C3-C7), 382–383
    vascular, 383
  in deep space infection, 353–355
  of lymph nodes, levels and nomenclature, 459–463
  penetrating injuries of the neck and, 395–397
  radiographic correlation with, **311–319**
    anatomy, 312
    imaging, 311–312
      CT, 311
      MRI, 311–312
    lymphatic system, 316–318
    spaces, 312–316
      infrahyoid, 315–316
      suprahyoid, 313–315

Angiography, in evaluation of neck masses, 326–327

Atlas (C1), anatomy of, 381–382
  fractures of, 385

Axis (C2), anatomy of, 382
  fractures of, 386–388
  traumatic spondylolisthesis of, 388

B

Ballistics, gunshot wounds to the neck, pathophysiology of, 397–399

Benign neoplastic masses, of neck, 329–330
  carotid body tumors, 329
  lipomas, 329
  thyroid nodules and goiters, 329–330

Biopsy, fine needle aspiration, in evaluation of neck masses, 323–324
  in evaluation of thyroid disorders, 438–441

Branchial cleft cysts, 327
  congenital neck masses due to, 345–348

C

Cancer, oral. *See* Oral cancer.

Carotid artery, involvement of, in node-positive oral cancer, 506–509

Carotid body tumors, benign neck masses due to, 329

Cat scratch disease, neck masses due to, 329

Cervical spine, injuries of, **381–391**
  anatomy, 381–383
  fractures and dislocations, 383–390
    atlas, 385
    axis, 386–388
    occiput C1 articulation, 383–385
    subaxial spine, 388–390
    penetrating, 410–411

Chemoradiotherapy, postoperative, for advanced-stage oral squamous cell carcinoma, 502–503

Computed tomography (CT), in evaluation of thyroid disorders, 437–438
  of neck, 311
  of neck masses, 325

Congenital neck masses, 327, **339–352**
  lateral, 345–351
    branchial cleft cyst, 345–348
    hemangioma, 350–351
    laryngocele, 348–349
    lymphangioma, 349–350
    thymic cyst, 345

Congenital (*continued*)
  midline, 339–345
    dermoid cyst, 341–342
    epidermoid cyst, 342–343
    plunging ranula, 343–344
    teratoma, 344–345
    thyroglossal duct cyst, 339–341

Cricothyroidectomy, elective, 519
  emergency, 517–518

Cystic hygroma, neck mass due to, 327

D

Deep spaces, of the neck, infections of, clinical considerations in aggressive disease, **367–380**
  surgical management of, **353–365**

Dermoid cysts, of neck, congenital, 341–342

Diagnosis, of deep space neck infections, 356–360
  of neck masses, **321–337**
  of penetrating injuries to the neck, 401–404

Dislocations, of cervical spine, 383–384

Dissection, of neck, **459–475**
  classification of, 463–464
  complications, 470–473
  lymph node levels, anatomy and nomenclature, 459–463
  sentinel node biopsy, 469–470
  technique, 464–468

E

Emergency care, tracheotomy, 517–519
  cricothyroidectomy, 517–518
    emergent re-opening of a trach site, 518
    slash tracheotomy, 518

Endocrine injuries, penetrating, 410

Endoscopy, in evaluation of neck masses, 322–323

Epidermoid cysts, of neck, congenital, 342–343

Esophageal injuries, penetrating, 409–410

Evaluation, of neck masses, **321–337**

Extended neck dissection, 464

F

Fine needle aspiration biopsy, in evaluation of neck masses, 323–324
  in evaluation of thyroid disorders, 438–441

Fractures, of cervical spine, 383–390
  atlas, 385

  axis, 386–388
    odontoid, 386–388
    traumatic spondylolisthesis of C2, 388
  occiput C1 articulation, 383–385
  subaxial spine, 388–390

G

Goiter, thyroid, benign neck masses due to, 329–330

Gunshot wounds, to the neck, pathophysiology of, 397–399

H

Hemangioma, congenital neck masses due to, 350–351

Heterotopic salivary gland disease, 445–446

History, patient, in aggressive deep neck infections, 370–371
  in evaluation of neck masses, 321
  in thyroid disorders, 432–433

Hygroma, cystic, neck mass due to, 327

I

Imaging, in deep neck infections, 372–373
  in evaluation of neck masses, 325–327
  in evaluation of thyroid disorders, 434–438
  radiographic correlation with neck anatomy, **311–319**
    anatomy, 312
    CT, 311
    lymphatic system, 316–318
    MRI, 311–312
    spaces, 312–316
      infrahyoid, 315–316
      suprahyoid, 313–315

Infections, neck masses due to, 328–329
  cat scratch disease, 329
  tuberculosis, 329
  of deep space of neck, clinical considerations in aggressive disease, **367–380**
    airway, 373–374
    etiology, 367–368
    examination, 371–372
    history, 370–371
    imaging, 372–373
    laboratory investigations, 374
    microbiology, 368–370
    pathogenesis of spread, 370
    role of systemic disease, 368
    surgical management, 374–379

medical management, 360
surgical management, **353–365**
  airway management, 361–363
  anatomy, 353–355
  complications, 363–364
  diagnosis, 356–360
  microbiology, 355–356

Infrahyoid spaces, of neck, 315–316

Injuries, of the neck, cervical spine, **381–391**
  anatomy, 381–383
  fractures and dislocations, 383–390
  penetrating, **393–414**
    anatomic considerations, 395–397
    diagnosis, 400–404
    historical perspective, 394–395
    management, cervical spine, 410–411
      endocrine, 410
      esophageal injury, 409–410
      extracranial vascular trauma, 407–409
      laryngotracheal injury, 410
    mechanism of, 399–400
    pathophysiology of gunshot wounds and ballistics, 397–399

L

Laryngeal trauma, **415–430**
  classification, 415–417
  evaluation, 417–420
  management, 420–428
    complications, 428
    historical perspective, 420–424
    nonsurgical treatment, 424–425
    surgical technique, 425–428

Laryngocele, congenital neck masses due to, 348–349

Laryngotracheal injuries, penetrating, 410

Lipoma, benign neck masses due to, 329

Lymph nodes, levels of, anatomy, and nomenclature, 459–463
  N0 neck in oral squamous cell carcinoma, **477–497**
    how to treat, 488–491
    when to treat, 477–488
  node-positive neck in oral cancer, **499–511**
    carotid artery treatment, 506–508
    in organ-preservation treatment regimens, 503–506
    postoperative chemoradiotherapy, 502
    surgical therapy, 499–502

Lymphangioma, congenital neck masses due to, 349–350
  neck mass due to, 327

Lymphatic system, cervical, imaging in evaluation of, 316–318
  radiographic-based classification of, 317–318

Lymphoma, neck masses due to, 334

M

Magnetic resonance imaging (MRI), in evaluation
  of thyroid disorders, 437–438
  of neck, 311–312
  of neck masses, 325–326

Masses, neck, common types of, 327–335
  benign neoplastic, 329–330
    carotid body tumors, 329
    lipomas, 329
    thyroid nodules and goiters, 329–330
  infectious, 328–329
    cat scratch disease, 329
    tuberculosis, 329
  malignant neoplastic, 330–335
    lymphoma, 334
    salivary gland tumors, 334
    skin cancer, 332–334
    thyroid cancer, 334
    unknown primaries, 334–335
    upper aerodigestive tract cancers, 330–332
  nonneoplastic, 327–328
    branchial cleft cysts, 327
    congenital, 327
    lymphangiomas, 327
    thyroglossal duct cysts, 327–328
    vascular lesions, 328
  congenital, 327, **339–352**
    lateral, 345–351
      branchial cleft cyst, 345–348
      hemangioma, 350–351
      laryngocele, 348–349
      lymphangioma, 349–350
      thymic cyst, 345
    midline, 339–345
      dermoid cyst, 341–342
      epidermoid cyst, 342–343
      plunging ranula, 343–344
      teratoma, 344–345
      thyroglossal duct cyst, 339–341
  evaluation and diagnostic approach, **321–337**
    clinical evaluation, 321

Masses *(continued)*
    differential diagnosis, 323
    endoscopy, 322–323
    fine needle aspiration biopsy, 323–324
    history and review of systems, 321
    imaging studies, 324–327
    pathologic assessment, 323
    physical examination, 322

Medical management, of deep space neck infections, 360

Metastases, of pleomorphic adenoma, 449–450

Microbiology, in deep neck abscesses, 355–356
    in aggressive disease, 368–370

Microvascular surgery, preparation of, for microvascular reconstruction of head and neck, **521–526**
    general considerations, 522
    microvascular anastomosis, 525
    planning for microsurgery, 522–525
    vessel-depleted neck, 525–526

Mixed tumors, of salivary gland, malignant, 450–451

Modified radical neck dissection, 463
    of node-positive neck in oral cancer, 500

N

Neck, clinical implications of, in salivary gland disease, **445–458**
    extraparotid Warthin's tumor, 447–449
    heterotopic disease, 445–446
    malignant mixed tumors, 450–451
    parotid carcinoma, 455–456
    pleomorphic adenoma, metastasizing, 449–450
    plunging ranula, 446–447
    submandibular gland tumors, 451–455
  dissection of, **459–475**
    classification of, 463–464
    complications, 470–473
    lymph node levels, anatomy and nomenclature, 459–463
    sentinel node biopsy, 469–470
    technique, 464–468
  in N0 oral squamous cell carcinoma, **477–497**
    how to treat, 488–491
    when to treat, 477–488
  in node-positive oral cancer, **499–511**
    carotid artery treatment, 506–508
    in organ-preservation treatment regimens, 503–506
    postoperative chemoradiotherapy, 502
    surgical therapy, 499–502
  infections, deep space, clinical considerations in aggressive disease, **367–380**
    airway, 373–374
    etiology, 367–368
    examination, 371–372
    history, 370–371
    imaging, 372–373
    laboratory investigations, 374
    microbiology, 368–370
    pathogenesis of spread, 370
    role of systemic disease, 368
    surgical management, 374–379
  medical management, 360
  surgical management, **353–365**
    airway management, 361–363
    anatomy, 353–355
    complications, 363–364
    diagnosis, 356–360
    microbiology, 355–356
injuries
  cervical spine, **381–391**
    anatomy, 381–383
    fractures and dislocations, 383–390
  laryngeal trauma, **415–430**
    classification, 415–417
    evaluation, 417–420
    management, 420–428
  penetrating, **393–414**
    anatomic considerations, 395–397
    diagnosis, 400–404
    historical perspective, 394–395
    management, 404–411
    mechanism of, 399–400
    pathophysiology of gunshot wounds and ballistics, 397–399
masses, congenital, **339–352**
  lateral, 345–351
  midline, 339–345
  evaluation and diagnostic approach, **321–337**
    clinical evaluation, 321
    common types of, 327–335
    differential diagnosis, 323
    endoscopy, 322–323
    fine needle aspiration biopsy, 323–324
    history and review of systems, 321
    imaging studies, 324–327
    pathologic assessment, 323
    physical examination, 322
preparation of, for microvascular reconstruction of head and neck, **521–526**

general considerations, 522
microvascular anastomosis, 525
planning for microsurgery, 522–525
vessel-depleted neck, 525–526
radiographic correlation with anatomy, **311–319**
anatomy, 312
imaging, 311–312
CT, 311
MRI, 311–312
lymphatic system, 316–318
radiographic classification of, 317–318
spaces, 312–316
infrahyoid, 315–316
suprahyoid, 313–315
thyroid disorders, **431–443**
diagnosis, 432–441
fine-needle aspiration, 438–441
history and physical examination, 432–433
imaging modalities, 434–438
laboratory evaluation, 433–434
tracheotomy, **513–520**
contraindications, 513
controversies, 519
elective, in adults, 513–516
complications, 514–516
emergency surgical airway, 517–519
cricothyroidectomy, 517–518
emergent re-opening of a trach site, 518
slash tracheotomy, 518
indications, 513
special considerations in elective, 516–517
in obese patients, 517
pediatric, 516–517
percutaneous dilational tracheotomy, 517

Neoplastic masses, of neck, benign, 329–330
carotid body tumors, 329
lipomas, 329
thyroid nodules and goiters, 329–330
malignant, 330–335
lymphoma, 334
salivary gland tumors, 334
skin cancer, 332–334
thyroid cancer, 334
unknown primaries, 334–335
upper aerodigestive tract cancers, 330–332

Nodules, thyroid, benign neck masses due to, 329–330

O

Obese patients, tracheotomy technique in, 517

Occipital condyles, anatomy of, 381

Occiput-C1 articulation, fractures and dislocations of, 383–385

Oral cancers, management of N0 neck in squamous cell carcinoma, **477–499**
how to treat, 488–491
extent of neck dissection, 489–491
when to treat, 477–488
assessing risk for occult metastases, 483
economic costs, 487–488
elective neck dissection vs. "wait and see," 480–483
future diagnostics using molecular biomarkers, 486–487
limitations of histopathologic grading, 485–486
limitations of imaging, 483–484
prospective trials evaluating treatment algorithms, 480
quality of life and, 478–480
staging and risk of occult metastases, 484
management of node-positive neck in, **499–511**
carotid artery treatment, 506–508
in organ-preservation treatment regimens, 503–506
postoperative chemoradiotherapy, 502
surgical therapy, 499–502

Organ preservation, in management of neck in node-positive oral cancer, 503–506

P

Parotid carcinoma, and the neck, 455–456

Pediatrics, tracheotomy technique in, 516–517

Penetrating injuries, of the neck, **393–414**
anatomic considerations, 395–397
diagnosis, 400–404
historical perspective, 394–395
management, cervical spine, 410–411
endocrine, 410
esophageal injury, 409–410
extracranial vascular trauma, 407–409
laryngotracheal injury, 410
mechanism of, 399–400
pathophysiology of gunshot wounds and ballistics, 397–399

Percutaneoius dilational tracheotomy, 517

Physical examination, in evaluation of neck masses, 322
  in evaluation of penetrating injuries to the neck, 400–401
  in thyroid disorders, 432–433

Pleomorphic adenoma, 449–450
  metastasizing, 449–450

Plunging ranula, 343–344, 446–447

Positron emission tomography (PET), in evaluation of neck masses, 326

R

Radical neck dissection, 463
  of node-positive neck in oral cancer, 499–500

Radiology, radiographic correlation with neck anatomy, **311–319**
  anatomy, 312
  CT, 311
  imaging, 311–312
  lymphatic system, 316–318
  MRI, 311–312
  spaces, 312–316
    infrahyoid, 315–316
    suprahyoid, 313–315

Radionuclide scintigraphy, in evaluation of thyroid disorders, 436–437

Ranula, plunging, 343–344, 446–447

Reconstructive surgery, preparation of, for microvascular reconstruction of head and neck, **521–526**
  general considerations, 522
  microvascular anastomosis, 525
  planning for microsurgery, 522–525
  vessel-depleted neck, 525–526

S

Salivary gland disease, clinical implications of neck in, **445–458**
  extraparotid Warthin's tumor, 447–449
  heterotopic disease, 445–446
  malignant mixed tumors, 450–451
  parotid carcinoma, 455–456
  pleomorphic adenoma, metastasizing, 449–450
  plunging ranula, 446–447
  submandibular gland tumors, 451–455

Salivary gland tumors, neck masses due to, 334

Scintigraphy, radionuclide, in evaluation of thyroid disorders, 436–437

Selective neck dissection, of node-positive neck in oral cancer, 500–502

Selective radical neck dissection, 463–464

Skin cancer, neck masses due to, 332–334

Slash tracheotomy, 518

Spaces, of neck, 312–316
  deep, infection of, aggressive disease, clinical considerations in, **367–380**
    surgical management, **353–365**
  infrahyoid, 315–316
  suprahyoid, 313–315

Spine, cervical. *See* Cervical spine.

Squamous cell carcinoma, management of N0 neck in, **477–499**
  how to treat, 488–491
    extent of neck dissection, 489–491
  when to treat, 477–488
    assessing risk for occult metastases, 483
    economic costs, 487–488
    elective neck dissection *vs.* "wait and see," 480–483
    future diagnostics using molecular biomarkers, 486–487
    limitations of histopathologic grading, 485–486
    limitations of imaging, 483–484
    prospective trials evaluating treatment algorithms, 480
    quality of life and, 478–480
    staging and risk of occult metastases, 484

Stay sutures, tracheal, in tracheotomy, controversies in, 519

Subaxial spine (C3-C7), anatomy of, 382–383
  injuries of, 388–390

Submandibular gland tumors, 451–455

Suprahyoid spaces, of neck, 313–315

Surgical management, neck dissection, **459–475**
  classification of, 463–464
  complications, 470–473
  lymph node levels, anatomy and nomenclature, 459–463
  sentinel node biopsy, 469–470
  technique, 464–468
  of deep space neck infections, **353–365**
    airway management, 361–363
    anatomy, 353–355
    complications, 363–364
    diagnosis, 356–360

in aggressive disease, 374–379
microbiology, 355–356
of laryngeal trauma, 425–428
of node-positive neck in oral cancer, 499–502
of penetrating injuries of the neck, cervical
spine, 410–411
endocrine, 410
esophageal injury, 409–410
extracranial vascular trauma, 407–409
laryngotracheal injury, 410
preparation of neck for for microvascular
reconstruction of head and neck, **521–526**
general considerations, 522
microvascular anastomosis, 525
planning for microsurgery, 522–525
vessel-depleted neck, 525–526

T

Teratoma, congenital neck masses due to, 344–345

Thymic cysts, congenital neck masses due to 345, 345

Thyroglossal duct cysts, 327–328, 339–341

Thyroid cancer, neck masses due to, 334

Thyroid disorders, evaluation and management of, **431–443**
fine-needle aspiration, 438–441
history and physical examination, 432–433
imaging modalities, 434–438
CT and MRI, 437–438
high-resolution ultrasound, 434–436
radionuclide scintigraphy, 436–437
laboratory evaluation, 433–434

Thyroid goiter, benign neck masses due to, 329–330

Thyroid nodules, benign neck masses due to, 329–330

Tracheotomy, **513–520**
contraindications, 513
controversies, 519
elective, in adults, 513–516
complications, 514–516
emergency surgical airway, 517–519
cricothyroidectomy, 517–518
emergent re-opening of a trach site, 518
slash tracheotomy, 518
indications, 513
special considerations in elective, 516–517
in obese patients, 517
pediatric, 516–517
percutaneous dilational tracheotomy, 517

Trauma. *See* Injuries.

Tuberculosis, neck masses due to, 329

U

Ultrasound, high-resolution, in evaluation of thyroid disorders, 434–436
in evaluation of neck masses, 326

Upper aerodigestive tract, cancer of, neck masses in, 330–331

V

Vascular anatomy, of cervical spine, 383

Vascular surgery, preparation of neck for microvascular reconstruction of head and neck, **521–526**

Vascular trauma, extracranial, in penetrating injuries to the neck, 407–409

Vesicular lesions, neck masses due to, 328

W

Warthin's tumor, extraparotid, 447–449

Moving?

Make sure your subscription moves with you!

To notify us of your new address, find your **Clinics Account Number** (located on your mailing label above your name), and contact customer service at:

E-mail: elspcs@elsevier.com

800-654-2452 (subscribers in the U.S. & Canada)
1-407-563-6020 (subscribers outside of the U.S. & Canada)

Fax number: 407-363-9661

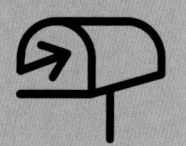

Elsevier Periodicals Customer Service
6277 Sea Harbor Drive
Orlando, FL 32887-4800

*To ensure uninterrupted delivery of your subscription, please notify us at least 4 weeks in advance of move.

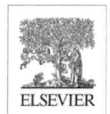